Breast Cancer

Breast Cancer Imaging and Therapy

Editor

Jean Seely

MDPI • Basel • Beijing • Wuhan • Barcelona • Belgrade • Manchester • Tokyo • Cluj • Tianjin

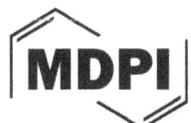

Editor
Jean Seely
University of Ottawa
Canada

Editorial Office
MDPI
St. Alban-Anlage 66
4052 Basel, Switzerland

This is a reprint of articles from the Special Issue published online in the open access journal *Current Oncology* (ISSN 1718-7729) (available at: https://www.mdpi.com/journal/curroncol/special_issues/BC_Image_Therapy).

For citation purposes, cite each article independently as indicated on the article page online and as indicated below:

LastName, A.A.; LastName, B.B.; LastName, C.C. Article Title. *Journal Name* **Year**, *Volume Number*, Page Range.

ISBN 978-3-0365-7930-6 (Hbk)
ISBN 978-3-0365-7931-3 (PDF)

Cover image courtesy of Jean Seely

© 2023 by the authors. Articles in this book are Open Access and distributed under the Creative Commons Attribution (CC BY) license, which allows users to download, copy and build upon published articles, as long as the author and publisher are properly credited, which ensures maximum dissemination and a wider impact of our publications.
The book as a whole is distributed by MDPI under the terms and conditions of the Creative Commons license CC BY-NC-ND.

Contents

About the Editor vii

Jean M. Seely
Progress and Remaining Gaps in the Early Detection and Treatment of Breast Cancer
Reprinted from: *Curr. Oncol.* **2023**, *30*, 242, doi:10.3390/curroncol30030242 1

Roberta Rosso, Marta D'Alonzo, Valentina Elisabetta Bounous, Silvia Actis, Isabella Cipullo, Elena Salerno and Nicoletta Biglia
Adherence to Adjuvant Endocrine Therapy in Breast Cancer Patients
Reprinted from: *Curr. Oncol.* **2023**, *30*, 112, doi:10.3390/curroncol30020112 7

Duke Appiah, Megan Mai and Kanak Parmar
A Prospective Population-Based Study of Cardiovascular Disease Mortality following Treatment for Breast Cancer among Men in the United States, 2000–2019
Reprinted from: *Curr. Oncol.* **2023**, *30*, 23, doi:10.3390/curroncol30010023 19

Alison Rusnak, Shawna Morrison, Erika Smith, Valerie Hastings, Kelly Anderson, Caitlin Aldridge, et al.
Feasibility Study and Clinical Impact of Incorporating Breast Tissue Density in High-Risk Breast Cancer Screening Assessment
Reprinted from: *Curr. Oncol.* **2022**, *29*, 688, doi:10.3390/curroncol29110688 33

Anna N. Wilkinson, Jean-Michel Billette, Larry F. Ellison, Michael A. Killip, Nayaar Islam and Jean M. Seely
The Impact of Organised Screening Programs on Breast Cancer Stage at Diagnosis for Canadian Women Aged 40–49 and 50–59
Reprinted from: *Curr. Oncol.* **2022**, *29*, 444, doi:10.3390/curroncol29080444 43

Ibrahim Hadadi, Jillian Clarke, William Rae, Mark McEntee, Wendy Vincent and Ernest Ekpo
Reducing Unnecessary Biopsies Using Digital Breast Tomosynthesis and Ultrasound in Dense and Nondense Breasts
Reprinted from: *Curr. Oncol.* **2022**, *29*, 435, doi:10.3390/curroncol29080435 61

Anfal Mohammed Alenezi, Ashokkumar Thirunavukkarasu, Farooq Ahmed Wani, Hadil Alenezi, Muhannad Faleh Alanazi, Abdulaziz Saud Alruwaili, et al.
Female Healthcare Workers' Knowledge, Attitude towards Breast Cancer, and Perceived Barriers towards Mammogram Screening: A Multicenter Study in North Saudi Arabia
Reprinted from: *Curr. Oncol.* **2022**, *29*, 344, doi:10.3390/curroncol29060344 71

Martin J. Yaffe and James G. Mainprize
Overdetection of Breast Cancer
Reprinted from: *Curr. Oncol.* **2022**, *29*, 311, doi:10.3390/curroncol29060311 87

Roberta Fusco, Elio Di Bernardo, Adele Piccirillo, Maria Rosaria Rubulotta, Teresa Petrosino, Maria Luisa Barretta, et al.
Radiomic and Artificial Intelligence Analysis with Textural Metrics Extracted by Contrast-Enhanced Mammography and Dynamic Contrast Magnetic Resonance Imaging to Detect Breast Malignant Lesions
Reprinted from: *Curr. Oncol.* **2022**, *29*, 159, doi:10.3390/curroncol29030159 105

Katarzyna Steinhof-Radwańska, Anna Grażyńska, Andrzej Lorek, Iwona Gisterek, Anna Barczyk-Gutowska, Agnieszka Bobola, et al.
Contrast-Enhanced Spectral Mammography Assessment of Patients Treated with Neoadjuvant Chemotherapy for Breast Cancer
Reprinted from: *Curr. Oncol.* **2021**, *28*, 298, doi:10.3390/curroncol28050298 . . . . **125**

Paula B. Gordon
The Impact of Dense Breasts on the Stage of Breast Cancer at Diagnosis: A Review and Options for Supplemental Screening
Reprinted from: *Curr. Oncol.* **2022**, *29*, 291, doi:10.3390/curroncol29050291 . . . . **141**

Daniel B. Kopans
Misinformation and Facts about Breast Cancer Screening
Reprinted from: *Curr. Oncol.* **2022**, *29*, 445, doi:10.3390/curroncol29080445 . . . . **183**

Shushiela Appavoo
How Did CNBSS Influence Guidelines for So Long and What Can That Teach Us?
Reprinted from: *Curr. Oncol.* **2022**, *29*, 313, doi:10.3390/curroncol29060313 . . . . **195**

Jennie Dale, Michelle Di Tomaso and Victoria Gay
Marrying Story with Science: The Impact of Outdated and Inconsistent Breast Cancer Screening Practices in Canada
Reprinted from: *Curr. Oncol.* **2022**, *29*, 286, doi:10.3390/curroncol29050286 . . . . **207**

About the Editor

Jean Seely

Jean Seely is a Professor in the Department of Radiology at the University of Ottawa, Head of the Breast Imaging Section at the Ottawa Hospital, and Regional Breast Imaging Lead for the Ontario Breast Screening Program in the Champlain region (Ottawa). She is the President of the Canadian Society of Breast Imaging. Her research interests include Breast MRI, breast cancer screening, quality in breast imaging, and patient experience. She is a volunteer on the Medical Advisory Board of densebreast-info.org. Her commitment is to reduce the mortality and morbidity of breast cancer and provide high quality breast imaging both nationally and internationally.

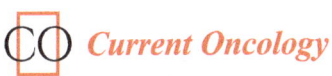

Editorial

Progress and Remaining Gaps in the Early Detection and Treatment of Breast Cancer

Jean M. Seely

Department of Radiology, The Ottawa Hospital, University of Ottawa, Ottawa, ON K1N 6N5, Canada; jeseely@toh.ca

1. Introduction

Breast cancer affects too many of us. The preventable loss of life of mothers, sisters, daughters, grandmothers, fathers and beloved friends must be addressed through science. Female breast cancer has now surpassed lung cancer as the most diagnosed cancer in the world [1]. Almost 2.3 million new cases were diagnosed in women in 2020 [1]. Survival from breast cancer has steadily increased, and in Canada, breast cancer mortality has decreased by 46% since its peak in 1986, where the age-standardized mortality rate fell from 42.7 deaths per 100,000 to a projected rate of 23.1 deaths per 100,000 in 2021 [2]. While 65% of women with breast cancer are diagnosed at early stage I or stage II (localized), there are still far too many women who present at a stage III (regional) (27%) or stage IV (de novo metastatic disease) (6%) [3]. These proportions vary according to race and ethnicity [3]. Unfortunately, the early-stage diagnosis of breast cancer still progresses to metastatic breast cancer in 20–30% of women [4]. Improved survival has been achieved through the early diagnosis of breast cancer with screening and more effective and targeted treatments. Significant gaps remain, however, where an early diagnosis of breast cancer in certain populations is not achieved, including women with dense breasts, those of Black, Asian, Indigenous, and Hispanic ethnicities, and in women aged 40–49 years who are not routinely included in screening mammography programs. In addition, women at high risk who are 30 years and older and men may not be detected at an early stage. In this Special Issue of *Current Oncology on Breast Cancer Imaging and Therapy*, the latest evidence is presented on the early detection of breast cancer and treatment of breast cancer, highlighting the areas where this may be improved.

2. Adjuvant Endocrine Therapy for Breast Cancer

Rosso et al. evaluated the importance of adjuvant endocrine therapy for hormone-receptor-positive breast cancer in a retrospective observational study of 373 women with breast cancer [5]. In this survey study of 64% postmenopausal women, 84% experienced side effects, the most common being arthralgia, hot flushes and vaginal dryness. Significantly higher rates of side effects were found among women who also received adjuvant chemotherapy compared with those who did not (84.8% vs. 78.6%; $p < 0.001$). Premenopausal women were also more likely to experience side effects than postmenopausal women (92% vs. 75%; $p < 0.001$). In their study, 12% of patients stopped the adjuvant endocrine therapy mostly due to the side effects; those who did discontinue treatment more often reported severe side effects compared to those who did not (44% vs. 15%; $p < 0.0001$).

3. Men and Breast Cancer

Appiah et al. reported a prospective study of breast cancer among men in the United States; the research investigated 5216 men with breast cancer aged ≥ 40 years from the Surveillance, Epidemiology, and End Results program from 2000–2019, and studied the relation between breast cancer treatment and cardiovascular disease mortality [6]. They investigated the impact of race/ethnicity. After a median follow-up of 5.6 years, 37%

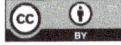

(1914) of deaths occurred, of which 25% were attributable to cardiovascular disease and 35% to breast cancer. In multivariable analysis, men who received chemotherapy had a significantly elevated risk for cardiovascular-related death (HR: 1.55, 95% CI: 1.18–2.04). There was a significant interaction between race and ethnicity and cancer treatment on the risk of cardiovascular-disease-related mortality ($p = 0.005$), with higher levels among Hispanic (HR: 3.96, 95% CI: 1.31–12.02) than Black and White men.

4. High Risk and Breast Tissue Density

Rusnak et al. performed a prospective study of 139 women who were 40–69 years of age with a strong family history of breast cancer and no genetic mutations and were referred for high-risk assessment in a population-based breast cancer screening program [7]. They evaluated the impact of incorporating breast tissue density into risk assessment and found that 5.8% women had never had a screening mammogram. Of those who had mammography, the eligibility of 16.8% (22/131) was affected by their breast tissue density; 7% women with dense breasts became eligible while 10% with non-dense tissue became ineligible. The incorporation of density into risk stratification allowed for improved access to supplemental screening with breast MRI in women with dense breast tissue.

5. Stage of Breast Cancer and Screening

Wilkinson et al. evaluated the stage of breast cancer at diagnosis in a study of 55,490 women aged 40–59 years in Canada from 2010 to 2017 [8]. Using the Canadian Cancer Registry, the authors found marked differences in the stages of breast cancer in women aged 40–49 years compared with those aged 50–59 years; there were significantly lower proportions of stage I BC (35.7 vs. 45.3%; $p < 0.001$), and greater proportions of stage II (42.6 vs. 36.7%, $p < 0.001$) and stage III (17.3 vs. 13.1%, $p < 0.001$) in women in their 40s compared with the 50s. The authors evaluated the impact of organised screening programs on the stage of breast cancer at diagnosis. Jurisdictions that included women in their 40s in population-based screening programs had higher proportions of stage I (39.9% vs. 33.3%, $p < 0.001$) and lower proportions of stages II (40.7% vs. 43.7%, $p < 0.001$), III (15.6% vs. 18.3%, $p < 0.001$) and IV (3.9 vs. 4.6%, $p = 0.001$) in women 40–49 years old compared with their peers in the urisdictions that did not include them. A downstream impact was also seen in women in the 50s where screening practices for women aged 40–49 affected women aged 50–59 years; jurisdictions that did not screen women in their 40s had higher proportions of stage II (37.2% vs. 36.0%, $p = 0.003$) and stage III (13.6% vs. 12.3%, $p < 0.001$) in women aged 50–59 years as compared with programs that included the women in their 40s.

6. Knowledge about Screening and the Overdetection of Breast Cancer

Alenezi et al. performed a cross-sectional study in Saudi Arabia among 414 randomly selected female healthcare workers to assess their level of knowledge, attitude to breast cancer and barriers to mammography screening [9]. A high rate of a lack of knowledge was found, with 48.6% of the health care workers having a very low knowledge of breast cancer, and there was a significant negative correlation between a lack of knowledge and barriers to screening. The most important barriers related to screening included apprehension about radiation exposure (57%), fear of pain related to the mammographic examination (55.8%), fear of discovering breast cancer (57.2%) and fear of not knowing the procedure (48%). Logistic regression analysis found that physicians ($p < 0.016$) and workers older than 30 years of age ($p < 0.03$) were significantly more likely to have higher awareness about mammograms. This information may help target educational programs to improve mammography screening.

One of the most cited harms of breast cancer screening is that caused by the overdiagnosis or the overdetection of a breast cancer that would not have otherwise been found without screening, and that would not have led to the harm or death of the woman. Yaffe and Mainprize [10], in an excellent review, explore the phenomenon of overdetection, the methods for accurate estimation and the reasons for the variability in published estimates, including the very high value used by the Canadian Breast Cancer Screening Studies (CNBSS) [11] that inform the Canadian Task Force on Preventive Health Guidelines for Breast Cancer Screening. They demonstrate unequivocally that in situ carcinomas are the most common cause of overdetection and should not be overtreated, and that overdetection is a far greater problem in older than younger women due to more competing causes of death in the older ages.

7. Contrast-Enhanced Mammography

The ability of contrast to detect cancers in dense breast tissue on mammograms is now well established with contrast-enhanced breast MRI and contrast-enhanced mammography (CEM). However, it is well recognized that many benign breast lesions will also enhance with contrast. In this special Issue, Fusco et al. performed a study to discriminate between benign and malignant breast lesions with radiomic metrics extracted from CEM and DCE-MRI images [12]. A total of 79 pathologically proven breast lesions (48 malignant and 31 benign lesions) in 54 patients were studied. Various features on both modalities were studied, with the two best predictors found with an Area Under the Curve (AUC) of 0.71 on the mediolateral oblique (MLO) image of CEM. When all 18 features derived from MRI and CEM were combined, the AUC reached 0.88. The use of morphological assessment was insufficient while the radiomic features allowed for a better discrimination of benign- from malignant-enhancing breast lesions. In another study of CEM, Steinhof-Radwanska et al. [13] studied its use on patients with breast cancer treated with neoadjuvant chemotherapy. In their retrospective study of 63 patients with breast cancer who underwent CEM to assess their chemotherapy response, they found that CEM was highly sensitive in detecting a complete response to chemotherapy (85.7%), but it tended to underestimate the correct tumor dimensions. Recognizing this morphological limitation, CEM is a viable alternative to contrast-enhanced MRI and is effective in the detection of a complete response to chemotherapy.

8. Dense Breast Tissue

In a comprehensive review, Gordon [14] summarizes the impact of dense breasts and the stage of breast cancer at diagnosis. In it, she cites the relative loss of breast cancer mortality reduction in screened women with dense compared with non-dense breasts (13% vs. 41%), and the increased breast cancer mortality relative risk of 1.91 in women with dense breasts. The various supplemental screening modalities are discussed, including those with the greatest ability to reduce the inequity of screening for breast cancer in dense breasts, and the balance of risks and benefits of each one.

In the study by Hadadi et al. [15] of 534 Australian women recalled from screening with mammographic abnormalities and subsequent digital breast tomosynthesis (DBT) and breast ultrasound, breast tissue density was found to correlate significantly with recall rates. Mammographic abnormalities were more likely to be recalled in women with dense breasts. Breast ultrasound was shown in this study to be more useful than DBT at reducing the rate of unnecessary breast benign biopsies.

9. Harms of Not Screening

The harms and benefits of screening mammography are not fully understood by many oncologists and physicians. World expert, Harvard Professor Kopans review, named, "Misinformation and Facts about Breast Cancer Screening", listed the 10 reasons that screening mammography is effective at saving lives from breast cancer by 40% or more [16]. Citing widely from the literature, he uncovers the myths that prevent women in their 40s from routinely being included in screening mammography programs. He summarizes the 1980 Canadian Breast Cancer Screening Studies' (CNBSS) significant flaws that include the subversion of the randomization allocation, poor image quality of the mammography, the inclusion of many symptomatic women and allocation of more to the so-called "screening" arm, and shows why the CNBSS are not credible to determine screening policies.

A review by Appavoo illustrates the influence of the CNBSS on national and international breast cancer screening guidelines [17]. She provides insight into how the flawed studies came to be included in reviews that inform guideline processes. Illustrating the lack of expertise in healthcare guideline processes and drawing on examples of epistemic trespassing, manufactured doubt, and the misuse of the evidence-based review principles, she lists many reasons for the ongoing inclusion of CNBSS in the body of mammography screening evidence. She suggests reforms for the creation of new breast cancer screening guidelines that include expert knowledge and sensitivity to context and the need for fundamental change.

In the last but potentially most clinically relevant article, Dale, Tomaso and Gay summarize the lived experiences of many patients with breast cancer, many of whom were impacted by outdated screening practices [18]. Told through eight stories of women personally affected by breast cancer, the authors depict variable screening practices across Canada for women in their 40s, contrasting the early stage of breast cancer in two different 40 year old women who were both detected by screening mammography in the provinces of British Columbia and Prince Edward island, while another woman in Alberta presented with stage IV breast cancer two years after being dismissed by her family physician when she requested to be screened with mammography, citing guidelines that she was too young. The healthcare costs and emotional and physical toll on women diagnosed at a later stage highlight the harms of not screening women for breast cancer. The authors call on the medical community to do everything possible to reduce advanced stage breast cancers by harmonizing and optimizing screening practices.

10. Conclusions

Breast cancer is the most frequently diagnosed cancer in women. However, information about breast cancer screening is still limited and affects our ability to diagnose breast cancer at an early stage. Knowledge and strong evidence are essential to provide the rationale for the early detection of breast cancer, and this Special Issue aims to highlight ways to further improve survival and quality of life in women diagnosed with breast cancer. As a physician and breast radiologist who sees the harm of advanced breast cancers at diagnosis, I dream of the ways that we can reduce the rate of advanced breast cancer. Marie Curie said, "I was taught that the way of progress was neither swift nor easy." As illustrated in this Special Issue, with improved screening practices that incorporate breast tissue density, we are making progress. Let us keep this in the realm of the possible and minimize the harm of breast cancer to our patients.

Conflicts of Interest: The authors declare no conflict of interest.

References

1. Sung, H.; Ferlay, J.; Siegel, R.L.; Laversanne, M.; Soerjomataram, I.; Jemal, A.; Bray, F. Global Cancer Statistics 2020: GLOBOCAN Estimates of Incidence and Mortality Worldwide for 36 Cancers in 185 Countries. CA. *Cancer J. Clin.* **2021**, *71*, 209–249. [CrossRef] [PubMed]
2. Canadian Cancer Statistics. Available online: https://www.cancer.ca/en/cancer-information/cancer-type/breast/statistics/?region=on (accessed on 24 May 2021).
3. American Cancer Society. *Breast Cancer Facts and Figures 2019–2020*; American Cancer Society: Atlanta, GA, USA, 2019.
4. Early Breast Cancer Trialists' Collaborative Group (EBCTCG). Effects of chemotherapy and hormonal therapy for early breast cancer on recurrence and 15-year survival: An overview of the randomised trials. *Lancet* **2005**, *365*, 1687–1717. [CrossRef] [PubMed]
5. Rosso, R.; D'Alonzo, M.; Bounous, V.E.; Actis, S.; Cipullo, I.; Salerno, E.; Biglia, N. Adherence to Adjuvant Endocrine Therapy in Breast Cancer Patients. *Curr. Oncol.* **2023**, *30*, 1461–1472. [CrossRef] [PubMed]
6. Appiah, D.; Mai, M.; Parmar, K. A Prospective Population-Based Study of Cardiovascular Disease Mortality following Treatment for Breast Cancer among Men in the United States, 2000–2019. *Curr. Oncol.* **2023**, *30*, 284–297. [CrossRef] [PubMed]
7. Rusnak, A.; Morrison, S.; Smith, E.; Hastings, V.; Anderson, K.; Aldridge, C.; Zelenietz, S.; Reddick, K.; Regnier, S.; Alie, E.; et al. Feasibility Study and Clinical Impact of Incorporating Breast Tissue Density in High-Risk Breast Cancer Screening Assessment. *Curr. Oncol.* **2022**, *29*, 8742–8750. [CrossRef] [PubMed]

8. Wilkinson, A.N.; Billette, J.-M.; Ellison, L.F.; Killip, M.A.; Islam, N.; Seely, J.M. The Impact of Organised Screening Programs on Breast Cancer Stage at Diagnosis for Canadian Women Aged 40–49 and 50–59. *Curr. Oncol.* **2022**, *29*, 5627–5643. [CrossRef] [PubMed]
9. Alenezi, A.M.; Thirunavukkarasu, A.; Wani, F.A.; Alenezi, H.; Alanazi, M.F.; Alruwaili, A.S.; Alashjaee, R.H.; Alashjaee, F.H.; Alrasheed, A.K.; Alshrari, B.D. Female Healthcare Workers' Knowledge, Attitude towards Breast Cancer, and Perceived Barriers towards Mammogram Screening: A Multicenter Study in North Saudi Arabia. *Curr. Oncol.* **2022**, *29*, 4300–4314. [CrossRef] [PubMed]
10. Yaffe, M.J.; Mainprize, J.G. Overdetection of Breast Cancer. *Curr. Oncol.* **2022**, *29*, 3894–3910. [CrossRef] [PubMed]
11. Baines, C.J.; To, T.; Miller, A.B. Revised estimates of overdiagnosis from the Canadian National Breast Screening Study. *Prev. Med.* **2016**, *90*, 66–71. [CrossRef] [PubMed]
12. Fusco, R.; Di Bernardo, E.; Piccirillo, A.; Rubulotta, M.R.; Petrosino, T.; Barretta, M.L.; Mattace Raso, M.; Vallone, P.; Raiano, C.; Di Giacomo, R.; et al. Radiomic and Artificial Intelligence Analysis with Textural Metrics Extracted by Contrast-Enhanced Mammography and Dynamic Contrast Magnetic Resonance Imaging to Detect Breast Malignant Lesions. *Curr. Oncol.* **2022**, *29*, 1947–1966. [CrossRef] [PubMed]
13. Steinhof-Radwańska, K.; Grażyńska, A.; Lorek, A.; Gisterek, I.; Barczyk-Gutowska, A.; Bobola, A.; Okas, K.; Lelek, Z.; Morawska, I.; Potoczny, J.; et al. Contrast-Enhanced Spectral Mammography Assessment of Patients Treated with Neoadjuvant Chemotherapy for Breast Cancer. *Curr. Oncol.* **2021**, *28*, 3448–3462. [CrossRef] [PubMed]
14. Gordon, P.B. The Impact of Dense Breasts on the Stage of Breast Cancer at Diagnosis: A Review and Options for Supplemental Screening. *Curr. Oncol.* **2022**, *29*, 3595–3636. [CrossRef] [PubMed]
15. Hadadi, I.; Clarke, J.; Rae, W.; McEntee, M.; Vincent, W.; Ekpo, E. Reducing Unnecessary Biopsies Using Digital Breast Tomosynthesis and Ultrasound in Dense and Nondense Breasts. *Curr. Oncol.* **2022**, *29*, 5508–5516. [CrossRef] [PubMed]
16. Kopans, D.B. Misinformation and Facts about Breast Cancer Screening. *Curr. Oncol.* **2022**, *29*, 5644–5654. [CrossRef] [PubMed]
17. Appavoo, S. How Did CNBSS Influence Guidelines for So Long and What Can That Teach Us? *Curr. Oncol.* **2022**, *29*, 3922–3932. [CrossRef] [PubMed]
18. Dale, J.; Di Tomaso, M.; Gay, V. Marrying Story with Science: The Impact of Outdated and Inconsistent Breast Cancer Screening Practices in Canada. *Curr. Oncol.* **2022**, *29*, 3540–3551. [CrossRef]

Disclaimer/Publisher's Note: The statements, opinions and data contained in all publications are solely those of the individual author(s) and contributor(s) and not of MDPI and/or the editor(s). MDPI and/or the editor(s) disclaim responsibility for any injury to people or property resulting from any ideas, methods, instructions or products referred to in the content.

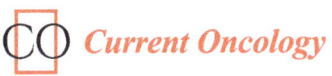

Article

Adherence to Adjuvant Endocrine Therapy in Breast Cancer Patients

Roberta Rosso, Marta D'Alonzo, Valentina Elisabetta Bounous *, Silvia Actis, Isabella Cipullo, Elena Salerno and Nicoletta Biglia

Division of Gynecology and Obstetrics, Department of Surgical Sciences, School of Medicine, University of Turin, 10100 Turin, Italy
* Correspondence: valentinaelisabetta.bounous@unito.it

Abstract: Background: Adjuvant endocrine therapy (AET) reduces breast cancer recurrence and mortality of women with hormone-receptor-positive tumors, but poor adherence remains a significant problem. The aim of this study was to analyze AET side effects and their impact on adherence to treatment. Methods: A total of 373 breast cancer patients treated with AET filled out a specific questionnaire during their follow up visits at the Breast Unit of our Centre. Results: Side effects were reported by 81% of patients, 84% of those taking tamoxifen and 80% of those taking aromatase inhibitors (AIs). The most common side effect in the tamoxifen group was hot flashes (55.6%), while in the AI group it was arthralgia (60.6%). The addition of GnRH agonists to both tamoxifen and AI significantly worsened all menopausal symptoms. Overall, 12% of patients definitively discontinued AET due to side effects, 6.4% during the first 5 years and 24% during extended therapy. Patients who had previously received chemotherapy or radiotherapy reported a significantly lower discontinuation rate. Conclusions: AET side effects represent a significant problem in breast cancer survivors leading to irregular assumption and discontinuation of therapy. Adherence to AET may be improved by trustful patient–physician communication and a good-quality care network.

Keywords: breast cancer; adjuvant endocrine therapy; adherence to treatment; side effects; tamoxifen; aromatase inhibitors; GnRH agonist; questionnaire

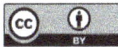

1. Introduction

Approximately 80% of breast cancer patients have hormone-receptor-positive tumors. In these patients, adjuvant endocrine therapy (AET) is widely used, which includes tamoxifen or aromatase inhibitors (AIs) with or without GnRH agonists, depending on tumor characteristics and menopausal state. In post-menopausal women, AIs represent the main adjuvant endocrine treatment, as they have demonstrated superior clinical outcomes compared to tamoxifen, while in premenopausal patients, different options are available, such as tamoxifen alone or tamoxifen plus GnRH agonists, with a switch to AIs alone when menopause occurs [1,2]. In particular, in young women with high-risk disease, the addition of GnRH agonists to the aromatase inhibitor exemestane significantly improves DFS and reduces the recurrence rate, as shown by SOFT and TEXT trials [3,4]. International guidelines agree with a standard treatment duration of 5 years, but a 10-year extended therapy may be suggested depending on tumor and patient individual characteristics with the support of specific algorithms such as CTS5 [5]. It has been demonstrated that AET reduces the risk of recurrence by 30% and mortality by 40% in patients with hormone-receptor-positive breast cancer and that extended therapy determines a further reduction, as shown by aTTom and ATLAS trials, as well as MA17R, DATA, IDEAL and NSABP B42 trials [6–14].

Despite these benefits, AET is burdened by considerable side effects and poor adherence to treatment, which represents a significant problem. Regarding side effects, the anti-estrogenic action of tamoxifen causes hot flashes, vaginal dryness, sexual dysfunction and dyspareunia, while its pro-estrogenic effect on endometrium increases the risk of endometrial hyperplasia, polyps and, rarely, endometrial cancer; moreover, it increases the risk of deep venous thrombosis and pulmonary thromboembolism. On the other side, AIs mostly determine arthralgia, joint pain and osteoporosis, as well as weight gain, headache, insomnia, mood changes and hypercholesterolemia [15,16]. Many clinical trials and epidemiological studies show that side effects have a significant impact on the quality of life and play a primary role in the suboptimal adherence to AET in breast cancer patients [17–20]. The discontinuation rate reported in the literature in the first 5 years of treatment is about 50% with a progressive decrease in adherence from the first year (87%) to the third (79%) and fifth (50%) [3,21–24].

It has been demonstrated that the early discontinuation of AET is related to a decline in survival, increased recurrence risk and reduced DFS, as well as increased medical costs and low quality of life due to disease progression and treatment [25–27].

Another significant element associated with non-adherence to AET is poor patient–physician communication, an inadequate explanation of the type and severity of side effects at the beginning of treatment and poor consideration of them during follow-up visits [28–31]. In fact, many studies highlighted the importance of discussing potential concerns and establishing a trustful patient–physician relationship in the acceptance of AET and adherence to treatment [32–35].

The aim of this study is to analyze the type, incidence and severity of AET side effects and determine their impact on adherence to treatment. We also intend to evaluate the importance of patient–physician communication and the benefit of medical and psychological support strategies.

2. Materials and Methods

In this retrospective observational study, we analyzed a population of 373 patients with hormone-receptor-positive breast cancer currently or previously treated with AET (tamoxifen, AI, GnRH agonists). A specific questionnaire was administered to these patients during one of their follow-up visits at the Breast Unit of "Mauriziano Umberto I" Hospital in Turin from January 2021 to December 2021.

The questionnaire was composed of 31 questions and 5 sections: AET tolerance and side effects; adherence to treatment (regularity of assumption, change or suspension of treatment due to intolerance); adherence and tolerance to extended therapy; patient–physician communication and strategies suggested to control side effects; and the importance and efficacy of medical and psychological support (Appendix A).

The study included patients with hormone-receptor-positive breast cancer (luminal A and luminal B) who underwent any type of surgery (mastectomy or conservative surgery) followed by AET (tamoxifen, AI, GnRH agonists) from at least 6 months, also including those in the extended therapy regimen. We did not include in our analysis patients on exclusive endocrine therapy and patients with breast cancer recurrence, nor did we include patients who used both tamoxifen and aromatase inhibitors because it could represent a confounding factor. We did not set any limit in terms of time from diagnosis or from the beginning of follow-up.

3. Results

3.1. Study Population

Patients' mean age at diagnosis was 59 years, while the mean age at the administration of the questionnaire was 66 years, on average 5.5 years after the beginning of AET. In our sample, premenopausal patients represented 36%, while postmenopausal ones represented 64%. At the time of the administration of the questionnaire, 292 patients (78.3%) had taken AIs, while 81 patients (21.7%) had taken tamoxifen. In total, 73 patients (19.6%) currently or previously used GnRH-agonists—55 of them in association with tamoxifen (75%) and 18 in association with AIs (25%). Seventy-nine patients had extended therapy—90% of them with AIs and 10% with tamoxifen. At the time of investigation, 178 patients (48%) had been taking AET for less than 5 years, while 195 patients (52%) had concluded the 5-year standard treatment.

Characteristics of patients included in our sample are reported in Table 1.

Table 1. Characteristics of the study population.

	n = 373
Mean age (years)	66.5 (33–90)
Mean age at surgery (years)	59.9 (28–86)
Menopausal state at surgery	
Premenopausal	134 (36%)
Postmenopausal	239 (64%)
Type of AET at time of administration of questionnaire	
Tamoxifen	81 (21.7%)
Aromatase inhibitors	292 (78.3%)
Association with GnRH-agonists	
Yes	73 (19.6%)
with tamoxifen	55 (75%)
with AI	18 (25%)
No	300 (80.4%)
Extended therapy	
Yes	79 (21%)
No	294 (79%)
Chemotherapy	
Yes	158 (42.4%)
No	215 (57.6%)
Radiotherapy	
Yes	256 (68.6%)
No	117 (31.4%)

3.2. Incidence of Side Effects

Eighty-one per cent of patients reported at least one side effect, and the majority of them reported more than one. Side effects were reported by 84% of patients taking tamoxifen and 80% of patients taking AI, and they were described as mild in 43% of cases, moderate in 34% and severe in 23% (Figure 1).

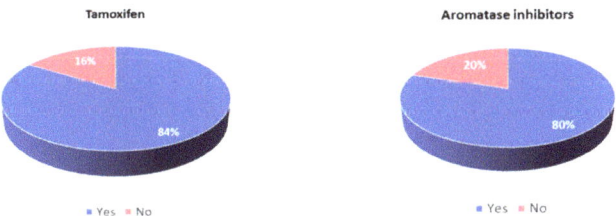

Figure 1. Incidence of side effects in patients taking tamoxifen and in patients taking aromatase inhibitors.

Overall, the most common side effects were arthralgia, hot flushes and vaginal dryness. The most common side effects among women taking tamoxifen were hot flushes, arthralgia and vaginal dryness, while they were arthralgia and hypercholesterolemia among women taking AI.

Side effects associated with each therapy and their incidence are reported in Table 2.

Table 2. Incidence of side effects of adjuvant endocrine therapy (overall, tamoxifen and aromatase inhibitors).

Side Effects	Overall 303 (81%)	Tamoxifen n = 81 (84%)	Aromatase Inhibitors n = 235 (80%)
Arthralgia	200 (53.6%)	26 (32.1%)	177 (60.6%)
Hot flushes	123 (33%)	45 (55.6%)	57 (19.5%)
Vaginal dryness	85 (23%)	21 (25.9%)	45 (15.4%)
Hypercholesterolemia	70 (18.7%)	3 (3.7%)	67 (22.9%)
Dyspareunia	45 (12%)	9 (11.1%)	23 (7.9%)
Asthenia	43 (11.5%)	7 (8.6%)	41 /14%)
Alopecia	33 (8.8%)	3 (3.7%)	28 (9.6%)
Weight gain	16 (4.2%)	7 (8.6%)	9 (3.2%)
CNS alterations	14 (3.7%)	3 (3.7%)	9 (3.1%)
Insomnia	14 (3.7%)	3 (3.7%)	10 (3.4%)
Itch	14 (3.7%)	3 (3.7%)	10 (3.4%)
Mood changes	11 (2.9%)	2 (2.5%)	8 (2.7%)
Liver function abnormalities	10 (2.9%)	4 (4.9%)	7 (2.4%)
Headache	10 (2.9%)	3 (3.7%)	5 (1.7%)
Decreased libido	9 (2.4%)	1 (1.2%)	5 (1.7%)
Dry skin	6 (1.6%)	2 (2.5%)	3 (1%)
Thromboembolism	5 (1.3%)	4 (4.9%)	1 (0.3%)
Anxiety	5 (1.3%)	3 (3.7%)	2 (0.6%)
Dizziness	4 (1.1%)	0 (0.0%)	3 (1%)

The addition of GnRH agonists to both tamoxifen and AIs significantly increased the incidence of side effects. In particular, patients taking tamoxifen plus GnRH agonists more often reported hot flushes, vaginal dryness, arthralgia and dyspareunia, while patients taking AIs plus GnRH agonists more often reported hot flushes, vaginal dryness, dyspareunia, mood changes, decreased libido and anxiety (Figure 2).

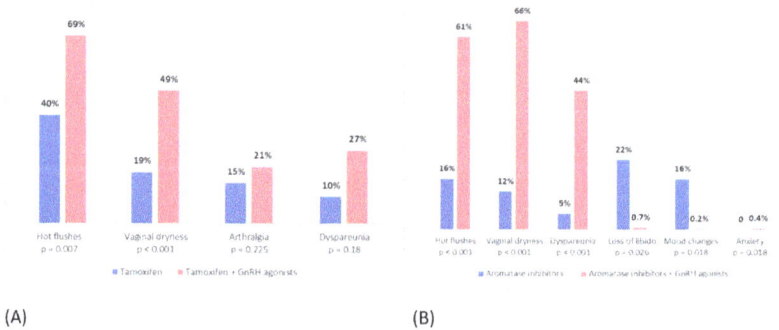

Figure 2. Incidence of side effects in: (**A**) patients taking tamoxifen vs. patients taking tamoxifen + GnRH agonists; (**B**) patients taking aromatase inhibitors alone vs. patients taking aromatase inhibitors + GnRH agonists.

Patients who received adjuvant chemotherapy before starting AET reported a significantly higher incidence of side effects (84.8% vs. 78.6%; $p < 0.001$), while no significant difference emerged between patients who received radiotherapy and those who did not receive it (81.6% vs. 80.3%; $p = 0.225$).

Premenopausal women were more likely to report side effects compared to those who were menopausal at diagnosis (92% vs. 75%; $p < 0.001$). Hot flushes, vaginal dryness, dyspareunia and decreased libido were more frequent and less tolerated by premenopausal women, while postmenopausal ones reported arthralgia as the most annoying side effect (Figure 3).

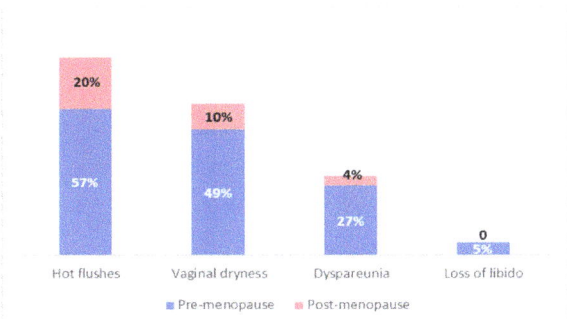

Figure 3. Adjuvant endocrine therapy side effects incidence in relation to menopausal status.

In total, 86 of our patients were offered to continue AET for a further 5 years in an extended therapy regimen, and 79 of them (91%) accepted, while 7 refused. Comparing these two groups of women, it emerged that those who refused the extended therapy regimen more often reported moderate and severe side effects during the first 5 years of treatment ($p < 0.001$). Among patients who accepted the extended therapy, 86% had side effects and 16% reported a worsening of them over time.

3.3. Adherence to Treatment and Discontinuation

Due to side effects, 79 patients (21%) considered discontinuing AET—57 (72%) taking AI and 22 (28%) taking tamoxifen. In addition, 33 patients (8.2%) reported an irregular assumption—23 (70%) taking AI and 10 (30%) taking tamoxifen. Fifty-nine patients (16%) replaced the treatment with another type of endocrine therapy due to intolerance, while forty-five patients (12%) definitively discontinued the treatment for this reason. The discontinuation rate was 6.4% during the first five years of treatment versus 24% during extended therapy, with no significant difference between different types of AET (14.8% among patients taking tamoxifen and 11.3% among patients taking AIs) (Figure 4).

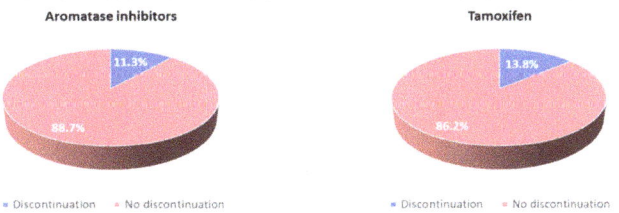

Figure 4. Discontinuation rate in patients taking tamoxifen and in patients taking aromatase inhibitors.

Among patients who definitively discontinued the treatment, 24 (53%) did it during the first 5 years, 7 (16%) did not accept extended therapy at the end of the first 5 years of treatment and 14 (31%) discontinued the therapy between the fifth and tenth year, due to intolerance (Figure 5).

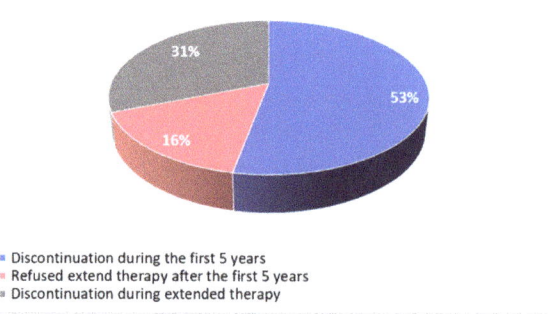

Figure 5. Time of discontinuation of adjuvant endocrine therapy.

Overall, 7/45 patients (16%) discontinued AET because of the appearance of severe pathologies, such as endometrial cancer, endometrial thickness or neurologic toxicity, while 38 patients (84%) discontinued because of intolerance to side effects, in particular, arthralgia (64%), hot flushes (4%) and mood alterations (2%), while 11% discontinued treatment for general intolerance, without specific symptoms.

Women who discontinued treatment more often reported severe side effects compared to those who did not discontinue it (44% vs. 15%; $p < 0.001$). Arthralgia was the principal side effect that caused patients to discontinue the treatment (64%).

Patients who had previously received adjuvant chemotherapy showed a lower discontinuation rate, despite a higher incidence of side effects. Even the patients who had received radiotherapy had a lower discontinuation rate compared to those who had not received it (Figure 6).

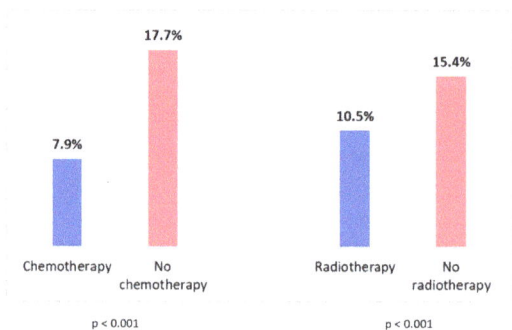

Figure 6. Discontinuation rate in patients who have received adjuvant chemotherapy or radiotherapy vs. patients who have not received adjuvant chemotherapy or radiotherapy.

We also stratified our patients by different breast cancer histological subtypes: ductal, lobular and others. The incidence of lobular breast cancer in our population was 10.5%, which is very similar to the incidence in the general population reported in the literature. We did not find any statistically significant difference in the incidence and severity of side effects nor in AET discontinuation rate between the different histological subtypes.

3.4. Patient–Physician Communication and Support Strategies

Eighty-eight per cent of patients who experienced AET side effects reported talking about it with the gynecologist during follow up visits. Overall, 77% of patients reported that the gynecologist asked them first about side effects and therapy compliance (Figure 7).

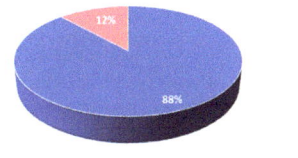
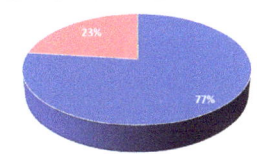

Figure 7. Patient–physician communication.

Among women who reported side effects, only 44% took medical treatments to overcome them, especially in the case of vaginal dryness (58.8%), arthralgia (26%) and hot flushes (16%), but 41.3% of them did not report any relief.

Only 9% of patients who experienced menopausal symptoms made regular visits to the dedicated menopause service of the Breast Unit.

Fifteen per cent of patients received psychological support from the dedicated psychology service of the Breast Unit, and ninety-four per cent of them reported that it was very useful and that they would have recommended it to other women diagnosed with breast cancer.

Overall, 94% of women felt well supported during follow-up visits and reported being correctly informed by gynecologists about adverse side effects of AET. On the other hand, 12% of patients who discontinued treatment reported that they would have continued it, if they were better informed about side effects and possible therapies to control them.

4. Discussion

The majority of breast cancers are represented by hormone-receptor-positive tumors, and treatment with AET has shown great advantages in terms of disease recurrence and mortality. Despite these widely demonstrated benefits, AET is burdened by considerable side effects, especially in young women. Many clinical trials and epidemiological studies have shown that these side effects significantly impact quality of life and play a primary role in suboptimal adherence to AET [6–13].

Some recent studies have demonstrated that about 90% of patients on AET report side effects, which are more frequent in women taking tamoxifen than in those taking AIs [36–38]. According to these data, side effects were reported by 82% of our patients overall and, in particular, by 84% of those taking tamoxifen and 80% of those taking AIs. Moreover, the literature shows that arthralgia is reported by about 40% of patients taking AIs and 28% of those taking tamoxifen [39]. In our study, arthralgia was the most common side effect, reported by 53% of patients overall and, in particular, by 60% of those taking AIs and 32% of those taking tamoxifen. A possible explanation for this difference is the higher adherence to treatment of our patients, as arthralgia is a symptom that persists and worsens over time during AET. Hot flushes are reported by about 60–70% of patients taking AET in the literature, while in our study, they were reported by only 33% of patients. This difference may also be attributed to the higher adherence to treatment of our patients, as hot flushes tend to decrease in intensity and be more tolerated by women over time [40,41].

In our study, we evaluated the impact of GnRH agonists on the tolerance of tamoxifen and AI. It emerged that the addition of GnRH agonists to both tamoxifen and AI in high-risk premenopausal women significantly increased all analyzed side effects and worsened the tolerance to treatment overall. In particular, the most reported and less tolerated side effects among patients taking tamoxifen or AIs plus GnRH agonists, compared to those taking tamoxifen or AIs alone, were hot flushes, vaginal dryness, dyspareunia, mood changes and decreased libido. Our results are similar to those that emerged from the SOFT156 trial, which demonstrated that the addition of GnRH agonists to both tamoxifen and AIs was related to a higher incidence of hot flushes, mood changes, vaginal dryness and decreased libido [42].

As there is consistent evidence of poorer AET tolerance in premenopausal women compared to postmenopausal ones, we evaluated side effects and tolerance in relation to the menopausal state [43]. The same results emerged from our study, as premenopausal women reported more side effects than those who were postmenopausal at the time of diagnosis (92% vs. 75%). Younger women more often reported hot flushes, vaginal dryness, decreased libido, dyspareunia and endometrial modifications.

In our study, the discontinuation rate was lower than that reported in the literature (12% vs. about 50%) [21,22,24,28]. It has to be considered that there are different methods of evaluation of adherence to AET in different studies. Self-assessment with a questionnaire or certified scales is the most used method, but in some cases, questionnaires include variables such as the percentage of tablets taken out of the total and consider as "non-adherents" those patients who take therapy irregularly or who simply report side effects [44], while we only considered non-adherent patients who definitively stopped the treatment. In fact, another study in which discontinuation is considered to be definitive suspension of treatment showed a discontinuation rate of 10%, although on a small sample of women [45].

Moreover, it emerged from our study that most of the patients who discontinued AET made this decision when extended therapy was proposed after the first five years of treatment or during extended therapy itself. The refusal of extended therapy may be explained not only by side effects, but also by the fact that patients could have perceived extended therapy as optional, without perceiving its real importance, maybe due to poor communication with the specialist. On the other hand, the discontinuation of AET during the extended therapy, after the initial acceptance, may also be explained by the worsening of the severity of side effects over time, as reported by 16% of our patients.

According to the literature, in our study, arthralgia was not only the most common side effect, but also the main reason for the discontinuation of therapy. A recent metanalysis, in fact, reported that the side effect most related to the discontinuation of AET was arthralgia, followed by weight gain and mood changes, while hot flushes, although very common, were considered physiological and generally did not lead patients to discontinue the treatment [36].

Moreover, from our analysis, it is evident that women who received adjuvant chemotherapy or radiotherapy had a lower discontinuation rate, despite a higher incidence of side effects in women who received chemotherapy. These data are in accordance with a recently published study and may be explained by a higher awareness of the severity of the disease, especially in patients who received chemotherapy, and of the importance of adjuvant treatments by these women [24].

It has been widely demonstrated that patient–physician communication plays a primary role in adherence to any medical treatment. Concerning AET, prior studies report that patients who have a referral specialist (gynecologist or oncologist) showed a higher compliance to AET than those followed up by a general practitioner, probably because the specialist can give the patients more detailed information about the importance of therapy and provide more specific medications to overcome side effects if needed, and this probably helps patients to continue the treatment [36,46,47]. In fact, the Necessity Concerns Framework (NCF) demonstrated that patients' adherence to treatment is related to their perception of the necessity and importance of treatment itself and the reduction of concerns about it more than to its side effects [48]. In fact, a recent study observed a meaningful difference in the necessity beliefs between women who accepted versus those who refused or discontinued AET, showing that women with ongoing AET intake had significantly higher trust in their treating physician and lower concerns regarding AET [35].

Concerning the evaluation of medical and psychological support, it emerged from our study that almost all of the patients taken in at our Breast Unit felt well supported. This may be attributed to a well-organized healthcare network, which allows us to take care of patients globally with regular follow-up visits and a direct communication channel managed by a breast nurse. Patients have the possibility to refer to them with their problems and organize an appointment with the gynecologist to manage side effects or evaluate the possibility of changing their treatment. All these elements encouraged patients to talk with the gynecologist about their difficulties and side effects and try to manage them together, before discontinuing therapy by themselves. In our Breast Unit, patients are regularly monitored by a gynecologist, who is probably more aware of gynecological and sexual AET side effects and could manage them more easily than another specialist. Moreover, the gynecologist who follows up breast cancer patients in our Breast Unit is often the same person who performed their surgery, and this may result in a stronger patient–physician relationship and continuity of care, which may contribute to the improvement of patients' adherence to treatment.

5. Conclusions

Despite its important advantages, AET is burdened by considerable side effects, which represent a significant problem in BC survivors leading to irregular assumption and discontinuation of therapy, especially in young premenopausal women and during extended therapy. Additionally, women who received adjuvant chemotherapy showed a higher incidence of AET side effects compared to those who did not receive it, but at the same time, they have a lower discontinuation rate, as well as women who received radiotherapy.

Moreover, it is evident from our study that adherence to AET may be improved by trustful physician–patient communication and a good-quality care network, which support women during each step of adjuvant therapy.

The challenge is to be more aware of treatment-related side effects reported by patients, to consider therapies to improve their tolerance and to provide patients with dedicated services, offering them adequate medical and psychological support.

The major strengths of our study are the large sample of patients and the fact that they were all taken in at our Breast Unit, thus limiting the differences in their follow-up and management. On the other hand, the main limitation is that our study is a one-time cross-sectional assessment, and our results came from self-reported information, even though complete anonymity was guaranteed to the patients to avoid untrue answers.

Author Contributions: All authors have made substantial contributions to the study conception and design. Material preparation, data collection and analysis were performed by E.S., S.A. and R.R. The first draft of the manuscript was written by R.R., I.C. and M.D., and all authors commented on previous versions of the manuscript. V.E.B. performed the revision of the final manuscript, which has been read and approved by all authors. The entire study was conducted under the supervision of N.B. All authors have read and agreed to the published version of the manuscript.

Funding: This research received no external funding.

Institutional Review Board Statement: Not applicable.

Informed Consent Statement: Informed consent was obtained from all subjects involved in the study.

Data Availability Statement: The datasets generated and analyzed during the current study are not publicly available due to privacy reasons but are available from the corresponding author on reasonable request.

Conflicts of Interest: The authors declare no conflict of interest.

Appendix A. Questionnaire

1. Did you experience any AET side effect? Yes—no.
2. What side effects did you experienced? Open answer.
3. How would you define your side effects? Mild—moderate—severe.
4. Have you ever considered to discontinue AET because of side effects? Yes—no.
5. Have you ever taken therapy irregularly because of side effects? Yes—no.
6. Have you ever changed your AET because of side effects? Yes- no. If yes, what? Open answer. Did you notice any improvement? Yes—no.
7. Did you stop AET because of side effects? Yes—no. If yes, when? Open answer. Did you stop therapy by yourself or under medical supervision? By myself—under medical supervision.
8. After the first 5 years of AET, was extended therapy suggested to you? Yes—no. If yes, did you accept? Yes—no.
9. Did you experience different or worse side effects during extended therapy? Yes—no. If yes, what? Open answer.
10. Did you stop extended therapy before 10 years of treatment because of side effects? Yes—no. If yes, when did you stop and why? Open answer.
11. If you did not accept extended therapy, it was because of side effects? Yes—no.
12. Have you ever talked to your gynecologist about these problems? Yes—no.
13. Have you ever taken any medication to overcome these symptoms? Yes—no. If yes, what? Open answer. Did you get relief? Yes—no.
14. If you had received more information about side effects by your gynecologist, would you have continued AET? Yes—no.
15. If you had received an effective therapy against your symptoms, would you have continued AET? Yes—no.
16. Have you ever used the menopause service of the Breast Unit? Yes—no. If yes, did you find it useful? Yes—no. Would you recommend it? Yes—no.
17. Have you ever received psychological support? Yes—no. If yes, did you find it useful? Yes—no. Would you recommend it? Yes—no.
18. Did you felt well supported by medical staff during your therapy? Yes—no.

References

1. Coates, A.S.; Keshaviah, A.; Thürlimann, B.; Mouridsen, H.; Mauriac, L.; Forbes, J.F.; Paridaens, R.; Castiglione-Gertsch, M.; Gelber, R.D.; Colleoni, M.; et al. Five years of letrozole compared with tamoxifen as initial adjuvant therapy for postmenopausal women with endocrine-responsive early breast cancer: Update of study BIG 1-98. *J. Clin. Oncol.* **2007**, *25*, 486–492. [CrossRef] [PubMed]
2. Forbes, J.F.; Cuzick, J.; Buzdar, A.; Howell, A.; Tobias, J.S.; Baum, M. ATAC/LATTE investigators. Effect of anastrozole and tamoxifen as adjuvant treatment for early-stage breast cancer: 100-month analysis of the ATAC trial. *Lancet Oncol.* **2008**, *9*, 45–53. [PubMed]
3. Aiello Bowles, E.J.; Boudreau, D.M.; Chubak, J.B.; Yu, O.; Fujii, M.; Chestnut, J.; Buist, D.S. Patient-reported discontinuation of endocrine therapy and related adverse effects among women with early-stage breast cancer. *J. Oncol. Pract.* **2012**, *8*, e149–e157. [CrossRef] [PubMed]
4. Pagani, O.; Francis, P.A.; Fleming, G.F.; Walley, B.A.; Viale, G.; Colleoni, M.; Láng, I.; Gómez, H.L.; Tondini, C.; Pinotti, G. SOFT and TEXT Investigators and International Breast Cancer Study Group. Absolute Improvements in Freedom from Distant Recurrence to Tailor Adjuvant Endocrine Therapies for Premenopausal Women: Results from TEXT and SOFT. *J. Clin. Oncol.* **2020**, *38*, 1293–1303. [CrossRef]
5. Burstein, H.J.; Curigliano, G.; Loibl, S.; Dubsky, P.; Gnant, M.; Poortmans, P.; Colleoni, M.; Denkert, C.; Piccart-Gebhart, M.; Regan, M.; et al. Members of the St. Gallen International Consensus Panel on the Primary Therapy of Early Breast Cancer 2019. Estimating the benefits of therapy for early-stage breast cancer: The St. Gallen International Consensus Guidelines for the primary therapy of early breast cancer 2019. *Ann. Oncol.* **2019**, *30*, 1541–1557.
6. Burstein, H.J.; Lacchetti, C.; Anderson, H.; Buchholz, T.A.; Davidson, N.E.; Gelmon, K.A.; Giordano, S.H.; Hudis, C.A.; Solky, A.J.; Stearns, V.; et al. Adjuvant Endocrine Therapy for Women with Hormone Receptor-Positive Breast Cancer: ASCO Clinical Practice Guideline Focused Update. *J. Clin. Oncol.* **2019**, *37*, 423–438. [CrossRef]
7. Early Breast Cancer Trialists' Collaborative Group (EBCTCG). Aromatase inhibitors versus tamoxifen in early breast cancer: Patient-level meta-analysis of the randomised trials. *Lancet* **2015**, *386*, 1341–1352. [CrossRef]

8. Gray, R. Early Breast Cancer Trialists' Collaborative Group. Abstract GS3-03: Effects of prolonging adjuvant aromatase inhibitor therapy beyond five years on recurrence and cause-specific mortality: An EBCTCG meta-analysis of individual patient data from 12 randomised trials including 24,912 women. *Cancer Res* **2019**, *79* (Suppl. 4), GS3-03.
9. Davies, C.; Pan, H.; Godwin, J.; Gray, R.; Arriagada, R.; Raina, V.; Abraham, M.; Medeiros Alencar, V.H.; Badran, A.; Bonfill, X.; et al. Adjuvant Tamoxifen: Longer Against Shorter (ATLAS) Collaborative Group. Long-term effects of continuing adjuvant tamoxifen to 10 years versus stopping at 5 years after diagnosis of oestrogen receptor-positive breast cancer: ATLAS, a randomised trial. *Lancet* **2013**, *381*, 805–816. [CrossRef]
10. Gray, R.; Rea, D.; Handley, K.; Bowden, S.J.; Perry, P.; Earl, H.M.; Poole, C.J.; Bates, T.; Chetiyawardana, S.; Dewar, J.A.; et al. aTTom Collaborative Group. aTTom: Long-term effects of continuing adjuvant tamoxifen to 10 years versus stopping at 5 years in 6,953 women with early breast cancer. *J. Clin. Oncol.* **2013**, *31* (Suppl. 18), 5. [CrossRef]
11. Goss, P.E.; Ingle, J.N.; Pritchard, K.I.; Robert, N.J.; Muss, H.; Gralow, J.; Gelmon, K.; Whelan, T.; Strasser-Weippl, K.; Rubin, S.; et al. Extending Aromatase-Inhibitor Adjuvant Therapy to 10 Years. *N. Engl. J. Med.* **2016**, *375*, 209–219. [CrossRef] [PubMed]
12. Tjan-Heijnen, V.C.G.; van Hellemond, I.E.G.; Peer, P.G.M.; Swinkels, A.C.P.; Smorenburg, C.H.; van der Sangen, M.J.C.; Kroep, J.R.; De Graaf, H.; Honkoop, A.H.; Erdkamp, F.L.G.; et al. Dutch Breast Cancer Research Group (BOOG) for the DATA Investigators. Extended adjuvant aromatase inhibition after sequential endocrine therapy (DATA): A randomised, phase 3 trial. *Lancet Oncol.* **2017**, *18*, 1502–1511. [CrossRef] [PubMed]
13. Blok, E.J.; Kroep, J.R.; Meershoek-Klein Kranenbarg, E.; Duijm-de Carpentier, M.; Putter, H.; van den Bosch, J.; Maartense, E.; van Leeuwen-Stok, A.E.; Liefers, G.J.; Nortier, J.W.R.; et al. IDEAL Study Group. Optimal Duration of Extended Adjuvant Endocrine Therapy for Early Breast Cancer; Results of the IDEAL Trial (BOOG 2006-05). *J. Natl. Cancer Inst.* **2018**, *110*, 40–48. [CrossRef] [PubMed]
14. Mamounas, E.P.; Bandos, H.; Lembersky, B.C.; Jeong, J.H.; Geyer, C.E., Jr.; Rastogi, P.; Fehrenbacher, L.; Graham, M.L.; Chia, S.K.; Brufsky, A.M.; et al. Use of letrozole after aromatase inhibitor-based therapy in postmenopausal breast cancer (NRG Oncology/NSABP B-42): A randomised, double-blind, placebo-controlled, phase 3 trial. *Lancet Oncol.* **2019**, *20*, 88–99. [CrossRef] [PubMed]
15. Garreau, J.R.; Delamelena, T.; Walts, D.; Karamlou, K.; Johnson, N. Side effects of aromatase inhibitors versus tamoxifen: The patients' perspective. *Am. J. Surg.* **2006**, *192*, 496–498. [CrossRef]
16. Awan, A.; Esfahani, K. Endocrine therapy for breast cancer in the primary care setting. *Curr. Oncol.* **2018**, *25*, 285–291. [CrossRef]
17. Harrow, A.; Dryden, R.; McCowan, C.; Radley, A.; Parsons, M.; Thompson, A.M.; Wells, M. A hard pill to swallow: A qualitative study of women's experiences of adjuvant endocrine therapy for breast cancer. *BMJ Open* **2014**, *4*, e005285. [CrossRef]
18. Brett, J.; Fenlon, D.; Boulton, M.; Hulbert-Williams, N.J.; Walter, F.M.; Donnelly, P.; Lavery, B.; Morgan, A.; Morris, C.; Watson, E. Factors associated with intentional and unintentional non-adherence to adjuvant endocrine therapy following breast cancer. *Eur. J. Cancer Care* **2018**, *27*, e12601. [CrossRef]
19. Cluze, C.; Rey, D.; Huiart, L.; Ben Diane, M.K.; Bouhnik, A.D.; Berenger, C.; Carrieri, M.P.; Giorgi, R. Adjuvant endocrine therapy with tamoxifen in young women with breast cancer: Determinants of interruptions vary over time. *Ann. Oncol.* **2012**, *23*, 882–890. [CrossRef]
20. Freedman, R.A.; Revette, A.C.; Hershman, D.L.; Silva, K.; Sporn, N.J.; Gagne, J.J.; Kouri, E.M.; Keating, N.L. Understanding Breast Cancer Knowledge and Barriers to Treatment Adherence: A Qualitative Study Among Breast Cancer Survivors. *Biores. Open Access* **2017**, *6*, 159–168. [CrossRef]
21. Murphy, C.C.; Bartholomew, L.K.; Carpentier, M.Y.; Bluethmann, S.M.; Vernon, S.W. Adherence to adjuvant hormonal therapy among breast cancer survivors in clinical practice: A systematic review. *Breast Cancer Res. Treat.* **2012**, *134*, 459–478. [CrossRef] [PubMed]
22. Peddie, N.; Agnew, S.; Crawford, M.; Dixon, D.; MacPherson, I.; Fleming, L. The impact of medication side effects on adherence and persistence to hormone therapy in breast cancer survivors: A qualitative systematic review and thematic synthesis. *Breast* **2021**, *58*, 147–159. [CrossRef] [PubMed]
23. Hadji, P.; Ziller, V.; Kyvernitakis, J.; Bauer, M.; Haas, G.; Schmidt, N.; Kostev, K. Persistence in patients with breast cancer treated with tamoxifen or aromatase inhibitors: A retrospective database analysis. *Breast Cancer Res. Treat.* **2013**, *138*, 185–191. [CrossRef] [PubMed]
24. Davies, S.; Voutsadakis, I.A. Adherence to adjuvant hormonal therapy in localised breast cancer. *Eur. J. Cancer Care* **2022**, e13729. [CrossRef] [PubMed]
25. Hershman, D.L.; Shao, T.; Kushi, L.H.; Buono, D.; Tsai, W.Y.; Fehrenbacher, L.; Kwan, M.; Gomez, S.L.; Neugut, A.I. Early discontinuation and non-adherence to adjuvant hormonal therapy are associated with increased mortality in women with breast cancer. *Breast Cancer Res. Treat.* **2011**, *126*, 529–537. [CrossRef] [PubMed]
26. McCowan, C.; Shearer, J.; Donnan, P.T.; Dewar, J.A.; Crilly, M.; Thompson, A.M.; Fahey, T.P. Cohort study examining tamoxifen adherence and its relationship to mortality in women with breast cancer. *Br. J. Cancer* **2008**, *99*, 1763–1768. [CrossRef] [PubMed]
27. Chalela, P.; Munoz, E.; Inupakutika, D.; Kaghyan, S.; Akopian, D.; Kaklamani, V.; Lathrop, K.; Ramirez, A. Improving adherence to endocrine hormonal therapy among breast cancer patients: Study protocol for a randomized controlled trial. *Contemp. Clin. Trials Commun.* **2018**, *12*, 109–115. [CrossRef]
28. Bright, E.E.; Petrie, K.J.; Partridge, A.H.; Stanton, A.L. Barriers to and facilitative processes of endocrine therapy adherence among women with breast cancer. *Breast Cancer Res. Treat.* **2016**, *158*, 243–251. [CrossRef]

29. Liu, Y.; Malin, J.L.; Diamant, A.L.; Thind, A.; Maly, R.C. Adherence to adjuvant hormone therapy in low-income women with breast cancer: The role of provider-patient communication. *Breast Cancer Res. Treat.* **2013**, *137*, 829–836. [CrossRef]
30. Stanton, A.L.; Petrie, K.J.; Partridge, A.H. Contributors to nonadherence and nonpersistence with endocrine therapy in breast cancer survivors recruited from an online research registry. *Breast Cancer Res. Treat.* **2014**, *145*, 525–534. [CrossRef]
31. Cahir, C.; Dombrowski, S.U.; Kelly, C.M.; Kennedy, M.J.; Bennett, K.; Sharp, L. Women's experiences of hormonal therapy for breast cancer: Exploring influences on medication-taking behaviour. *Support Care Cancer* **2015**, *23*, 3115–3130. [CrossRef] [PubMed]
32. Piette, J.D.; Heisler, M.; Krein, S.; Kerr, E.A. The role of patient-physician trust in moderating medication nonadherence due to cost pressures. *Arch. Intern. Med.* **2005**, *165*, 1749–1755. [CrossRef] [PubMed]
33. Pellegrini, I.; Sarradon-Eck, A.; Soussan, P.B.; Lacour, A.C.; Largillier, R.; Tallet, A.; Tarpin, C.; Julian-Reynier, C. Women's perceptions and experience of adjuvant tamoxifen therapy account for their adherence: Breast cancer patients' point of view. *Psychooncology* **2010**, *19*, 472–479. [CrossRef]
34. Kirk, M.C.; Hudis, C.A. Insight into barriers against optimal adherence to oral hormonal therapy in women with breast cancer. *Clin. Breast Cancer* **2008**, *8*, 155–161. [CrossRef]
35. Constanze, E.; Uwe, G.; Christoph, T.; Kavitha, D.; Dominik, R.; Urte, S.; Walter, B. The role of trust in the acceptance of adjuvant endocrine therapy in breast cancer patients. *Psychooncology* **2022**, *31*, 2122–2131. [CrossRef] [PubMed]
36. Toivonen, K.I.; Williamson, T.M.; Carlson, L.E.; Walker, L.M.; Campbell, T.S. Potentially Modifiable Factors Associated with Adherence to Adjuvant Endocrine Therapy among Breast Cancer Survivors: A Systematic Review. *Cancers* **2020**, *13*, 107. [CrossRef] [PubMed]
37. Mouridsen, H.T. Incidence and management of side effects associated with aromatase inhibitors in the adjuvant treatment of breast cancer in postmenopausal women. *Curr. Med. Res. Opin.* **2006**, *22*, 1609–1621. [CrossRef]
38. Jones, S.E.; Cantrell, J.; Vukelja, S.; Pippen, J.; O'Shaughnessy, J.; Blum, J.L.; Brooks, R.; Hartung, N.L.; Negron, A.G.; Richards, D.A.; et al. Comparison of menopausal symptoms during the first year of adjuvant therapy with either exemestane or tamoxifen in early breast cancer: Report of a Tamoxifen Exemestane Adjuvant Multicenter trial substudy. *J. Clin. Oncol.* **2007**, *25*, 4765–4771. [CrossRef]
39. Coombes, R.C.; Kilburn, L.S.; Snowdon, C.F.; Paridaens, R.; Coleman, R.E.; Jones, S.E.; Jassem, J.; Van de Velde, C.J.; Delozier, T.; Alvarez, I.; et al. Intergroup Exemestane Study. Survival and safety of exemestane versus tamoxifen after 2-3 years' tamoxifen treatment (Intergroup Exemestane Study): A randomised controlled trial. *Lancet* **2007**, *369*, 559–570. [CrossRef]
40. Antoine, C.; Vandromme, J.; Fastrez, M.; Carly, B.; Liebens, F.; Rozenberg, S. A survey among breast cancer survivors: Treatment of the climacteric after breast cancer. *Climacteric* **2008**, *11*, 322–328. [CrossRef]
41. Fenlon, D.; Morgan, A.; Khambaita, P.; Carly, B.; Liebens, F.; Rozenberg, S. NCRI CSG Breast Cancer Symptom Working Party. Management of hot flushes in UK breast cancer patients: Clinician and patient perspectives. *J. Psychosom. Obstet. Gynaecol.* **2017**, *38*, 276–283. [CrossRef] [PubMed]
42. Francis, P.A.; Regan, M.M.; Fleming, G.F.; Láng, I.; Ciruelos, E.; Bellet, M.; Bonnefoi, H.R.; Climent, M.A.; Da Prada, G.A.; Burstein, H.J. SOFT Investigators; International Breast Cancer Study Group. Adjuvant ovarian suppression in premenopausal breast cancer. *N. Engl. J. Med.* **2015**, *372*, 436–446. [CrossRef]
43. Verbrugghe, M.; Verhaeghe, S.; Lauwaert, K.; Beeckman, D.; Van Hecke, A. Determinants and associated factors influencing medication adherence and persistence to oral anticancer drugs: A systematic review. *Cancer Treat. Rev.* **2013**, *39*, 610–621. [CrossRef] [PubMed]
44. Chlebowski, R.T.; Kim, J.; Haque, R. Adherence to endocrine therapy in breast cancer adjuvant and prevention settings. *Cancer Prev. Res.* **2014**, *7*, 378–387. [CrossRef] [PubMed]
45. Hagen, K.B.; Aas, T.; Kvaløy, J.T.; Søiland, H.; Lind, R. Adherence to adjuvant endocrine therapy in postmenopausal breast cancer patients: A 5-year prospective study. *Breast* **2019**, *44*, 52–58. [CrossRef]
46. Fink, A.K.; Gurwitz, J.; Rakowski, W.; Guadagnoli, E.; Silliman, R.A. Patient beliefs and tamoxifen discontinuance in older women with estrogen receptor–positive breast cancer. *J. Clin. Oncol.* **2004**, *22*, 3309–3315. [CrossRef]
47. Horne, R.; Weinman, J. Patients' beliefs about prescribed medicines and their role in adherence to treatment in chronic physical illness. *J. Psychosom. Res.* **1999**, *47*, 555–567. [CrossRef] [PubMed]
48. Hershman, D.L.; Kushi, L.H.; Shao, T.; Buono, D.; Kershenbaum, A.; Tsai, W.Y.; Fehrenbacher, L.; Gomez, S.L.; Miles, S.; Neugut, A.I. Early discontinuation and nonadherence to adjuvant hormonal therapy in a cohort of 8769 early-stage breast cancer patients. *J. Clin. Oncol.* **2010**, *28*, 4120–4128. [CrossRef]

Disclaimer/Publisher's Note: The statements, opinions and data contained in all publications are solely those of the individual author(s) and contributor(s) and not of MDPI and/or the editor(s). MDPI and/or the editor(s) disclaim responsibility for any injury to people or property resulting from any ideas, methods, instructions or products referred to in the content.

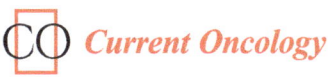

Article

A Prospective Population-Based Study of Cardiovascular Disease Mortality following Treatment for Breast Cancer among Men in the United States, 2000–2019

Duke Appiah [1,*], Megan Mai [2] and Kanak Parmar [3]

1 Department of Public Health, Texas Tech University Health Sciences Center, Lubbock, TX 79430, USA
2 School of Medicine, Texas Tech University Health Sciences Center, Lubbock, TX 79430, USA
3 Department of Internal Medicine, Texas Tech University Health Sciences Center, Lubbock, TX 79430, USA
* Correspondence: duke.appiah@ttuhsc.edu; Tel.: 806-743-9472; Fax: 325-677-1108

Abstract: Male breast cancer is rare but its incidence and mortality are increasing in the United States, with racial/ethnic disparities in survival reported. There is limited evidence for cardiotoxicity of cancer treatment among men with breast cancer. We evaluated the relation between breast cancer treatment and cardiovascular disease (CVD) mortality among men and investigated the salient roles that race/ethnicity play on this relation. Data were from 5216 men with breast cancer aged ≥ 40 years from the Surveillance, Epidemiology, and End Results program who were diagnosed from 2000 to 2019 and underwent surgery. Competing risk models were used to estimate hazards ratios (HR) and 95% confidence intervals (CI). During a median follow-up of 5.6 years, 1914 deaths occurred with 25% attributable to CVD. In multivariable-adjusted models, men who received chemotherapy had elevated risk for CVD (HR: 1.55, 95%CI: 1.18–2.04). This risk was higher among Hispanic men (HR: 3.96, 95%CI: 1.31–12.02) than non-Hispanic Black and non-Hispanic White men. There was no significant association between radiotherapy and CVD deaths. In this population-based study, treatment with chemotherapy was associated with elevated risk of CVD mortality in men with breast cancer. Racial/ethnic disparities in the association of chemotherapy and CVD mortality were observed.

Keywords: breast cancer; cardiovascular disease; chemotherapy; radiotherapy; mortality

Citation: Appiah, D.; Mai, M.; Parmar, K. A Prospective Population-Based Study of Cardiovascular Disease Mortality following Treatment for Breast Cancer among Men in the United States, 2000–2019. *Curr. Oncol.* **2023**, *30*, 284–297. https://doi.org/10.3390/curroncol30010023

Received: 2 December 2022
Revised: 19 December 2022
Accepted: 23 December 2022
Published: 25 December 2022

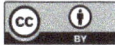

Copyright: © 2022 by the authors. Licensee MDPI, Basel, Switzerland. This article is an open access article distributed under the terms and conditions of the Creative Commons Attribution (CC BY) license (https:// creativecommons.org/licenses/by/ 4.0/).

1. Introduction

Male breast cancer (MBC) is a rare and understudied cancer that accounts for about 1% of all breast cancer cases in the United States [1]. Over the past few decades, the incidence of MBC has been on the rise. In 2022, it was estimated that 2710 new cases and 530 deaths from MBC will occur, representing an increase of 94% and 33%, respectively from estimates for 2000 [2,3]. While substantial efforts have been made in the past 20 years to understand the biologic features, effective treatment modalities, and outcomes for breast cancer, MBC remains largely understudied compared to female breast cancer (FBC) [4,5].

Due to its rarity, most MBC patients in the past have not been included in therapeutic studies, therefore, treatment strategies for MBC have largely been extrapolated from evidence from FBC patients [4–7]. While MBC share similar characteristics with FBC, it has distinct features that may influence treatment outcomes [1,8]. For example, MBC usually occurs at older ages and approximately occur 5 years before FBC [1]. While young MBC patients tend to have better overall survival than older male patients diagnosed with breast cancer, young MBC patients have worse survival outcomes than young FBC patients [9]. The lack of established screening guidelines for breast cancer in men often results in delays in the diagnosis of MBC of about 21 months after the onset of symptoms [6]. Furthermore, MBC patients are less likely to receive conventional treatments that may partly be due to low compliance among MBC patients [10]. Other clinicopathological differences include

MBC patients having higher frequency of mutations in BRCA2 tumor suppressor gene compared to BRCA1, having more frequent lymph node metastases, and having a higher proportion of estrogen-receptor positive tumors [1,5,6].

Although inconclusive, several studies have reported worse prognosis for MBC patients compared to FBC patients [4]. Recent registry-based studies have reported lower overall and 5-year survival in MBC compared to FBC patients, with the risk of death in MBC patients being 19% to 43% higher than FBC after controlling for potential confounding factors [4,10]. Clinical characteristics and undertreatments are reported to explain about 63% of the excess mortality for MBC patients [10]. Among MBC patients, racial and ethnic disparities in survival and other clinicopathological characteristics have also been reported with racial and ethnic minority men having lower overall survival compared to non-Hispanic White men [11].

Noncancer death, especially cardiovascular disease (CVD)-related deaths, accounts for a large proportion of deaths in MBC survivors as these two conditions share in common several risk factors [6,12]. Only a few studies have evaluated CVD outcomes in MBC patients [6,12,13]. A recent population-based epidemiologic study reported higher CVD mortality among MBC patients than would have been expected compared to the general population, with the mortality being highest among younger MBC patients aged 35–44 years at diagnosis [6].

Tremendous changes in treatment modalities for breast cancer have occurred over the past five decades that has been suggested to influence cardiovascular outcomes among breast cancer survivors [5,14,15]. The etiology of cardiotoxicity has been reported to vary by the type of cancer therapy. For example, HER2-directed therapeutics and chemotherapeutics such as anthracyclines that are standard-of-care treatment in high-risk individuals have been reported to increase the risk for cardiomyopathy and heart failure [16,17]. However, there is limited evidence on the pertinent roles that treatment for breast cancer plays on CVD outcomes in men. Recent ASCO guidelines on MBC recommend conducting post-treatment surveillance studies to provide evidence-based data for the management of breast cancer in men [18]. Therefore, the primary aim of this study was to evaluate the relation between breast cancer treatment and CVD mortality among men in the United States. The secondary aim was to investigate racial and ethnic disparities in the relation of breast cancer treatment and CVD mortality.

2. Materials and Methods

2.1. Study Population

Data for this registry-based prospective cohort study were obtained from National Cancer Institute's Surveillance, Epidemiology, and End Results (SEER) program which covers about 34% of the US population and obtains information from 17 population-based cancer registries located in the following states: Alaska, California, Connecticut, Georgia, Hawaii, Iowa, Kentucky, Louisiana, New Mexico, New Jersey, Utah. and Washington [19]. Men aged $\geq$ 40 years who were diagnosed with histologically confirmed stage I–III primary breast cancer from 1 January 2000 to 31 December 2019 were eligible for the current study. Of the 5508 eligible samples whose diagnosis was not made only at autopsy or via death certificates, the following exclusions were made: 219 persons that did not undergo surgery, 72 persons with no follow-up information or unknown cause of death, and 1 person with no information on tumor laterality. This resulted in an analytic sample of 5216 MBC patients. Institutional review board approval was not required for this study as the SEER registry is a de-identified publicly available database.

2.2. Definition of Study Variables

Information obtained from the SEER database included age at diagnosis, year of diagnosis, race and ethnicity, geographic region, location (rural or urban), marital status, annual median household income of the county of patient's residence, disease stage, tumor grade, tumor size, laterality, number of regional lymph nodes examined, hormone (estrogen and progesterone) receptor status, cancer therapy, cause of death, and survival time.

The main exposure of interest in the current study was first course of cancer therapy. For the current analysis, both radiotherapy and chemotherapy were classified as received or not received. The reported sensitivity, specificity, and positive predictive value of the SEER database correctly identifying individuals with breast cancer who received therapy are 69%, 98%, and 91% for chemotherapy and 80%, 98%, and 98% for radiotherapy [20]. Breast cancer was defined using International Classification of Diseases for Oncology, 3rd edition (ICD-O-3) codes C500-C509. Race and ethnicity were defined as non-Hispanic White, non-Hispanic Black, Hispanic, and other which includes American Indians/Alaska Native, Asian or Pacific Islander, and other race or ethnic groups. Cancer stage at time of diagnosis was defined using the American Joint Committee on Cancer's staging manual that uses information on tumor size, regional lymph node involvement, and the presence of metastasis [21]. Editions of the manual that were applicable during the period of the current study were used.

Cause of death information was classified using the World Health Organization's International Classification of Diseases, Tenth Revision codes. CVD mortality was defined as deaths due to diseases of heart (I00–I09, I11, I13, I20–I51), hypertensive heart disease (I10–I15), cerebrovascular diseases (I60–I69), atherosclerosis (I70), aortic aneurysm and dissection (I71), or other diseases of arteries, arterioles, or capillaries (I72–I78).

2.3. Statistical Analysis

Characteristics of men at the time of cancer diagnosis were described and compared among cancer treatment groups using chi-square test. Competing risk analyses were conducted using cause-specific hazard models, with deaths from all other causes besides CVD considered as competing risk events. Because the incidence of MBC and CVD mortality rates increase with advancing age, attained age in years was used as the time scale for all time-to-event analyses. Thus, estimates from such model are age-adjusted [22]. The validity of the proportional hazards assumption was tested and confirmed using weighted Schoenfeld residuals as well as using formal statistical test of non-proportionality.

Covariate selection for multivariable models was based on variables that were significant in bivariable analyses at an alpha of 0.2. Variables evaluated in bivariate models were year of diagnosis, race and ethnicity, geographic region, location, marital status, income, disease stage, estrogen and progesterone receptor status, tumor grade, tumor size, laterality, and number of regional lymph nodes examined. Because the impact of radiation on overall survival among MBC patients is not the same between breast conservation surgery and mastectomy [23], and radiation to the left side of the breast is associated with a higher risk of CVD than on the right breast [24], additional analyses were performed to evaluate the role of type of surgery and tumor laterality on the association of radiotherapy with CVD mortality among men who did not receive chemotherapy.

Finally, interaction between race and ethnicity with cancer therapy was tested. The SEER*Stat version 8.4.0.1 software (Information Management Systems, Rockville, MD, USA) and the SAS software version 9.4 (SAS Institute, Inc., Cary, NC, USA) were used to conduct the statistical analyses with statistical significance determined with a two-tailed test p value of less than 0.05.

3. Results

Over the study period, there was an increase in the number men diagnosed with cancer. Approximately 20% of men with breast cancer were diagnosed in 2000–2004 compared to 28% in 2015–2019. The mean age at diagnosis was 66.1 (standard deviation: 11.7; median 66) years, with more than half of them (52%) living in the west region of the United States at the time of cancer diagnosis. The racial and ethnic distribution of the sample are as follows: non-Hispanic White, 75%; non-Hispanic Black, 12%; and Hispanic, 7%. Only 12% of men diagnosed with breast cancer lived in counties with median household incomes of less than $50,000. With regards to receipt of cancer treatment, 38.8% and 28.4% of men reported receiving chemotherapy and radiotherapy, respectively, with the median time from diagnosis to treatment being 1 month. Characteristics of participants according to the first course of cancer therapy received are reported in Table 1.

Table 1. Characteristics of men at the time of breast cancer diagnosis according to cancer therapy, SEER program (n = 5216).

Characteristics, %	Cancer Treatment Groups				p Value
	No Chemotherapy, No Radiotherapy (n = 2653)	Chemotherapy, No Radiotherapy (n = 1083)	No Chemotherapy, Radiotherapy (n = 541)	Chemotherapy and Radiotherapy (n = 939)	
Age, years					<0.001
40–64	34.7	61.6	34.2	60.7	
65–74	30.5	29.1	29.6	30.8	
≥75	34.8	9.3	36.2	8.5	
Year of diagnosis					<0.001
2000–2004	22.2	20.4	17.2	19.5	
2005–2009	24.3	26.5	18.9	20.9	
2010–2014	26.8	28.7	28.5	26.2	
2015–2019	26.7	24.4	35.5	33.4	
Race and ethnicity					0.447
Non-Hispanic White	76.10	73.80	74.70	73.80	
Non-Hispanic Black	11.70	12.20	12.60	13.50	
Hispanic	6.50	7.70	8.50	7.00	
Other	5.70	6.40	4.30	5.60	
Region					0.003
Midwest	4.3	3.9	4.6	5.1	
Northeast	20.0	21.9	20.9	16.5	
South	20.8	23.7	24.2	26.6	
West	54.9	50.5	50.3	51.8	
Marital status, married	68.5	69.3	68.2	69.0	0.947
Median household income					0.992
<$50,000	12.2	12.2	12.4	12.8	
$50,000–$75,000	54.2	53.2	53.0	53.7	
>$75,000	33.5	34.6	34.6	33.5	
Location, rural	12.6	13.2	9.2	11.5	0.103
Stage					<0.001
I	51.5	27.1	41.6	11.9	
II	41.0	54.8	39.7	41.7	
III	7.6	18.1	18.7	46.3	
Tumor grade					<0.001
I/II	68.7	53.70	65.10	54.10	
III/IV	24.6	42.50	27.70	42.20	
Unknown	6.7	3.8	7.2	3.7	
Lymph nodes examined					<0.001
0	9.1	2.0	7.6	1.8	
≥1	90.9	98.0	92.4	98.2	
Tumor size (cm)					<0.001
<2	46.3	35.6	44.4	26.9	
≥2	35.3	48.0	41.4	57.1	
Unknown	18.4	16.3	14.2	16.0	

Table 1. Cont.

Characteristics, %	Cancer Treatment Groups				p Value
	No Chemotherapy, No Radiotherapy (n = 2653)	Chemotherapy, No Radiotherapy (n = 1083)	No Chemotherapy, Radiotherapy (n = 541)	Chemotherapy and Radiotherapy (n = 939)	
ER status					<0.001
Yes	89.9	91.7	94.5	92.8	
No	1.9	3.7	2.0	4.8	
Unknown	8.1	4.6	3.5	2.4	
PR status					<0.001
Yes	82.9	80.0	89.1	82.9	
No	7.5	13.7	6.7	14.2	
Unknown	9.6	6.4	4.3	3.0	
Type of surgery					<0.001
Breast conservation surgery	9.4	7.1	35.2	12.2	
Mastectomy	90.6	92.9	64.8	87.8	

ER: estrogen receptor, PR: progesterone receptor status.

Over the period of the study, the proportion of patients who received radiotherapy (with or without chemotherapy) increased while the proportion of patients who received chemotherapy reduced with age. Additionally, a greater proportion of patients who received both chemotherapy and radiotherapy had stage III cancer while the proportion of patients with mastectomy was lowest among those who received radiotherapy alone.

During a median follow-up of 5.6 years (interquartile range: 2.6 to 9.8), 1914 deaths occurred with 25% and 35% attributable to CVD and breast cancer, respectively. Characteristics of patients at the time of diagnosis according to cardiovascular disease mortality status are presented in Table 2. Of the 485 CVD deaths, 64.5% occurred among patients who received neither chemotherapy or radiation, 14.6% occurred among those who received chemotherapy but not radiation, 11.8% occurred among patients who received radiation but not chemotherapy, and 9.1% occurred among patients who received both chemotherapy and radiotherapy. Similarly, among the 1914 all-cause mortality cases, 55.7% occurred among patients who received neither chemotherapy nor radiation, 19.1% occurred among those who received chemotherapy but not radiation, 10.2% occurred among patients who received radiation but not chemotherapy, and 15.0% occurred among patients who received both chemotherapy and radiotherapy.

Table 2. Characteristics of men at the time of breast cancer diagnosis according to cardiovascular disease mortality status at the end of follow-up, SEER registry (n = 5216).

Characteristics, %	CVD Mortality		p Value
	No (n = 4731)	Yes (n = 485)	
Age, years			<0.001
40–64	47.6	18.6	
65–74	30.4	27.6	
≥75	22.0	53.8	
Year of diagnosis			<0.001
2000–2004	19.2	37.1	
2005–2009	22.5	34.0	
2010–2014	27.9	20.6	
2015–2019	30.4	8.2	

Table 2. Cont.

Characteristics, %	CVD Mortality		p Value
	No (n = 4731)	Yes (n = 485)	
Race and ethnicity			0.087
Non-Hispanic White	74.6	79.4	
Non-Hispanic Black	12.4	10.7	
Hispanic	7.1	6.2	
Other	5.9	3.7	
Region			0.002
Midwest	4.2	6.2	
Northeast	20.1	17.3	
South	23.4	17.7	
West	52.3	58.8	
Marital status, married	69.0	66.2	0.217
Median household income			0.825
<$50,000	12.4	11.5	
$50,000–$75,000	53.7	54.8	
>$75,000	33.9	33.6	
Location, rural	12.1	12.8	0.662
Stage			0.001
I	39.0	30.5	
II	43.1	51.5	
III	17.9	17.9	
Tumor grade			0.780
I/II	62.7	61.4	
III/IV	31.7	33.2	
Unknown	5.6	5.4	
Lymph nodes examined			<0.001
0	5.4	13.4	
≥1	94.6	86.6	
Tumor size (mm)			<0.001
<2	41.4	30.5	
≥2	42.7	40.4	
Unknown	15.9	29.1	
ER status			<0.001
Yes	91.6	88.0	
No	3.0	1.4	
Unknown	5.4	10.5	
PR status			<0.001
Yes	83.2	80.6	
No	10.1	7.4	
Unknown	6.7	12	
Type of surgery			0.380
Breast conservation surgery	12.2	10.8	
Mastectomy	87.8	89.2	
Cancer therapy			<0.001
No chemotherapy, no radiotherapy	49.5	64.5	
Chemotherapy, no radiation	21.4	14.6	
Radiation, no chemotherapy	10.2	11.8	
Chemotherapy and radiotherapy	18.9	9.1	

ER: estrogen receptor, PR: progesterone receptor status.

Multivariable models were adjusted for age, year of cancer diagnosis, race and ethnicity, disease stage, tumor size, and number of lymph nodes examined as these variables were found to be statistically significant in bivariable analyses. In these models, men with breast cancer who received chemotherapy as part of their first course of treatment had elevated risk for CVD (Hazard ratio (HR): 1.32, 95% CI: 1.05–1.66)), with the risk being higher among those who received chemotherapy alone (HR: 1.55, 95% CI: 1.18–2.04) (Table 3).

Table 3. Hazard ratios and 95% confidence intervals for the association of cancer treatment with CVD mortality in men diagnosed with breast cancer, SEER registry (2000–2019).

Treatment	Model 1		Model 2	
	HR (95% CI)	p Value	HR (95% CI)	p Value
Chemotherapy		<0.001		0.019
No	1		1	
Yes	1.56 (1.25–1.94)		1.32 (1.05–1.66)	
Radiotherapy		0.385		0.848
No	1		1	
Yes	1.10 (0.88–1.38)		0.98 (0.77–1.24)	
Radiotherapy and/or chemotherapy		<0.001		0.018
No chemotherapy or radiotherapy	1		1	
No radiotherapy, chemotherapy	1.80 (1.38–2.35)		1.55 (1.18–2.04)	
Radiotherapy, no chemotherapy	1.15 (0.86–1.52)		1.08 (0.81–1.45)	
Radiotherapy and chemotherapy	1.34 (0.97–1.85)		1.07 (0.76–1.52)	

Model 1: age adjusted model. Model 2: adjusted for age, year of cancer diagnosis, race and ethnicity, disease stage, tumor size, and number of lymph nodes examined. CI: confidence interval, HR: hazard ratio.

There was no significant association between radiotherapy (with or without chemotherapy) and CVD deaths. There was a significant interaction between race and ethnicity and cancer treatment on the risk of CVD mortality ($p = 0.005$). The risk of CVD mortality was observed to be highest among Hispanic men (HR: 3.96, 95% CI: 1.31–12.02) (Figure 1).

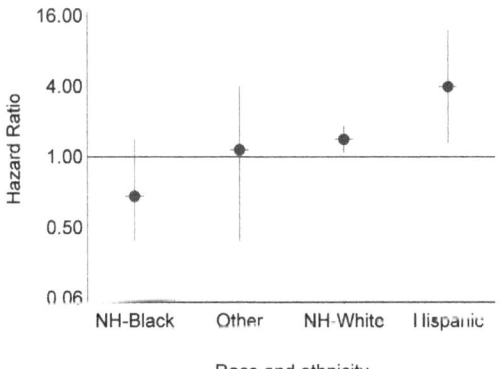

Figure 1. The association of cancer treatment with cardiovascular disease mortality in men diagnosed with breast cancer according to race and ethnicity, SEER registry (2000–2019). NH: Non-Hispanic. p value for interaction = 0.005.

Among persons who received radiotherapy, there was no significant influence of laterality or the association of radiotherapy and CVD mortality ($p = 0.672$). Similarly, the relation of radiotherapy and CVD mortality was not significantly influenced by the type of surgery, thus breast conservation surgery or mastectomy ($p = 0.206$).

4. Discussion

In this population-based study of men diagnosed with breast cancer in the United States over a 20-year period, treatment with chemotherapy was associated with elevated risk of CVD mortality, while no significant association was observed between radiation therapy and deaths due to CVD. Racial and ethnic disparities in the association of chemotherapy and CVD mortality were observed, with Hispanic men having higher risk of CVD deaths compared to non-Hispanic Black and non-Hispanic White men. To our knowledge, this is the first study to comprehensively characterize CVD mortality due to cancer treatment among men diagnosed with breast cancer.

Some breast cancer therapeutics have been reported to result in early or delayed cardiotoxicity comprising of hypertension, arrhythmias, pericarditis, thromboembolism, valvular disease, left ventricular dysfunction, heart failure, and myocardial infarction [14,15]. Accordingly, it has been estimated that the cumulative incidence of treatment-related cardiotoxic outcomes among breast cancer patients may be as high as 33% [25]. There are limited prospective investigations of the relation of neoadjuvant or adjuvant chemotherapy on CVD morality in MBC patients. Results from the current study of elevated risk of CVD mortality among MBC patients who received chemotherapy is supported by several pieces of evidence of the cardiotoxic effects of chemotherapy in murine models and studies conducted among FBC patients [14,26–30]. The most widely reported cardiotoxic effect of chemotherapy is left ventricular dysfunction that manifests as overt heart failure over time [14,25], although other cardiac events such as thrombosis, arrhythmias, myocarditis, pericarditis, and myocardial infarction have also been reported [31]. For instance, Yang et al. [32] reported a 74% elevated risk of heart failure among breast cancer patients who received chemotherapy. Conversely, as seen in some studies among women [33], a few studies conducted mostly among small samples of men with breast cancer have also reported lower mortality in men who received adjuvant chemotherapy [34–36]. However, these studies did not specifically evaluate cardiovascular-related mortality.

There are several mechanisms by which chemotherapy may influence cardiovascular health in breast cancer patients. Anthracyclines, such as doxorubicin interacts with deoxyribonucleic acids, intercalating and inhibiting macromolecular biosynthesis of cardiac myocytes that eventually leads to apoptosis of myocytes and permanent damage to the myocardium [14,31]. Additionally, chemotherapeutics fosters the generation of reactive oxygen species which damage deoxyribonucleic acids, proteins, and mitochondrial membrane of myocytes [14,31]. In light of this, finding avenues to reduce the risk of CVD events among MBC patients is of great importance. With adjuvant chemotherapy not improving overall or breast cancer-specific survival among MBC patients with stage I and IIA cancer, the risk of CVD mortality may be reduced in this population by perhaps skipping chemotherapy for MBC patients with early-stage disease [37]. In addition, more consideration may be given to administering adjuvant trastuzumab which often, but not always, results in reversible LV dysfunction together with chemotherapy for patients with HER2-positive early-stage breast due to the reported marked improvement in survival and reoccurrence of cancer with this treatment regimen [14,38]. Finally, the risk-benefit profile of each MBC patient should be taken into consideration when choosing chemotherapy especially for those who are at high risk for CVD [14]. For those who have a risk-benefit profile in favor of chemotherapy, early detection and interception of cardiotoxicity remains important for clinicians.

Emerging evidence suggests that there are declining CVD mortality trends by radiation therapy among breast cancer patients [16,39]. Vo et al. [16] evaluating trends in heart disease mortality in the United States among women with invasive breast cancer from 1975 to 2017 observed significant declines in heart disease mortality for breast cancer survivors treated with radiotherapy alone compared to the general population, while an increasing trend in heart disease mortality was seen for regional stage patients treated with chemotherapy alone. From 1975–1984 to 2005–2016, the 10-year cumulative heart disease mortality declined from 6.35% to 2.94% among breast cancer survivors treated with radiotherapy alone while the 10-year cumulative heart disease mortality reduced from 1.78% to 1.21% [16]. Similarly, Hooning et al. [39] studying 7425 patients in the Netherlands treated for early breast cancer from 1970 to 1986 and followed through to 2000 found no increased CVD mortality for post-lumpectomy radiation, with the risk estimates for CVD mortality highest for post-lumpectomy radiation administered before 1979. Studies conducted in the modern era of breast cancer therapy have largely found no association between radiation therapy and CVD outcomes [31,39]. Similar to the current study where no association between radiotherapy (with or without chemotherapy) and CVD mortality, regardless of tumor laterality, was observed among MBC patients, Onwudiwe et al. using data from women aged 66 years and older with stage 0–III breast cancer diagnosed between 2000 and 2005 in the SEER-Medicare database also observed no association between radiation therapy and combined endpoints of death or cardiovascular disease [40]. Another register-based matched cohort study of Swedish breast cancer patients diagnosed from 2001 to 2008 and followed up until 2017 also observed no elevated risk of heart disease following locoregional radiotherapy [32].

The lack of a positive association of radiotherapy with CVD mortality observed in the current study as well as other studies of cancer therapy administered in the 21st century reflects the impact of changes in radiotherapy procedures [5,14]. However, it should be noted that radiation-associated cardiotoxicity often appears about 10 to 30 years after treatment and most studies including the current study did not have any individuals with follow-up beyond 20 years [41]. Increasing clinical guidelines about the adverse cardiac effects of radiation therapy has advanced cardio-protection strategies to minimize radiation-related damage to the cardiovascular system [14]. For example, reduction in radiation doses to the left side of the chest during radiotherapy, positioning patients to displace the heart during radiotherapy administration, the use of more precise radiotherapy using imaging and brachytherapy, and alternative radiotherapy options have all gone a long way to reduce the effects of radiation therapy on cardiac damage during cancer treatment [16,32,42–45]. Alternatively, the null association between radiotherapy and CVD mortality in MBC patients may be due to patients with left-sided breast cancer being less likely to be selected for radiotherapy due to the proximity of the tumor to the heart [32,45]. Future studies evaluating dosages of radiation to the heart and CVD mortality will enhance our understanding of a safe threshold of radiation that enhances cancer treatment response and at the same time reduce the risk for CVD outcomes in breast cancer patients.

Another interesting observation from the current study is the racial and ethnic disparities in the relation of chemotherapy with CVD mortality in MBC patients. The risk of CVD mortality in Hispanic men was more than twice the risk in non-Hispanic White men with no association observed between chemotherapy and CVD mortality among non-Hispanic Black men with breast cancer. While reasons for these findings are largely unknown, it is possible that differences in sociodemographic, socioeconomic, behavioral, and biological factors as well as differences in access to cancer treatment may partly explain these findings. For instance, compared to non-Hispanic White individuals, Hispanic populations are less likely to partake in mammography screening and adhere to cancer screening recommendations [46–48]. Thus, they often experience longer times to diagnosis of cancer resulting in them being likely to be diagnosed with advanced staged cancer [46]. Furthermore, they often experience poor quality of life following diagnosis of cancer than non-Hispanic White individuals [46]. Due to language barriers among low-acculturated Hispanic individuals, they often receive limited communication about cancer diagnosis and treatment which hinders the decision-making processes concerning cancer treatments [46,49]. A few studies among men [50] and several studies among women with breast cancer consistently report longer delays in receipt of chemotherapy among Hispanic and non-Hispanic Black individuals [51–53]. Taken together, it is possible that all these factors may contribute to the high risk of CVD mortality due to chemotherapy among Hispanic population.

With non-Hispanic Black individuals also experiencing delays in chemotherapy treatment [54,55] despite rates of oncologic consultation being similar between Black and White cancer patients [56], it would have been expected that this population would also experience high CVD risk due to chemotherapy. However, this was not the case in the current study. We speculate that the greater proportion of early discontinuation of chemotherapy of non-Hispanic Black patients mostly due to negative beliefs about efficacy of chemotherapy often due to concern about adverse effects [55,57,58], coupled with Black patients having lower pathologic complete response to neoadjuvant chemotherapy than Hispanic and other racial groups [59] may result in them having reduced exposure to the cardiotoxic effect of chemotherapeutics. With delays and interruptions in breast cancer treatment being positively related to breast cancer-specific mortality [60], this explanation is further supported by the observation that Black MBC patients have greater breast cancer-related mortality than CVD mortality compared to MBC patients of other racial and ethnic groups [12,50,61].

Currently, most treatment options for breast cancer in men are based on evidence from trials among women with breast cancer [62]. Although some reports show that treatment options in men produce comparable results to FBC patients [63], overall survival in MBC patients is lower than those for FBC patients [64] with some studies reporting excess mortality rates of about 60% in men when compared to women [10]. The lack of evidence-based treatment recommendations and screening guidelines for breast cancer in men, coupled with limited reports on treatment-associated complications continue to impact treatment choices and care for men with breast cancer [62]. Some studies report that screening mammography yields similar cancer detection rates between men and women at high risk for breast cancer [65]. Therefore, interventions focusing on increasing awareness and promoting breast cancer education in men, together with enhancing access to care among high-risk groups regardless of race and ethnicity will go a long way to increase early-stage cancer diagnosis and reduce racial and ethnic disparities in survival outcomes [66]. Furthermore, the few clinical trials among male breast cancer patients [18,67,68] currently underway will provide comprehensive data on the long-term management of MBC to inform treatment recommendations and guidelines on regimens that optimize cancer therapy and at the same time limit the risk of CVD [15].

The strength of the current study includes the use of a large population-based sample of MBC patients selected within a modern timeframe of cancer treatment. Limitations of the study include the lack of detailed information on specific drugs or hormone therapy not being available in the SEER registry for most of the period of observation for this study. HER2 positivity status was not evaluated in the current study as such information was only available after 2010. Furthermore, information on CVD risk factors at the time of cancer diagnosis as well as information on other comorbid noncancer diseases were not collected by SEER program. Finally, the chance of misclassification bias influencing the results of the study due to the use of death certificates to identify deaths attributable to CVD cannot be entirely ruled out. However, cause-of-death information in the SEER registry have been reported to have good validity [69].

5. Conclusions

In this population-based study of men with breast cancer, treatment with chemotherapy was significantly associated with elevated risk of CVD mortality, with the highest risk observed among Hispanic men. These findings have important implications for cardio-oncology care as well as extending research in the context of noncancerous outcomes in men with breast cancer. With the proportion of cancer patients receiving radiation therapy and chemotherapy increasing over the past few decades [16], future studies on cardiovascular outcomes due to cancer treatment regimens among racially and ethnically diverse MBC patients are warranted to enhance the clinical management of breast cancer in men.

Author Contributions: Conceptualization, D.A., M.M. and K.P.; methodology, D.A., M.M. and K.P.; formal analysis, D.A.; investigation, D.A.; resources, D.A., M.M. and K.P.; data curation, D.A.; writing—original draft preparation, D.A.; writing—review and editing, D.A., M.M. and K.P.; supervision, D.A. All authors have read and agreed to the published version of the manuscript.

Funding: This research received no external funding.

Institutional Review Board Statement: Institutional review board approval was not required for this study as the SEER registry is a de-identified publicly available database.

Informed Consent Statement: Not applicable.

Data Availability Statement: Data used for this study are publicly available from the National Cancer Institute at https://seer.cancer.gov/, accessed on 20 November 2022.

Conflicts of Interest: The authors declare no conflict of interest.

References

1. Giordano, S.H. Breast Cancer in Men. *N. Engl. J. Med.* **2018**, *378*, 2311–2320. [CrossRef] [PubMed]
2. Greenlee, R.T.; Murray, T.; Bolden, S.; Wingo, P.A. Cancer statistics, 2000. *CA Cancer J. Clin.* **2000**, *50*, 7–33. [CrossRef]
3. Siegel, R.L.; Miller, K.D.; Fuchs, H.E.; Jemal, A. Cancer statistics, 2022. *CA Cancer J. Clin.* **2022**, *72*, 7–33. [CrossRef] [PubMed]
4. Liu, N.; Johnson, K.J.; Ma, C.X. Male Breast Cancer: An Updated Surveillance, Epidemiology, and End Results Data Analysis. *Clin. Breast Cancer* **2018**, *18*, e997–e1002. [CrossRef] [PubMed]
5. Yadav, S.; Karam, D.; Bin Riaz, I.; Xie, H.; Durani, U.; Duma, N.; Giridhar, K.V.; Hieken, T.J.; Boughey, J.C.; Mutter, R.W.; et al. Male breast cancer in the United States: Treatment patterns and prognostic factors in the 21st century. *Cancer* **2020**, *126*, 26–36. [CrossRef] [PubMed]
6. Zheng, G.; Leone, J.P. Male Breast Cancer: An Updated Review of Epidemiology, Clinicopathology, and Treatment. *J. Oncol.* **2022**, *2022*, 1734049. [CrossRef] [PubMed]
7. Invasive Breast Cancer. Special Considerations for Breast Cancer in Males (Sex Assigned at Birth). NCCN Guidelines Version 4. 2022. Available online: https://www.nccn.org/guidelines/guidelines-detail?category=1&id=1419 (accessed on 1 December 2022).
8. Fox, S.; Speirs, V.; Shaaban, A.M. Male breast cancer: An update. *Virchows Arch.* **2022**, *480*, 85–93. [CrossRef]
9. Li, N.; Wang, X.; Zhang, H.; Wang, H. Young male breast cancer, a small crowd, the survival, and prognosis?: A population-based study. *Medicine* **2018**, *97*, e12686. [CrossRef]
10. Wang, F.; Shu, X.; Meszoely, I.; Pal, T.; Mayer, I.A.; Yu, Z.; Zheng, W.; Bailey, C.E.; Shu, X.O. Overall Mortality After Diagnosis of Breast Cancer in Men vs Women. *JAMA Oncol.* **2019**, *5*, 1589–1596. [CrossRef]
11. Sun, H.F.; Zhao, Y.; Gao, S.P.; Li, L.D.; Fu, W.Y.; Jiang, H.L.; Chen, M.T.; Yang, L.P.; Jin, W. Clinicopathological characteristics and survival outcomes of male breast cancer according to race: A SEER population-based study. *Oncotarget* **2017**, *8*, 69680–69690. [CrossRef] [PubMed]
12. Zhang, H.; Lin, W.; Chen, D.; Wang, K.; Tu, W.; Lin, H.; Li, K.; Ye, S.; Guan, T.; Chen, Y. Cardiovascular and Other Competing Causes of Death in Male Breast Cancer Patients: A Population-Based Epidemiologic Study. *Clin. Interv. Aging* **2021**, *16*, 1393–1401. [CrossRef] [PubMed]
13. Reiner, A.S.; Navi, B.B.; DeAngelis, L.M.; Panageas, K.S. Increased risk of arterial thromboembolism in older men with breast cancer. *Breast Cancer Res. Treat.* **2017**, *166*, 903–910. [CrossRef] [PubMed]
14. Mehta, L.S.; Watson, K.E.; Barac, A.; Beckie, T.M.; Bittner, V.; Cruz-Flores, S.; Dent, S.; Kondapalli, L.; Ky, B.; Okwuosa, T.; et al. Cardiovascular Disease and Breast Cancer: Where These Entities Intersect: A Scientific Statement From the American Heart Association. *Circulation* **2018**, *137*, e30–e66. [CrossRef] [PubMed]
15. Cherukuri, S.P.; Chikatimalla, R.; Dasaradhan, T.; Koneti, J.; Gadde, S.; Kalluru, R. Breast Cancer and the Cardiovascular Disease: A Narrative Review. *Cureus* **2022**, *14*, e27917. [CrossRef] [PubMed]
16. Vo, J.B.; Ramin, C.; Barac, A.; Berrington de Gonzalez, A.; Veiga, L. Trends in heart disease mortality among breast cancer survivors in the US, 1975–2017. *Breast Cancer Res. Treat.* **2022**, *192*, 611–622. [CrossRef] [PubMed]
17. Hader, S.N.; Zinkevich, N.; Toro, L.E.N.; Kriegel, A.J.; Kong, A.; Freed, J.K.; Gutterman, D.D.; Beyer, A.M. Detrimental effects of chemotherapy on human coronary microvascular function. *Am. J. Physiol. -Heart Circ. Physiol.* **2019**, *317*, H705–H710. [CrossRef]
18. Hassett, M.J.; Somerfield, M.R.; Baker, E.R.; Cardoso, F.; Kansal, K.J.; Kwait, D.C.; Plichta, J.K.; Ricker, C.; Roshal, A.; Ruddy, K.J.; et al. Management of Male Breast Cancer: ASCO Guideline. *J. Clin. Oncol. Off. J. Am. Soc. Clin. Oncol.* **2020**, *38*, 1849–1863. [CrossRef] [PubMed]
19. National Cancer Institute. Overview of the Surveillance, Epidemiology, and End Results Program. Available online: https://seer.cancer.gov/about/overview.html (accessed on 12 September 2020).
20. Noone, A.M.; Lund, J.L.; Mariotto, A.; Cronin, K.; McNeel, T.; Deapen, D.; Warren, J.L. Comparison of SEER Treatment Data with Medicare Claims. *Med. Care* **2016**, *54*, e55–e64. [CrossRef] [PubMed]
21. Amin, M.B.; Greene, F.L.; Edge, S.B.; Compton, C.C.; Gershenwald, J.E.; Brookland, R.K.; Meyer, L.; Gress, D.M.; Byrd, D.R.; Winchester, D.P. The Eighth Edition AJCC Cancer Staging Manual: Continuing to build a bridge from a population-based to a more "personalized" approach to cancer staging. *CA Cancer J. Clin.* **2017**, *67*, 93–99. [CrossRef]
22. Lamarca, R.; Alonso, J.; Gomez, G.; Munoz, A. Left-truncated data with age as time scale: An alternative for survival analysis in the elderly population. The journals of gerontology. *Ser. A Biol. Sci. Med. Sci.* **1998**, *53*, M337–M343. [CrossRef] [PubMed]
23. He, Y.; Gao, X.; Wu, J.; Li, X.; Ma, Z. Effect of Breast Conservation Therapy vs Mastectomy on Overall Survival and Breast Cancer-Specific Survival Among Men With Stage I-II Breast Cancer: Analysis of SEER, 2000–2018. *Clin. Breast Cancer* **2022**, *22*, 410–417. [CrossRef] [PubMed]

24. Gkantaifi, A.; Papadopoulos, C.; Spyropoulou, D.; Toumpourleka, M.; Iliadis, G.; Kardamakis, D.; Nikolaou, M.; Tsoukalas, N.; Kyrgias, G.; Tolia, M. Breast Radiotherapy and Early Adverse Cardiac Effects. The Role of Serum Biomarkers and Strain Echocardiography. *Anticancer Res.* **2019**, *39*, 1667–1673. [CrossRef] [PubMed]
25. Schmitz, K.H.; Prosnitz, R.G.; Schwartz, A.L.; Carver, J.R. Prospective surveillance and management of cardiac toxicity and health in breast cancer survivors. *Cancer* **2012**, *118*, 2270–2276. [CrossRef] [PubMed]
26. Barish, R.; Lynce, F.; Unger, K.; Barac, A. Management of Cardiovascular Disease in Women With Breast Cancer. *Circulation* **2019**, *139*, 1110–1120. [CrossRef] [PubMed]
27. Smith, L.A.; Cornelius, V.R.; Plummer, C.J.; Levitt, G.; Verrill, M.; Canney, P.; Jones, A. Cardiotoxicity of anthracycline agents for the treatment of cancer: Systematic review and meta-analysis of randomised controlled trials. *BMC Cancer* **2010**, *10*, 337. [CrossRef] [PubMed]
28. Bowles, E.J.; Wellman, R.; Feigelson, H.S.; Onitilo, A.A.; Freedman, A.N.; Delate, T.; Allen, L.A.; Nekhlyudov, L.; Goddard, K.A.; Davis, R.L.; et al. Risk of heart failure in breast cancer patients after anthracycline and trastuzumab treatment: A retrospective cohort study. *J. Natl. Cancer Inst.* **2012**, *104*, 1293–1305. [CrossRef] [PubMed]
29. Du, X.L.; Xia, R.; Liu, C.C.; Cormier, J.N.; Xing, Y.; Hardy, D.; Chan, W.; Burau, K. Cardiac toxicity associated with anthracycline-containing chemotherapy in older women with breast cancer. *Cancer* **2009**, *115*, 5296–5308. [CrossRef]
30. Doyle, J.J.; Neugut, A.I.; Jacobson, J.S.; Grann, V.R.; Hershman, D.L. Chemotherapy and cardiotoxicity in older breast cancer patients: A population-based study. *J. Clin. Oncol. Off. J. Am. Soc. Clin. Oncol.* **2005**, *23*, 8597–8605. [CrossRef]
31. Shakir, D.K.; Rasul, K.I. Chemotherapy induced cardiomyopathy: Pathogenesis, monitoring and management. *J. Clin. Med. Res.* **2009**, *1*, 8–12. [CrossRef]
32. Yang, H.; Bhoo-Pathy, N.; Brand, J.S.; Hedayati, E.; Grassmann, F.; Zeng, E.; Bergh, J.; Bian, W.; Ludvigsson, J.F.; Hall, P.; et al. Risk of heart disease following treatment for breast cancer—Results from a population-based cohort study. *eLife* **2022**, *11*, e71562. [CrossRef]
33. Guan, T.; Zhang, H.; Yang, J.; Lin, W.; Wang, K.; Su, M.; Peng, W.; Li, Y.; Lai, Y.; Liu, C. Increased Risk of Cardiovascular Death in Breast Cancer Patients Without Chemotherapy or (and) Radiotherapy: A Large Population-Based Study. *Front. Oncol.* **2021**, *10*, 619622. [CrossRef]
34. Izquierdo, M.A.; Alonso, C.; De Andres, L.; Ojeda, B. Male breast cancer. Report of a series of 50 cases. *Acta Oncol.* **1994**, *33*, 767–771. [CrossRef]
35. Patel, H.Z., 2nd; Buzdar, A.U.; Hortobagyi, G.N. Role of adjuvant chemotherapy in male breast cancer. *Cancer* **1989**, *64*, 1583–1585. [CrossRef] [PubMed]
36. Konduri, S.; Singh, M.; Bobustuc, G.; Rovin, R.; Kassam, A. Epidemiology of male breast cancer. *Breast* **2020**, *54*, 8–14. [CrossRef] [PubMed]
37. Li, W.P.; Gao, H.F.; Ji, F.; Zhu, T.; Cheng, M.Y.; Yang, M.; Yang, C.Q.; Zhang, L.L.; Li, J.Q.; Zhang, J.S.; et al. The role of adjuvant chemotherapy in stage I-III male breast cancer: A SEER-based analysis. *Ther. Adv. Med. Oncol.* **2020**, *12*, 1758835920958358. [CrossRef] [PubMed]
38. Suter, T.M.; Procter, M.; van Veldhuisen, D.J.; Muscholl, M.; Bergh, J.; Carlomagno, C.; Perren, T.; Passalacqua, R.; Bighin, C.; Klijn, J.G.; et al. Trastuzumab-associated cardiac adverse effects in the herceptin adjuvant trial. *J. Clin. Oncol. Off. J. Am. Soc. Clin. Oncol.* **2007**, *25*, 3859–3865. [CrossRef] [PubMed]
39. Hooning, M.J.; Aleman, B.M.; van Rosmalen, A.J.; Kuenen, M.A.; Klijn, J.G.; van Leeuwen, F.E. Cause-specific mortality in long-term survivors of breast cancer: A 25-year follow-up study. *Int. J. Radiat. Oncol. Biol. Phys.* **2006**, *64*, 1081–1091. [CrossRef] [PubMed]
40. Onwudiwe, N.C.; Kwok, Y.; Onukwugha, E.; Sorkin, J.D.; Zuckerman, I.H.; Shaya, F.T.; Daniel Mullins, C. Cardiovascular event-free survival after adjuvant radiation therapy in breast cancer patients stratified by cardiovascular risk. *Cancer Med.* **2014**, *3*, 1342–1352. [CrossRef]
41. Belzile-Dugas, E.; Eisenberg, M.J. Radiation-Induced Cardiovascular Disease: Review of an Underrecognized Pathology. *J. Am. Heart Assoc.* **2021**, *10*, e021686. [CrossRef]
42. Darby, S.C.; Ewertz, M.; McGale, P.; Bennet, A.M.; Blom-Goldman, U.; Brønnum, D.; Correa, C.; Cutter, D.; Gagliardi, G.; Gigante, B.; et al. Risk of ischemic heart disease in women after radiotherapy for breast cancer. *N. Engl. J. Med.* **2013**, *368*, 987–998. [CrossRef]
43. Taylor, C.W.; Kirby, A.M. Cardiac Side-effects From Breast Cancer Radiotherapy. *Clin. Oncol.* **2015**, *27*, 621–629. [CrossRef] [PubMed]
44. Taylor, C.; Correa, C.; Duane, F.K.; Aznar, M.C.; Anderson, S.J.; Bergh, J.; Dodwell, D.; Ewertz, M.; Gray, R.; Jagsi, R.; et al. Estimating the Risks of Breast Cancer Radiotherapy: Evidence From Modern Radiation Doses to the Lungs and Heart and From Previous Randomized Trials. *J. Clin. Oncol. Off. J. Am. Soc. Clin. Oncol.* **2017**, *35*, 1641–1649. [CrossRef] [PubMed]

45. Darby, S.C.; McGale, P.; Taylor, C.W.; Peto, R. Long-term mortality from heart disease and lung cancer after radiotherapy for early breast cancer: Prospective cohort study of about 300,000 women in US SEER cancer registries. *Lancet Oncol.* **2005**, *6*, 557–565. [CrossRef] [PubMed]
46. Yanez, B.; McGinty, H.L.; Buitrago, D.; Ramirez, A.G.; Penedo, F.J. Cancer Outcomes in Hispanics/Latinos in the United States: An Integrative Review and Conceptual Model of Determinants of Health. *J. Lat. Psychol.* **2016**, *4*, 114–129. [CrossRef] [PubMed]
47. Gonzalez, P.; Castaneda, S.F.; Mills, P.J.; Talavera, G.A.; Elder, J.P.; Gallo, L.C. Determinants of breast, cervical and colorectal cancer screening adherence in Mexican-American women. *J. Community Health* **2012**, *37*, 421–433. [CrossRef]
48. Wells, K.J.; Roetzheim, R.G. Health disparities in receipt of screening mammography in Latinas: A critical review of recent literature. *Cancer Control* **2007**, *14*, 369–379. [CrossRef]
49. Janz, N.K.; Mujahid, M.S.; Hawley, S.T.; Griggs, J.J.; Hamilton, A.S.; Katz, S.J. Racial/ethnic differences in adequacy of information and support for women with breast cancer. *Cancer* **2008**, *113*, 1058–1067. [CrossRef]
50. Crew, K.D.; Neugut, A.I.; Wang, X.; Jacobson, J.S.; Grann, V.R.; Raptis, G.; Hershman, D.L. Racial disparities in treatment and survival of male breast cancer. *J. Clin. Oncol. Off. J. Am. Soc. Clin. Oncol.* **2007**, *25*, 1089–1098. [CrossRef]
51. Zhang, L.; King, J.; Wu, X.C.; Hsieh, M.C.; Chen, V.W.; Yu, Q.; Fontham, E.; Loch, M.; Pollack, L.A.; Ferguson, T. Racial/ethnic differences in the utilization of chemotherapy among stage I-III breast cancer patients, stratified by subtype: Findings from ten National Program of Cancer Registries states. *Cancer Epidemiol.* **2019**, *58*, 1–7. [CrossRef]
52. Vandergrift, J.L.; Niland, J.C.; Theriault, R.L.; Edge, S.B.; Wong, Y.N.; Loftus, L.S.; Breslin, T.M.; Hudis, C.A.; Javid, S.H.; Rugo, H.S.; et al. Time to adjuvant chemotherapy for breast cancer in National Comprehensive Cancer Network institutions. *J. Natl. Cancer Inst.* **2013**, *105*, 104–112. [CrossRef]
53. Fedewa, S.A.; Ward, E.M.; Stewart, A.K.; Edge, S.B. Delays in adjuvant chemotherapy treatment among patients with breast cancer are more likely in African American and Hispanic populations: A national cohort study 2004–2006. *J. Clin. Oncol. Off. J. Am. Soc. Clin. Oncol.* **2010**, *28*, 4135–4141. [CrossRef] [PubMed]
54. He, X.; Ye, F.; Zhao, B.; Tang, H.; Wang, J.; Xiao, X.; Xie, X. Risk factors for delay of adjuvant chemotherapy in non-metastatic breast cancer patients: A systematic review and meta-analysis involving 186982 patients. *PLoS ONE* **2017**, *12*, e0173862. [CrossRef] [PubMed]
55. Green, A.K.; Aviki, E.M.; Matsoukas, K.; Patil, S.; Korenstein, D.; Blinder, V. Racial disparities in chemotherapy administration for early-stage breast cancer: A systematic review and meta-analysis. *Breast Cancer Res. Treat.* **2018**, *172*, 247–263. [CrossRef] [PubMed]
56. Bickell, N.A.; Wang, J.J.; Oluwole, S.; Schrag, D.; Godfrey, H.; Hiotis, K.; Mendez, J.; Guth, A.A. Missed opportunities: Racial disparities in adjuvant breast cancer treatment. *J. Clin. Oncol. Off. J. Am. Soc. Clin. Oncol.* **2006**, *24*, 1357–1362. [CrossRef] [PubMed]
57. Hershman, D.; McBride, R.; Jacobson, J.S.; Lamerato, L.; Roberts, K.; Grann, V.R.; Neugut, A.I. Racial disparities in treatment and survival among women with early-stage breast cancer. *J. Clin. Oncol. Off. J. Am. Soc. Clin. Oncol.* **2005**, *23*, 6639–6646. [CrossRef] [PubMed]
58. Shelton, R.C.; Clarke Hillyer, G.; Hershman, D.L.; Leoce, N.; Bovbjerg, D.H.; Mandelblatt, J.S.; Kushi, L.H.; Lamerato, L.; Nathanson, S.D.; Ambrosone, C.B.; et al. Interpersonal influences and attitudes about adjuvant therapy treatment decisions among non-metastatic breast cancer patients: An examination of differences by age and race/ethnicity in the BQUAL study. *Breast Cancer Res. Treat.* **2013**, *137*, 817–828. [CrossRef]
59. Killelea, B.K.; Yang, V.Q.; Wang, S.Y.; Hayse, B.; Mougalian, S.; Horowitz, N.R.; Chagpar, A.B.; Pusztai, L.; Lannin, D.R. Racial Differences in the Use and Outcome of Neoadjuvant Chemotherapy for Breast Cancer: Results From the National Cancer Data Base. *J. Clin. Oncol. Off. J. Am. Soc. Clin. Oncol.* **2015**, *33*, 4267–4276. [CrossRef] [PubMed]
60. Williams, F. Assessment of Breast Cancer Treatment Delay Impact on Prognosis and Survival: A Look at the Evidence from Systematic Analysis of the Literature. *J. Cancer Biol. Res.* **2015**, *3*, 1071.
61. Ellington, T.D.; Henley, S.J.; Wilson, R.J.; Miller, J.W. Breast Cancer Survival Among Males by Race, Ethnicity, Age, Geographic Region, and Stage—United States, 2007–2016. *MMWR Morb. Mortal. Wkly. Rep.* **2020**, *69*, 1481–1484. [CrossRef]
62. Arzanova, E.; Mayrovitz, H.N. Male Breast Cancer: Treatment Trends, Reported Outcomes, and Suggested Recommendations. *Cureus* **2021**, *13*, e18337. [CrossRef]
63. Kiluk, J.V.; Lee, M.C.; Park, C.K.; Meade, T.; Minton, S.; Harris, E.; Kim, J.; Laronga, C. Male breast cancer: Management and follow-up recommendations. *Breast J.* **2011**, *17*, 503–509. [CrossRef] [PubMed]
64. Sabih, Q.A.; Young, J.; Takabe, K. Management of Male Breast Cancer: The Journey so Far and Future Directions. *World J. Oncol.* **2021**, *12*, 206–213. [CrossRef] [PubMed]
65. Marino, M.A.; Gucalp, A.; Leithner, D.; Keating, D.; Avendano, D.; Bernard-Davila, B.; Morris, E.A.; Pinker, K.; Jochelson, M.S. Mammographic screening in male patients at high risk for breast cancer: Is it worth it? *Breast Cancer Res. Treat.* **2019**, *177*, 705–711. [CrossRef] [PubMed]
66. Moadel, A.B.; Morgan, C.; Dutcher, J. Psychosocial needs assessment among an underserved, ethnically diverse cancer patient population. *Cancer* **2007**, *109*, 446–454. [CrossRef] [PubMed]

67. Khan, N.A.J.; Tirona, M. An updated review of epidemiology, risk factors, and management of male breast cancer. *Med. Oncol.* **2021**, *38*, 39. [CrossRef] [PubMed]
68. Corti, C.; Crimini, E.; Criscitiello, C.; Trapani, D.; Curigliano, G. Adjuvant treatment of early male breast cancer. *Curr. Opin. Oncol.* **2020**, *32*, 594–602. [CrossRef] [PubMed]
69. Hu, C.; Xing, Y.; Cormier, J.N.; Chang, G.J. The validity of cause of death coding within the Surveillance, Epidemiology, and End Results (SEER) Registry. *J. Clin. Oncol.* **2009**, *27*, 6544. [CrossRef]

Disclaimer/Publisher's Note: The statements, opinions and data contained in all publications are solely those of the individual author(s) and contributor(s) and not of MDPI and/or the editor(s). MDPI and/or the editor(s) disclaim responsibility for any injury to people or property resulting from any ideas, methods, instructions or products referred to in the content.

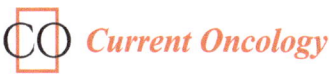

Article

Feasibility Study and Clinical Impact of Incorporating Breast Tissue Density in High-Risk Breast Cancer Screening Assessment

Alison Rusnak [1], Shawna Morrison [2], Erika Smith [2], Valerie Hastings [2], Kelly Anderson [2], Caitlin Aldridge [2], Sari Zelenietz [2], Karen Reddick [3], Sonia Regnier [3], Ellen Alie [4], Nayaar Islam [5], Rutaaba Fasih [6], Susan Peddle [6], Erin Cordeiro [7], Eva Tomiak [8] and Jean M. Seely [6,*]

[1] Inherited Cancer Program, Children's Hospital of Eastern Ontario, 401 Smyth Road, Ottawa, ON K1H 8L1, Canada
[2] Regional Genetics Program, Children's Hospital of Eastern Ontario, Ottawa, ON K1H 8L1, Canada
[3] The High-Risk OBSP Program Nurse Navigator, The Ottawa Hospital, Ottawa, ON K1H 8L6, Canada
[4] Previously High-Risk OBSP Program Screening Manager, The Ottawa Hospital, Ottawa, ON K1H 8L6, Canada
[5] School of Epidemiology and Public Health, The Ottawa Hospital, University of Ottawa, Ottawa, ON K1N 6N5, Canada
[6] Department of Radiology, The Ottawa Hospital, University of Ottawa, Ottawa, ON K1N 6N5, Canada
[7] Department of Surgery, University of Ottawa, Ottawa, ON K1N 6N5, Canada
[8] Department of Genetics, Children's Hospital of Eastern Ontario, University of Ottawa, Ottawa, ON K1N 6N5, Canada
* Correspondence: jeseely@toh.ca

Abstract: Breast tissue density (BTD) is known to increase the risk of breast cancer but is not routinely used in the risk assessment of the population-based High-Risk Ontario Breast Screening Program (HROBSP). This prospective, IRB-approved study assessed the feasibility and impact of incorporating breast tissue density (BTD) into the risk assessment of women referred to HROBSP who were not genetic mutation carriers. All consecutive women aged 40–69 years who met criteria for HROBSP assessment and referred to Genetics from 1 December 2020 to 31 July 2021 had their lifetime risk calculated with and without BTD using Tyrer-Cuzick model version 8 (IBISv8) to gauge overall impact. McNemar's test was performed to compare eligibility with and without density. 140 women were referred, and 1 was excluded (*BRCA* gene mutation carrier and automatically eligible). Eight of 139 (5.8%) never had a mammogram, while 17/131 (13%) did not have BTD reported on their mammogram and required radiologist review. Of 131 patients, 22 (16.8%) were clinically impacted by incorporation of BTD: 9/131 (6.9%) became eligible for HROBSP, while 13/131 (9.9%) became ineligible ($p = 0.394$). It was feasible for the Genetics clinic to incorporate BTD for better risk stratification of eligible women. This did not significantly impact the number of eligible women while optimizing the use of high-risk supplemental MRI screening.

Keywords: breast screening; high-risk breast screening; dense breasts; supplemental breast screening; breast MRI

Key Points:

1. Breast cancer risk assessment should be performed for all women ≥25–30 years of age to optimize early detection of breast cancer.
2. Women considered at high risk of breast cancer ≥40 years old must undergo screening mammography prior to referral to improve risk assessment.
3. Incorporating BTD into risk assessment was feasible, did not increase the overall number of women eligible for B-MRI and optimized supplemental B-MRI screening in women with dense breasts.

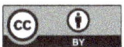

1. Introduction

Breast tissue density (BTD) decreases mammographic sensitivity by masking underlying cancers. It is also a well-established independent risk factor for breast cancer (BC) [1–4]. Mammographically dense breasts are very common and may contribute more cancer risk than other significant but less common risk factors [3] including obesity [5] and mitochondrial mutations [6,7].

In order to maximally benefit from early detection of breast cancer, international guidelines recommend that risk assessment for all women begin at 25–30 years of age [8,9]. Risk assessment models have been shown to increase their diagnostic accuracy with incorporation of BTD [10]. The High-Risk Ontario Breast Screening Program (HROBSP) is a population-based program for women who have a lifetime risk (LTR) of BC ≥25% or who carry a genetic mutation for BC [11]. Lifetime risk of BC is assessed by Tyrer-Cuzick model version 8 (IBISv8) [12] or Breast and Ovarian Analysis of Disease Incidence of Carrier Estimation Algorithm (BOADICEA) model (incorporated within the CanRisk tool 1 May 2021). Within HROBSP, a woman aged 30–69 years determined to have LTR assessed to be ≥25% is invited to participate in annual mammographic and B-MRI screening.

In the Genetics Clinic, prior to the introduction of the CanRisk model, IBISv8 was the predominant instrument used to assess BC risk for eligible women who had never been diagnosed with BC and who were not known genetic mutation carriers (unaffected). Version 8 incorporates BTD (for woman age 40+) and other personal risk factors along with family history of breast and ovarian cancer and is considered the most reliable model for assessing BC risk [12]. However, BTD was not included by our clinic before the study as it was not available at time of risk assessment. To assess the impact of incorporating BTD into the IBISv8 calculation, our group performed a retrospective review of 156 unaffected, 40–69-year-old women who had already undergone high-risk BC assessment from 1 November 2019 to 31 March 2020. We determined that 93.4% (146/156) had a prior mammogram and calculated that if BTD had been incorporated in the IBISv8, it would have changed the eligibility of 14.4% (21/146) with overall 4% (5/146) fewer women qualifying for annual screening MRI and mammography. Based on this preliminary work demonstrating the importance of including BTD we set out to prospectively determine the feasibility of incorporating this metric for all women undergoing HROBSP assessment at our centre and study the impact on program eligibility for women requiring B-MRI (B-MRI).

2. Methods

In this Research Ethics Board approved study from 1 December 2020 to 31 July 2021, genetic counsellors [GCs] performed risk assessments for all women who met Category B criteria for HROBSP screening eligibility (APPENDIX). All patients received one-on-one meeting with a GC. All appointments were virtual (by video or phone) due to the COVID-19 pandemic. Women were excluded from this study if they were under 40 years of age, as incorporation of BTD in IBISv8 is not validated for this age group. Women known to carry a hereditary BC risk gene were automatically eligible for high-risk screening and were excluded.

GCs completed the usual HROBSP assessments using IBISv8 and calculated lifetime risk (to age 80) with and without including BTD. The calculated risk with density included was used for determination of eligibility to the HROBSP program. For the purpose of the study, both numbers were recorded, along with information regarding the length of time it took to access the BTD.

At our centre, most referrals for HROBSP were sent directly to the OBSP nurse navigator (NN) for triage. The NN ensured that the referral met criteria for HROBSP assessment and then forwarded it to the Genetics clinic. For the study, the NN included the report of the most recent available mammogram with the referral. BTD was assesed visually on mammograms in the region and reported using BI-RADS® categories A, B, C, or D [13] (Figure 1). If BTD was not included on this report, the NN contacted the radiologist (JS or SP) to determine the BTD by reviewing the mammogram and/or report so that this could be included with the referral. In other instances, referrals for HROBSP came directly to the Genetics clinic and when the GC could not access their mammogram reports from the electronic medical record, the study radiologist (JS or SP) was contacted. Patients who reported having a prior mammogram within the province of Ontario could have their reports and/or actual mammogram images accessed through the electronic medical record and/or the picture archiving computer software (PACS) for review by the radiologist. BTD was not obtained for women with mammograms from outside of Ontario and for those who never had a mammogram; their risk assessment was calculated only without incorporating density. The McNemar's test was performed to compare the number of patients who were eligible with density versus the number of patients who were eligible without density; $p < 0.05$ was used to determine significance.

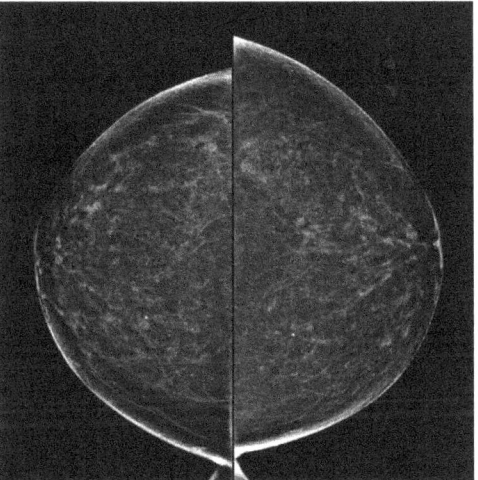

(**A**) ACR BI-RADS category A—fatty replaced breast tissue density.

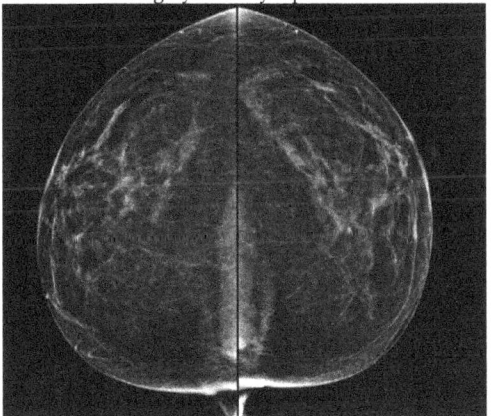

(**B**) ACR BI-RADS category B—scattered breast tissue densities breast tissue density.

Figure 1. *Cont.*

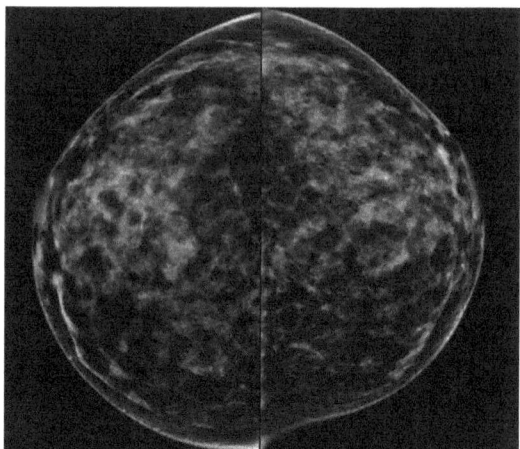

(C) ACR BI-RADS category C–heterogeneously dense breast tissue density.

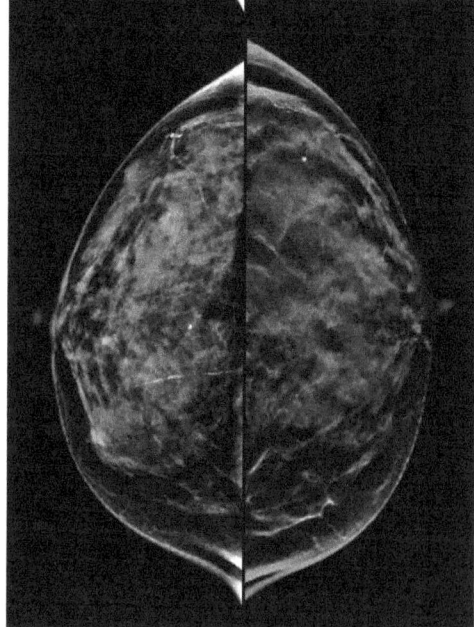

(D) ACR BI-RADS category D–extremely dense breast tissue density.

Figure 1. ACR BI-RADS categories (**A**–**D**) for craniocaudal mammogram views in 4 different women. As density increases from Categories (**A**) to (**D**), the masking effect increases, and the sensitivity of the mammograms decreases accordingly.

3. Results

3.1. Impact on Eligibility for B-MRI through the HROBSP Program

During the study interval, 140 women age 40–69 (average 51.4 years) with no prior history of BC underwent HROBSP assessment. One was excluded from this study as she was a known carrier of a *BRCA* gene pathogenic variant and automatically eligible for HR OBSP. Eight of the remaining 139 women (5.8%) never had a mammogram in the past 10 years (7) or only had a mammogram from another country (1) (Table 1).

Table 1. The impact on risk assessment and determination of clinical eligibility on addition of breast tissue density according to age groups 40–49 and 50–69.

Age Groups in Years (Total)	Patient Did Not Have a MG or Was Not Available *	Number of Patients (%) with MG and Density Available	Number of Patients (%) Where Density Increased Calculated Risk ^	Number of Patients (%) Where Density Decreased Calculated Risk ^^	Number of Patients (%) Where Density Made Patient Eligible **	Number of Patients (%) Where Density Made Patient Ineligible	Radiologist Input Required to Assess Density on MG
40–49 (65)	5 (7.7%)	60 (92.3%)	24 (40.0%)	27 (45.0%)	6 (10.0%)	10 (16.7%)	6 (10.0%)
50–69 (74)	3 (4.1%)	71 (95.9%)	26 (37.1%)	34 (47.9%)	3 (4.2%)	3 (4.2%)	11 (15.5%)
Total (139)	8 (5.8%)	131 (94.2%)	50 (38.5%)	61 (46.5%)	9 (6.9%)	13 (9.9%)	17 (13.0%)

MG = mammogram. * Women age 40–49 y had never undergone a mammogram while those 50–69 had mammograms in another province or country and the report was not available. ** eligibility was determined if calculated lifetime risk ≥25%. ^ Increase of calculated risk ≥1%. ^^ Decrease of calculated risk ≤1%.

Excluding the genetic mutation carrier, 139 women were assessed, 94.2% (131/139) of whom had a mammogram available and 13% (17/131) of whom required review by a radiologist to determine BTD on the mammogram. The incorporation of BTD impacted 16.8% (22/131). When reported BTD was incorporated into the risk assessment, 6.9% (9/131) became eligible for HROBSP and MRI screening; 9.9% (13/131) became ineligible, for a net 3.1% (4/131) fewer eligible patients (Table 2, Figure 2).

Table 2. Eligibility according to ACR BI-RADS categories of breast tissue density.

Density Category	Total Women with Mammograms (% of Total)	Became Eligible (% of Women with Density Category) *	Became Ineligible (% of Women with Density Category)
Density A	10 (7.6%)	0 (0%)	2 (20.0%)
Density B	40 (30.5%)	0(0%)	6 (15.0%)
Density C	58 (44.3%)	5 (8.6%)	5 (8.6%)
Density D	23 (17.7%)	4 (17.4%)	0 (0%)
Total	131	9 (6.9%)	13 (9.9%)

* Eligibility determined if calculated lifetime risk ≥25%.

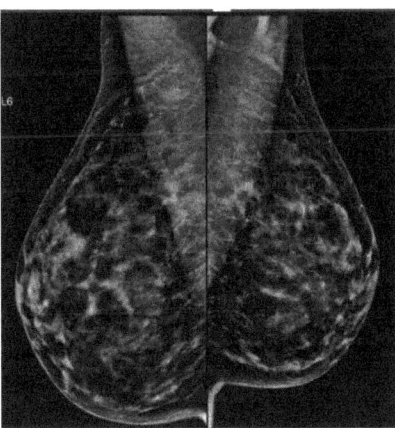

Figure 2. 42-year-old woman with a strong family history of BC shown to have BI-RADS category C breast tissue on screening mammograms. When BTD was incorporated into IBISv8 calculation, the lifetime risk increased from 24.2% to 32.4%, and she became eligible for HROBSP screening with B-MRI.

When comparing the number of patients who were eligible with reported BTD versus the number of patients who were eligible without including density, no significant difference was identified ($p = 0.3938$); even when considering the McNemar's exact test to account for the relatively small sample size ($p = 0.5235$). Based on these results, the proportion of eligible individuals was not significantly different between the two assessment methods.

As predicted, the 10 women who became eligible had the highest BTD as measured by BI-RADS (C or D) while 61.5% (8/13) who became ineligible had non-dense breasts (A or B). Five women who had never had a mammogram were 40–49 years old. Three women who had no mammogram available were 50–69 years and had it done outside of Ontario or remotely.

3.2. Feasibility of Incorporating BTD into the IBISv8 Calculation

When it became routine practice for the HROBSP NN to include the mammogram report in the referral to Genetics, it took no extra time for the GC to add BTD (BI-RADS A, B, C or D) with the other risk factors and family history information routinely collected from the patient in the risk calculation. This occurred in 87% (114/131) of assessed patients. For 13% (17/131) patients that required contact with the radiologist to help obtain the BI-RADS density score, both the GC/nurse navigator and radiologist estimated that it took about 5 min each, or 10 min in addition to the assessment, because the images were readily available for viewing. In total, for 17 patients at 10 min each, took 170 min.

4. Discussion

Our results demonstrated that it was feasible to incorporate BTD in high-risk assessment for BC. Including BTD in risk assessment optimized supplemental high-risk screening. No patients with non-dense tissue became eligible and 16% (8/50) ineligible, while 12% (10/81) with dense BTD became eligible, only 6% (5/81) (category C) ineligible. More patients with dense BTD were eligible while fewer with non-dense BTD required B-MRI, with an overall reduction of 3.1% (4/131) HROBSP eligible women. Although including density impacted eligibility for 17% women, the overall number of eligible women with vs. without density was not significantly different ($p = 0.3938$). Despite having been referred for a high-risk assessment for BC, 5.8% (8/139) women, and the *BRCA* carrier, had never undergone mammography.

It is well known that sensitivity of mammography is reduced in women with dense breasts, decreasing as BTD increases, 81–93% for fatty (A), 84–90% for scattered fibroglandular densities (B), 69–81% for heterogeneously dense (C) and 57–71% for extremely dense (D) breasts in women 40–74 years of age [14]. The interval cancer rate (BC detected after a normal screening study) is significantly higher in women with the most dense breasts when screened every 2 years versus every year [15]. B-MRI screening every 3–4 years in addition to mammography is cost-effective in average risk women who have the most dense breasts [16]. For women at high-risk, B-MRI is essential to permit early stage detection of BC and to reduce BC mortality. Our study found that more women with dense BTD became eligible for B-MRI while more with non-dense became ineligible, with no overall impact on use of B-MRI. Because of the masking effect of BTD, where BCs are obscured by dense tissue on mammography, contrast-enhanced B-MRI is required for early detection of BC in women with dense BTD [17].

Initial IBIS models did not incorporate BTD (v7,2004) but were updated in 2018 (v8), when BTD was shown to be more accurate in long-term assessment of BC risk [12]. Recently, researchers showed that risk stratification is improved when adding volumetric and visual mammographic density [18]. Destounis found a significantly higher proportion of high-risk women (defined as LTR $\geq 20\%$) when incorporating BI-RADS into IBISv8 compared with v7 (11.4% vs. 8.3% $p < 0.001$) [19]. In this study, fewer women with non-dense BTD were included in the high-risk category. A case–control study in 2019 of 474 patient participants and 2243 healthy control participants) of women aged 40–79 years found more women were included in the high-risk category, using IBISv8 instead of IBISv7 (7.1% vs. 4.8%) [20]. The

Brentnall study defined high risk as 8% 10-year or >20% lifetime risk while our study used the OBSP definition of high-risk as ≥25%. It would have been interesting to compare the impact using a similar risk assessment of ≥20%. In their study, BI-RADS assessment was a better predictor of risk than volumetric assessment of mammographic density. Our study however was a prospective evaluation of women already referred for high-risk assessment. IBISv8 is used by the HROBSP but the BTD information had not been widely incorporated as it was not being provided to the GCs performing the assessment. We showed that the HROBSP NN could provide available mammogram reports with the referral for HROBSP genetics' assessment. This occurred with 94.2% (130/138) patients assessed, which allowed for easy incorporation of BTD. Only 13.1% (17/130) of women had a prior mammogram but the report was unavailable to the GC and required radiologist input. In this instance, in took about 5 min for the GC and the radiologist to converse with each other to obtain this information.

Recently, as of October 2021, OBSP has made it mandatory for all mammograms reported through the OBSP to include the BTD according to BI-RADS categories. However, at present there is no mandatory requirement for BTD to be reported in diagnostic mammograms or screening mammogram done outside the OBSP program. BTD reporting should be mandatory for all mammograms done in Canada. In future, given these mandatory reporting requirements, it is expected that input from the radiologist will further decrease over time. In this prospective study, 16.9% (22/130) of women were clinically impacted by the incorporation of BTD with 4 fewer women requiring B-MRI. These results were consistent with the retrospective data (14.4% impacted and 4% fewer eligible women).

It is notable that 8 women from our prospective study and 8 from the retrospective data had never had a mammogram. In Ontario, population screening for BC with biennial mammograms begins at age 50. Women eligible for HROBSP assessment have a strong family history of breast and/or ovarian cancer and it is generally recommended that these women start annual mammograms (outside of OBSP) beginning at age 40 or 5–10 years prior to the earliest BC diagnosis in the family [21]. It should be noted that women considered at high risk are not included in the 2018 Canadian Task Force Preventive Health Care Guidelines [22]. Requiring a baseline mammogram prior to acceptance for HROBSP assessment would help to educate primary care providers and allow all women the opportunity to have BTD incorporated into their HROBSP assessment.

We recognize several limitations in our study. Inter-observer variation is well known in visual categorizing of BTD, and automated BTD was not used in our study. The 2013 BI-RADS 5th ed. density classification is based on the masking effect of BTD, while the 2003 BI-RADS 4th ed. [23] was based on visually estimated percentage BTD; both are associated with high rates of inter- and intra-observer variability [24,25]. Future considerations for OBSP include whether women's BC risk needs to be reassessed at some point, for example after menopause when many women's BTD decreases. There are also many women aged 30–39 y who were referred for HROBSP assessment to our centre. Neither IBISv8 or CanRisk are validated for inclusion of BTD for this age group and it is unknown whether they would benefit from reassessment after age 40. In May 2021, the BOADICEA tool was incorporated into the CanRisk tool which can now be used for unaffected women and includes similar personal risk factors as IBISv8 including BTD. The CanRisk tool provides some advantages to the genetic clinic assessment. For example, It allows for incorporation affected relatives with pancreatic and prostate cancer in addition to breast and ovarian and provides a mutation carrier likelihood for five BC risk genes (*BRCA1*, *BRCA2*, *PALB2*, *ATM*, *CHEK2*), and three ovarian cancer risk genes (*RAD51C*, *RAD51D*, *BRIP1*) compared to *BRCA1* and *BRCA2* only with IBISv8 ([26]). Unlike IBIS, CanRisk, does not however, allow for incorporation of benign breast disease such as atypical ductal hyperplasia and lobular carcinoma in situ, which are significant risk factors for BC. Which tool should be used for calculating HROBSP for unaffected women in our population is an ongoing question. Our study is limited by the small sample size but comparison with our retrospective data showed consistent results that are also in keeping with the recent larger data sets from

Brentnall and Destounis' studies [19,20]. Lastly, our study was limited by the lack of an outcomes audit and information about the stage of breast cancer in women previously assessed for eligibility in HROBSP. Including outcome information might prompt further evaluation of the eligibility threshold.

5. Conclusions

Our results provide support for inclusion of BTD into IBISv8 tool for purposes of HROBSP assessment of unaffected women, aged 40–69 y as it impacted the eligibility for MRI in 17% of women. The overall number of patients eligible for B-MRI was not significantly different when density was included, implying that there would not be a substantial impact to the resource requirements of the HR-OBSP. Family physicians are instrumental in assessing patient's risk for BC. If aware of a family history of BC in a woman 40 years or older, family physicians should order a mammogram to obtain BTD, as incorporating BTD will help to refine and improve risk assessment.

Author Contributions: Conceptualization, J.M.S., E.T., E.C., S.P. and A.R.; methodology, A.R., J.M.S., S.P., E.A. and E.T.; software, S.R., R.F. and K.R.; validation, E.A., V.H., E.S., K.A., S.Z., S.M., and C.A.; formal analysis, N.I., J.M.S. and R.F.; investigation, S.R., K.R., V.H., E.S., K.A., S.Z., C.A., S.M., S.P., J.M.S., E.T. and A.R.; resources, E.A. and J.M.S.; data curation, R.F. and J.M.S.; writing—original draft preparation, J.M.S.; writing—review and editing, A.R., E.T., S.P., E.C., V.H., E.S., K.A., S.Z., S.M., and C.A.; visualization, J.M.S. and A.R.; supervision, E.A., E.T. and A.R.; project administration, E.A.; funding acquisition, E.A. All authors have read and agreed to the published version of the manuscript.

Funding: This research received no external funding.

Institutional Review Board Statement: Ethical review and approval were waived for this study due to Ottawa Hospital Research Institute approved as QI project.

Informed Consent Statement: Patient consent was waived due to approved QI project.

Data Availability Statement: Data Availability upon request in Dataverse.

Conflicts of Interest: The authors declare no conflict of interest.

References

1. Boyd, N.F.; Guo, H.; Martin, L.J.; Sun, L.; Stone, J.; Fishell, E.; Jong, R.A.; Hislop, G.; Chiarelli, A.; Minkin, S.; et al. Mammographic density and the risk and detection of breast cancer. *N. Engl. J. Med.* **2007**, *356*, 227–236. [CrossRef] [PubMed]
2. Boyd, N.F.; Dite, G.S.; Stone, J.; Gunasekara, A.; English, D.R.; McCredie, M.R.; Giles, G.G.; Tritchler, D.; Chiarelli, A.; Yaffe, M.J.; et al. Heritability of mammographic density, a risk factor for breast cancer. *N. Engl. J. Med.* **2002**, *347*, 886–894. [CrossRef]
3. Engmann, N.J.; Golmakani, M.K.; Miglioretti, D.L.; Sprague, B.L.; Kerlikowske, K.; Breast Cancer Surveillance, C. Population-Attributable Risk Proportion of Clinical Risk Factors for Breast Cancer. *JAMA Oncol.* **2017**, *3*, 1228–1236. [CrossRef] [PubMed]
4. McCormack, V.A.; dos Santos Silva, I. Breast density and parenchymal patterns as markers of breast cancer risk: A meta-analysis. *Cancer Epidemiol. Biomarkers Prev.* **2006**, *15*, 1159–1169. [CrossRef] [PubMed]
5. Chen, K.; Zhang, J.; Beeraka, N.M.; Tang, C.; Babayeva, Y.V.; Sinelnikov, M.Y.; Zhang, X.; Zhang, J.; Liu, J.; Reshetov, I.V.; et al. Advances in the Prevention and Treatment of Obesity-Driven Effects in Breast Cancers. *Front. Oncol.* **2022**, *12*, 820968. [CrossRef] [PubMed]
6. Chen, K.; Lu, P.; Beeraka, N.M.; Sukocheva, O.A.; Madhunapantula, S.V.; Liu, J.; Sinelnikov, M.Y.; Nikolenko, V.N.; Bulygin, K.V.; Mikhaleva, L.M.; et al. Mitochondrial mutations and mitoepigenetics: Focus on regulation of oxidative stress-induced responses in breast cancers. *Semin. Cancer Biol.* **2022**, *83*, 556–569. [CrossRef]
7. Liu, Y.; Chen, C.; Wang, X.; Sun, Y.; Zhang, J.; Chen, J.; Shi, Y. An Epigenetic Role of Mitochondria in Cancer. *Cells* **2022**, *11*, 2518. [CrossRef]
8. Daly, M.B.; Pal, T.; Berry, M.P.; Buys, S.S.; Dickson, P.; Domchek, S.M.; Elkhanany, A.; Friedman, S.; Goggins, M.; Hutton, M.L.; et al. Genetic/Familial High-Risk Assessment: Breast, Ovarian, and Pancreatic, Version 2.2021, NCCN Clinical Practice Guidelines in Oncology. *J. Natl. Compr. Cancer Netw.* **2021**, *19*, 77–102. [CrossRef]
9. Monticciolo, D.L.; Malak, S.F.; Friedewald, S.M.; Eby, P.R.; Newell, M.S.; Moy, L.; Destounis, S.; Leung, J.W.T.; Hendrick, R.E.; Smetherman, D. Breast Cancer Screening Recommendations Inclusive of All Women at Average Risk: Update from the ACR and Society of Breast Imaging. *J. Am. Coll. Radiol.* **2021**, *18*, 1280–1288. [CrossRef]

10. Vilmun, B.M.; Vejborg, I.; Lynge, E.; Lillholm, M.; Nielsen, M.; Nielsen, M.B.; Carlsen, J.F. Impact of adding breast density to breast cancer risk models: A systematic review. *Eur. J. Radiol.* **2020**, *127*, 109019. [CrossRef]
11. Chiarelli, A.M.; Prummel, M.V.; Muradali, D.; Majpruz, V.; Horgan, M.; Carroll, J.C.; Eisen, A.; Meschino, W.S.; Shumak, R.S.; Warner, E.; et al. Effectiveness of screening with annual magnetic resonance imaging and mammography: Results of the initial screen from the ontario high risk breast screening program. *J. Clin. Oncol.* **2014**, *32*, 2224–2230. [CrossRef] [PubMed]
12. Brentnall, A.R.; Cuzick, J.; Buist, D.S.M.; Bowles, E.J.A. Long-term Accuracy of Breast Cancer Risk Assessment Combining Classic Risk Factors and Breast Density. *JAMA Oncol.* **2018**, *4*, e180174. [CrossRef] [PubMed]
13. Sickles, E.; D'Orsi, C.; Bassett, L.W. ACR BI-RADS®Mammography. In *ACR BI-RADS®Atlas, Breast Imaging Reporting and Data System*; American College of Radiology: Reston, VA, USA, 2013.
14. Kerlikowske, K.; Zhu, W.; Tosteson, A.N.; Sprague, B.L.; Tice, J.A.; Lehman, C.D.; Miglioretti, D.L.; Breast Cancer Surveillance, C. Identifying women with dense breasts at high risk for interval cancer: A cohort study. *Ann. Intern. Med.* **2015**, *162*, 673–681. [CrossRef] [PubMed]
15. Seely, J.M.; Peddle, S.E.; Yang, H.; Chiarelli, A.M.; McCallum, M.; Narasimhan, G.; Zakaria, D.; Earle, C.C.; Fung, S.; Bryant, H.; et al. Breast Density and Risk of Interval Cancers: The Effect of Annual Versus Biennial Screening Mammography Policies in Canada. *Can. Assoc. Radiol. J.* **2021**, *73*, 90–100. [CrossRef] [PubMed]
16. Geuzinge, H.A.; Bakker, M.F.; Heijnsdijk, E.A.M.; van Ravesteyn, N.T.; Veldhuis, W.B.; Pijnappel, R.M.; de Lange, S.V.; Emaus, M.J.; Mann, R.M.; Monninkhof, E.M.; et al. Cost-Effectiveness of Magnetic Resonance Imaging Screening for Women With Extremely Dense Breast Tissue. *J. Natl. Cancer Inst.* **2021**, *113*, 1476–1483. [CrossRef] [PubMed]
17. Bakker, M.F.; de Lange, S.V.; Pijnappel, R.M.; Mann, R.M.; Peeters, P.H.M.; Monninkhof, E.M.; Emaus, M.J.; Loo, C.E.; Bisschops, R.H.C.; Lobbes, M.B.I.; et al. Supplemental MRI Screening for Women with Extremely Dense Breast Tissue. *N. Engl. J. Med.* **2019**, *381*, 2091–2102. [CrossRef] [PubMed]
18. Destounis, S.; Arieno, A.; Morgan, R.; Roberts, C.; Chan, A. Qualitative Versus Quantitative Mammographic Breast Density Assessment: Applications for the US and Abroad. *Diagnostics* **2017**, *7*, 30. [CrossRef]
19. Destounis, S. Impact on risk categorization with inclusion of mammographic density in the tyrer-cuzick model. In Proceedings of the Radiological Society of North America, Abstract Presentation, Chicago, IL, USA, 28 November–2 December 2021.
20. Brentnall, A.R.; Cohn, W.F.; Knaus, W.A.; Yaffe, M.J.; Cuzick, J.; Harvey, J.A. A Case-Control Study to Add Volumetric or Clinical Mammographic Density into the Tyrer-Cuzick Breast Cancer Risk Model. *J Breast Imaging* **2019**, *1*, 99–106. [CrossRef]
21. Appavoo, S.; Aldis, A.; Causer, P.; Crystal, P.; Mesurolle, B.; Mundt, Y.; Panu, N.; Seely, J.M.; Wadden, N. *Canadian Association of Radiologists (CAR) Practice Guidelines and Technical Standards for Breast Imaging and Intervention*; Canadian Association of Radiologists: Ottawa, ON, Canada; Available online: https://car.ca/wp-content/uploads/Breast-Imaging-and-Intervention-2016.pdf (accessed on 17 September 2016).
22. Klarenbach, S.; Sims-Jones, N.; Lewin, G.; Singh, H.; Theriault, G.; Tonelli, M.; Doull, M.; Courage, S.; Garcia, A.J.; Thombs, B.D.; et al. Recommendations on screening for breast cancer in women aged 40-74 years who are not at increased risk for breast cancer. *CMAJ* **2018**, *190*, E1441–E1451. [CrossRef]
23. American College of Radiology. *ACR BI-RADS Atlas—Mammography*, 4th ed.; American College of Radiology: Reston, VA, USA, 2003.
24. Pesce, K.; Tajerian, M.; Chico, M.J.; Swiecicki, M.P.; Boietti, B.; Frangella, M.J.; Benitez, S. Interobserver and intraobserver variability in determining breast density according to the fifth edition of the BI-RADS(R) Atlas. *Radiologia* **2020**, *62*, 481–486. [CrossRef]
25. Sprague, B.L.; Conant, E.F.; Onega, T.; Garcia, M.P.; Beaber, E.F.; Herschorn, S.D.; Lehman, C.D.; Tosteson, A.N.; Lacson, R.; Schnall, M.D.; et al. Variation in Mammographic Breast Density Assessments Among Radiologists in Clinical Practice: A Multicenter Observational Study. *Ann. Intern. Med.* **2016**, *165*, 457–464. [CrossRef] [PubMed]
26. Carver, T.; Hartley, S.; Lee, A.; Cunningham, A.P.; Archer, S.; Babb de Villiers, C.; Roberts, J.; Ruston, R.; Walter, F.M.; Tischkowitz, M.; et al. CanRisk Tool-A Web Interface for the Prediction of Breast and Ovarian Cancer Risk and the Likelihood of Carrying Genetic Pathogenic Variants. *Cancer Epidemiol. Biomarkers Prev.* **2021**, *30*, 469–473. [CrossRef] [PubMed]

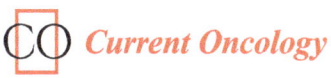

Article

The Impact of Organised Screening Programs on Breast Cancer Stage at Diagnosis for Canadian Women Aged 40–49 and 50–59

Anna N. Wilkinson [1,*], Jean-Michel Billette [2], Larry F. Ellison [2], Michael A. Killip [3], Nayaar Islam [4] and Jean M. Seely [5]

1. Department of Family Medicine, Faculty of Medicine, University of Ottawa, Ottawa, ON K1H 8L6, Canada
2. Centre for Population Health Data at Statistics Canada, Ottawa, ON K1A 0T6, Canada
3. School of Medicine, University of Limerick, V94 T9PX Limerick, Ireland
4. Clinical Epidemiology Program, The Ottawa Hospital Research Institute, Ottawa, ON K1H 8L6, Canada
5. Department of Radiology, The Ottawa Hospital Research Institute, University of Ottawa, Ottawa, ON K1H 8L6, Canada
* Correspondence: anwilkinson@toh.ca

Abstract: The relationship between Canadian mammography screening practices for women 40–49 and breast cancer (BC) stage at diagnosis in women 40–49 and 50–59 years was assessed using data from the Canadian Cancer Registry, provincial/territorial screening practices, and screening information from the Canadian Community Health Survey. For the 2010 to 2017 period, women aged 40–49 were diagnosed with lesser relative proportions of stage I BC (35.7 vs. 45.3%; $p < 0.001$), but greater proportions of stage II (42.6 vs. 36.7%, $p < 0.001$) and III (17.3 vs. 13.1%, $p < 0.001$) compared to women 50–59. Stage IV was lower among women 40–49 than 50–59 (4.4% vs. 4.8%, $p = 0.005$). Jurisdictions with organised screening programs for women 40–49 with annual recall (screeners) were compared with those without (comparators). Women aged 40–49 in comparator jurisdictions had higher proportions of stages II (43.7% vs. 40.7%, $p < 0.001$), III (18.3% vs. 15.6%, $p < 0.001$) and IV (4.6% vs. 3.9%, $p = 0.001$) compared to their peers in screener jurisdictions. Based on screening practices for women aged 40–49, women aged 50–59 had higher proportions of stages II (37.2% vs. 36.0%, $p = 0.003$) and III (13.6% vs. 12.3%, $p < 0.001$) in the comparator versus screener groups. The results of this study can be used to reassess the optimum lower age for BC screening in Canada.

Keywords: breast cancer; screening mammography; stage shift; registries; prevention; recommendations; clinical practice

Citation: Wilkinson, A.N.; Billette, J.-M.; Ellison, L.F.; Killip, M.A.; Islam, N.; Seely, J.M. The Impact of Organised Screening Programs on Breast Cancer Stage at Diagnosis for Canadian Women Aged 40–49 and 50–59. *Curr. Oncol.* **2022**, *29*, 5627–5643. https://doi.org/10.3390/curroncol29080444

Received: 23 June 2022
Accepted: 3 August 2022
Published: 9 August 2022

Publisher's Note: MDPI stays neutral with regard to jurisdictional claims in published maps and institutional affiliations.

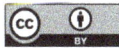

Copyright: © 2022 by the authors. Licensee MDPI, Basel, Switzerland. This article is an open access article distributed under the terms and conditions of the Creative Commons Attribution (CC BY) license (https://creativecommons.org/licenses/by/4.0/).

1. Introduction

Early detection of breast cancer through screening mammography and advances in technology and treatments have led to improved breast cancer (BC) survival [1]. Technology improvements such as breast ultrasound and magnetic resonance imaging have also markedly improved the ability of radiologists to diagnose breast cancer and profound changes in treatment have contributed to a 46% reduction in breast cancer mortality since screening mammography began in 1989 in Canada [2]. Treatment advances for breast cancer may raise questions about the relative importance of screening. Yet despite these advances, BC is still expected to be responsible for a quarter of all new cancer diagnoses in Canadian women and 14% of all cancer deaths in women in 2022 [3]. BC is the leading cause of non-accidental death in women younger than 50, and 30% of life years lost to BC are among women diagnosed in their 40s [4].

Mammographic screening for women in their 40s is contentious. The Canadian Task Force on Preventive Health Care (CTFPHC) recommended against routine screening of women aged 40–49 in their 2011 and 2018 guidelines and suggested that care providers should engage in discussion with these patients around screening [5,6]. The eight randomised controlled trials (RCTs) considered in these guidelines were performed between

1963 and 1991, prior to advances such as digital mammography and trastuzumab, and had screening intervals of up to 33 months [7–14]. Meta-analysis of these eight trials showed a BC mortality reduction of 15–18% for women 40–49 [15]. The Canadian National Breast Screening Study was the only trial that did not show a significant mortality reduction with screening [16]; however, the validity of randomisation and image quality in this trial have since been called into question [17,18]. A meta-analysis of the remaining seven trials showed a BC mortality reduction of 24% for the number of women invited to screen [19], and 29% for the combined five Swedish RCTs for women aged 40–49 at entry into screening [15].

Several observational studies exist which contribute valuable population-level insight and more accurately reflect actual screening practices, such as a yearly screening interval. The Pan Canadian trial involved 2.8 million women in Canadian screening programs over a 20-year period and showed a 44% BC mortality reduction in women aged 40–49 who were screened with mammography [20]. A similar rate of 41% reduction in mortality was seen in Sweden in 550,000 women after 10 years of participation in an organised screening program, as well as a 25% reduction in the rate of advanced cancers [21,22].

The goal of BC screening is to detect earlier, more treatable stages of BC. Although some studies postulate that the rate of advanced stage BC has not changed since the introduction of screening in the late 1980s [23–25], these studies have been criticised because tumor registry data were not linked to exposure to screening, and the annual increase in BC incidence of 1% from 1950 until 2001 was not accounted for [26–28]. It is clear that women in organised breast screening programs are more likely to have a lower-stage disease at diagnosis [29]. Early stage BC typically involves treatments with lower morbidity, including the decreased need for mastectomy, axillary dissection, chemotherapy, and radiation therapy, ultimately providing cost savings [30]. Stage-shift with screen detection has been shown to translate into survival benefits and is not merely a reflection of lead-time bias [31,32].

The relationship between breast cancer screening and overdiagnosis has garnered increasing attention, particularly given the improvements in treatments for breast cancer [33]. A recent review by Yaffe and Mainprize demonstrated that overdiagnosis is better-termed overdetection and may occur in the context of screening when cancers that are slow growing or indolent are detected and would not have surfaced clinically or caused the patient's death [34]. This may be an important harm from screening if treatment is not tailored to the affected individual. Using Canadian modelling data, Yaffe and Mainprize found that rates of overdetection were much lower than estimated by the CTFPHC and were more likely to occur in older women than younger women due to competing causes of death [34]. A very recent Belgian modelling study similarly confirmed that overdiagnosis was much more likely in older women and found that estimates of overdiagnosis were much more accurate with a follow-up of 10 years or more [35].

BC screening programs for women aged 40–49 are considered most effective when they are organised, (i.e., population-based) and when they include annual reminders [4,36]. Active recruitment is generally employed to achieve a target participation rate of 70%. Opportunistic programs where women are required to take an active role in arranging their screening have been shown to have significantly lower screening rates [37]. Annual screening is important as the growth of BC in premenopausal women is more rapid [38]. Younger women aged 40–49 are more likely to have dense breasts, which among other factors increase the risk of BC [39]. It has been shown that mammography in women with extremely dense breasts is more effective if it is performed yearly [40,41].

This study assesses the relationship between Canadian mammography screening practices for women aged 40–49 on the stage of BC at diagnosis in women aged 40–49 and 50–59 years using incidence data from the Canadian Cancer Registry (CCR) and screening information from the Canadian Community Health Survey (CCHS) as well as provincial and territorial screening practices. Variations in jurisdictional screening policies in Canada allow this unique opportunity to evaluate the impact of different programmatic screening policies on the stages of breast cancer at diagnosis in women 40–49 and 50–59 years old. To our knowledge, this work has not been performed before in Canada or elsewhere in another country.

2. Methods

The CCR is a population-based database comprised of data annually collected and reported to Statistics Canada by each provincial and territorial cancer registry. Demographic information regarding the individual diagnosed with cancer, and characteristics of the cancer itself, are available for each new primary case. Cancer-specific information, including stage at diagnosis, is available for common cancers, including BC [42]. Individual provinces and territories have varying practices for screening women aged 40–49, ranging from organised screening programs with annual recall to recommendations against screening in several provinces [43]. The Canadian Community Health Survey (CCHS) is a national cross-sectional survey that allows the determination of screening mammography activity [44] with acknowledged inherent bias [45]. Because health care in Canada is publicly funded, regular screening activity was mostly captured in the population-based screening programs, unless screens were performed outside of the organised programs or recorded as diagnostic mammograms. Although information about the method of detection of BC is not available, combining provincial-level BC data with the presence of organised programs and screening activity allows for a comparison of screening policies on stage at diagnosis in age cohorts 40–49 and 50–59.

This study was a secondary analysis of nationally de-identified data collected by Statistics Canada, and as such, ethics approval was not required. Female BC incidence data were obtained from the CCR file released on 19 May 2021 [46]. This version of the CCR included primary invasive cancer cases diagnosed among Canadian residents from 1992 to 2018, although cases diagnosed in Quebec from 2011 onward had not yet been submitted. The analytic file used followed the multiple primary coding rules of the International Agency for Research on Cancer (IARC) [47]. Full staging data were available from 2010 to 2017. Stage data used collaborative stage; a comprehensive standardised system sponsored by the American Joint Committee on Cancer (AJCC) which is compatible with the other staging systems in use during that period [48]. Unstaged BC cases were excluded from our analysis. There was no information on breast density or ethnicity.

Results for women aged 40–49 at diagnosis were compared to those for women aged 50–59 to assess the impact of screening policies in younger women. The 50–59 age group was chosen because it is the closest age group to 40–49 for which women in all jurisdictions may undergo regular screening mammography

Provincial and territorial screening practices varied across the country (Table 1). Those jurisdictions with screening programs that allowed women to access BC screening in their 40s by self-referral, and subsequently followed these women with annual recall, were designated as screeners [19,50]. Five screener jurisdictions were identified: Nova Scotia, British Columbia, Alberta, Prince Edward Island, and Northwest Territories. Alberta allowed self-referral in 2007, but by 2012 required a physician referral for the first screen. BC changed from annual to biennial recall in 2014. The other jurisdictions collectively formed the comparator group. Quebec was necessarily excluded from this group due to the absence of incidence data from this province in the CCR for the study period. Manitoba had biennial recall, and after the study period Yukon began to send anual reminder letters. In provinces that required a physician referral, some 40–49-year-old women screened may have had a family history of breast cancer that led to the referral. Data from Statistics Canada's nationally representative CCHS were used to determine the percentage of women aged 40–49 who reported having a screening mammogram in the previous two years [51]. This yielded screening participation rates that were independent of provincial/territorial screening programs. Despite this, these jurisdictions were not included in the "screener" group based on the a priori definition.

Table 1. Breast cancer screening information and participation rates by province and territory, women aged 40–49, Canada, selected years.

Province/Territory	Screening Programmatic Information (2007–2008)		Screening Participation Rates			
	Referral 40–49	Recall	2003	2008	2012	2017
British Columbia *	Self	Annual	44.2	47.4	45.7	39.0
Alberta **	Self	Annual	43.2	52.9	48.5	44.1
Saskatchewan	No	None	26.6	27.9	30.3	32.6
Manitoba	MD	Biennial	24.5	21.8	35.5	18.1
Ontario	MD-High Risk only	High Risk-Annual	33.1	37.5	38.1	27.0
Quebec	MD	None	26.0	31.4	25.2	21.4
New Brunswick	MD	None	42.2	41.4	31.0	20.8
Nova Scotia	Self	Annual	50.2	50.7	47.6	45.5
Prince Edward Island	Self	Annual	31.2	35.2	58.6	45.4
Newfoundland and Labrador	No	None	41.9	51.8	50.0	51.3
Northwest Territories	Self	Annual	43.9	42.7	63.6	n/a
Yukon	Self	None	10.0	32.6	11.4	n/a
Nunavut	n/a	n/a	12.2	13.2	41.0	n/a

n/a = no screening data available. Note: screening percentage rates refer to the percentage of women 40–49 with a screening mammogram in the previous two years, based on data from the Canadian Community Health Survey. Shaded provinces and territories denote screeners while the non-shaded ones are the comparators. Source: Canadian Community Health Survey, Cycle 2.1 (2003), Annual Component (2008, 2012, 2017); provincial and territorial screening practices [49,50]. Screening program information changed in some jurisdictions throughout the study period: * BC changed from annual to biennial recall in 2014. ** Alberta changed from self-referral to requiring an MD referral for the first screen in 2012.

Annual average percent changes in age- and stage-specific female BC incidence rates between 2011 and 2017 were calculated using JoinPoint 4.9.0.0 [52], which fit a piecewise-linear regression model that assumed a constant rate of change in the logarithm of the annual incidence rate. The year 2011 was chosen as the starting point for this trend analysis because it corresponded with the CTFPHC recommendation against screening women aged 40–49 years. Because the incidence of BC is lower in women in their 40s than in their 50s, the relative proportions of BC stages at diagnosis for the period from 2010 to 2017 were compared between screener and comparator jurisdictions, and statistical significance was calculated using z-tests. Standard errors for incidence rates were derived directly from the Poisson distribution, whereas those for proportions were calculated using the Agresti–Coull method [53].

A linear regression analysis was used to assess the relationship between self-reported jurisdictional screening percentages for 2012 and BC incidence rates for the period from 2011 to 2013. The analysis was restricted to early stage BC, defined by TMIST (AJCC 8th ed) as stage I, and the most advanced BC as stage IV. This time period encompasses the 2012 two-year time frame for reported mammography. Stage migration in women aged 50–59 was investigated by using provincial screening status for women aged 40–49 and comparing proportions of BC stage at diagnosis for women aged 50–59 in screener and comparator provinces. P-values correspond to two-sided tests of the null hypothesis that there was no difference in stage distribution, with a significance level of 0.05.

3. Results

Female BC incidence rates increased with age until a peak in the 70–74 year age group (Figure 1). Between 2010 and 2017, less than half (46.1%) of all new primary BC cases were diagnosed in women aged 50–74, the age range recommended by current screening guidelines. This percentage increased by almost 9 percentage points to 54.6% when women in their forties are included. The number of BC cases diagnosed in women aged 40–49 was equivalent to 18.5% of the total number of BC cases in screened women aged 50–74. The incidence rate ratio between cases diagnosed in the 40s and those diagnosed in their 50s was 0.63.

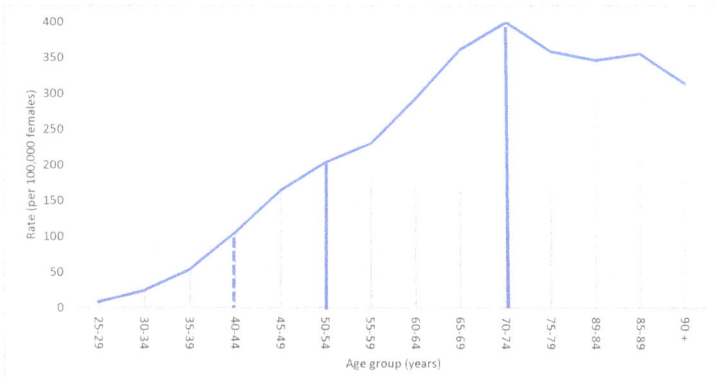

Figure 1. Age–specific female breast cancer incidence rate, by five–year age group, Canada excluding Quebec, 2010 to 2017 period. Note: Quebec is excluded because cases diagnosed in Quebec from 2011 onward had not been submitted to the Canadian Cancer Registry. Solid lines display current ages included in screening; dashed line indicates the age threshold where screening is being explored. Source: Canadian Cancer Registry (1992 to 2018) at Statistics Canada [42].

The proportion of women diagnosed with stage I BC was observed to be greater among those aged 50–74 at diagnosis—for whom screening is currently recommended—than among those diagnosed outside of this age range (Figure 2). Canadian women aged 50–74 had a proportionally higher incidence of stage I BC, and lower relative proportions of stage II and III BC, compared with younger and older women who fall outside the CTFPHC recommended screening age.

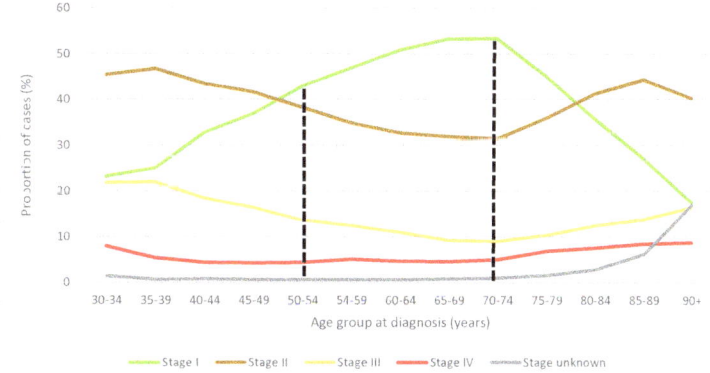

Figure 2. Stage–specific distribution of female breast cancer cases by age group at diagnosis, Canada excluding Quebec, 2010 to 2017 period. Note: Quebec is excluded because cases diagnosed in Quebec from 2011 onward had not been submitted to the Canadian Cancer Registry. The ages between the dashed lines represent those age groups for which mammogram screening is currently recommended. Source: Canadian Cancer Registry (1992 to 2018) at Statistics Canada [42].

The distribution of BC stage at diagnosis was significantly different between women aged 50–59 and their 40–49 year counterparts not targeted by screening programs (Figure 3, Table 2). Except for stage IV, Canadian women aged 40–49 had BC diagnosed at significantly later stages than those aged 50–59 who had higher relative proportions of stage I BC (45.3% vs. 35.7%; $p < 0.001$), and lower proportions of stage II (36.7% vs. 42.6%, $p < 0.001$), and III (13.1% vs. 17.3%, $p < 0.001$) BC. The proportion of stage IV at diagnosis in women aged 40–49 was significantly lower than in women aged 50–59 years old (4.4% vs. 4.8%, $p = 0.005$).

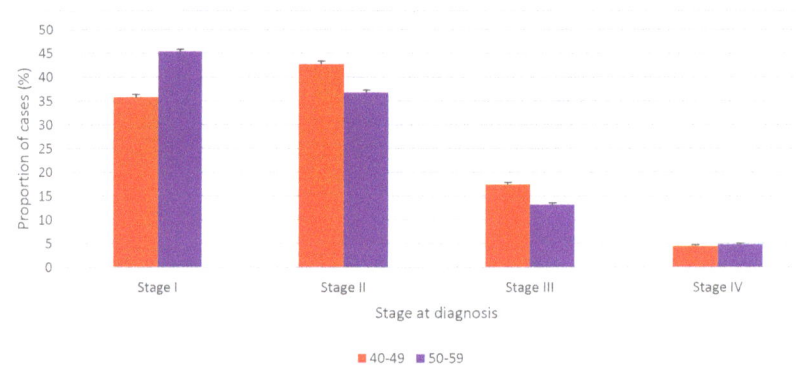

Figure 3. Stage–specific distribution of female breast cancer cases, ages 40 to 49 years versus ages 50 to 59 years, Canada excluding Quebec, 2010 to 2017. Note: Quebec is excluded because cases diagnosed in Quebec from 2011 onward had not been submitted to the Canadian Cancer Registry. Vertical error bars indicate 95% confidence intervals. Source: Canadian Cancer Registry (1992 to 2018) at Statistics Canada [42].

Table 2. Number and proportion of women diagnosed with breast cancer by stage at diagnosis, ages 40 to 49 years versus 50 to 59 years, Canada excluding Quebec, 2010 to 2017 period.

Stage at Diagnosis	40 to 49 Years			50 to 59 Years			p-Value for Differences in Stage-Specific Proportions
	Number	Proportion of Cases Diagnosed at Stages I to IV (%)	95% CI of the Proportion	Number	Proportion of Cases Diagnosed at Stages I to IV (%)	95% CI of the Proportion	
Stage I	7200	35.7	(35.0, 36.3)	15,125	45.3	(44.8, 45.8)	<0.001
Stage II	8600	42.6	(41.9, 43.3)	12,265	36.7	(36.2, 37.3)	<0.001
Stage III	3500	17.3	(16.8, 17.9)	4385	13.1	(12.8, 13.5)	<0.001
Stage IV	880	4.4	(4.1, 4.7)	1610	4.8	(4.6, 5.1)	0.005
Unknown	140	NA	NA	210	NA	NA	NA
Unstaged	645	NA	NA	930	NA	NA	NA
Total	20,965	NA	NA	34,525	NA	NA	NA

NA = not applicable, CI = confidence interval. Note: Quebec is excluded because cases diagnosed in Quebec from 2011 onward had not been submitted to the Canadian Cancer Registry. Counts have been randomly rounded to a multiple of five in accordance with Statistics Canada's disclosure-avoidance guidelines. Source: Canadian Cancer Registry (1992 to 2018) at Statistics Canada [42].

3.1. Screening Participation

From 2003 to 2017, reported BC screening participation generally declined among women aged 40–49, with the largest decrease (21.4 percentage points) occurring in New Brunswick (Table 1). Even in comparator jurisdictions, some screening occurred among women aged 40–49, ranging from 10.0% in Yukon in 2003 to 51.8% in Newfoundland and Labrador in 2008.

3.2. Stage Distribution of BC Related to Screening Guidelines for Women 40–49 Years Old

The rate of diagnosis of stage I disease decreased by a non-statistically significant average of 1.5% per year from 2011 to 2017 ($p = 0.147$) for women 40–49 years old (Figures 4 and 5). The corresponding rate of diagnosis of stage II BC in women in their forties increased by an average of 2.1% per year ($p = 0.001$). The increasing trend for stage II cases was more pronounced among screening jurisdictions (3.0% annual average) than among comparators (1.6% annual average). Stage III BC incidence rates decreased by an average of 2.5% per year ($p = 0.012$) over this same time period. This reduction was driven by a 5.7% annual decrease in the rate of diagnosis of stage III cases in screener jurisdictions ($p = 0.007$) (Figure 5A). Stage IV BC rates increased by an annual average of 1.8% per year ($p = 0.103$); 2.4% among comparators ($p = 0.244$) and 1.4% among screeners ($p = 0.707$).

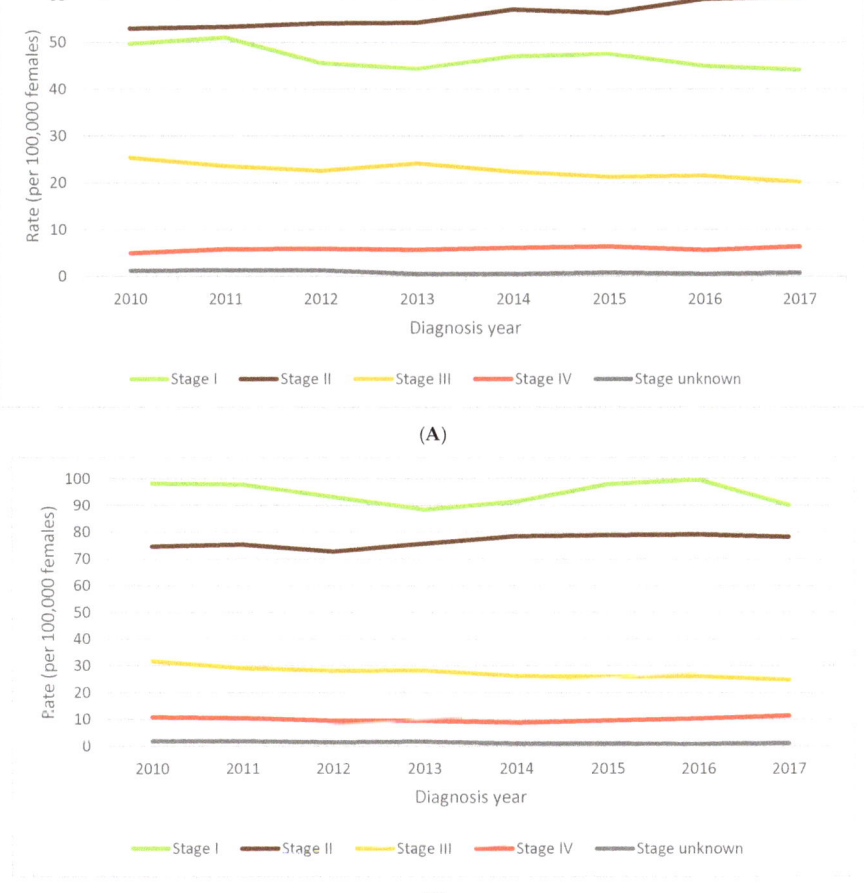

Figure 4. (**A**). Stage-specific female breast cancer incidence rates, ages 40 to 49 years, Canada excluding Quebec, 2010 to 2017. (**B**). Stage-specific female breast cancer incidence rates, ages 50 to 59 years, Canada excluding Quebec, 2010 to 2017. Note: Quebec is excluded because cases diagnosed in Quebec from 2011 onward had not been submitted to the Canadian Cancer Registry. Source: Canadian Cancer Registry (1992 to 2018) at Statistics Canada [42].

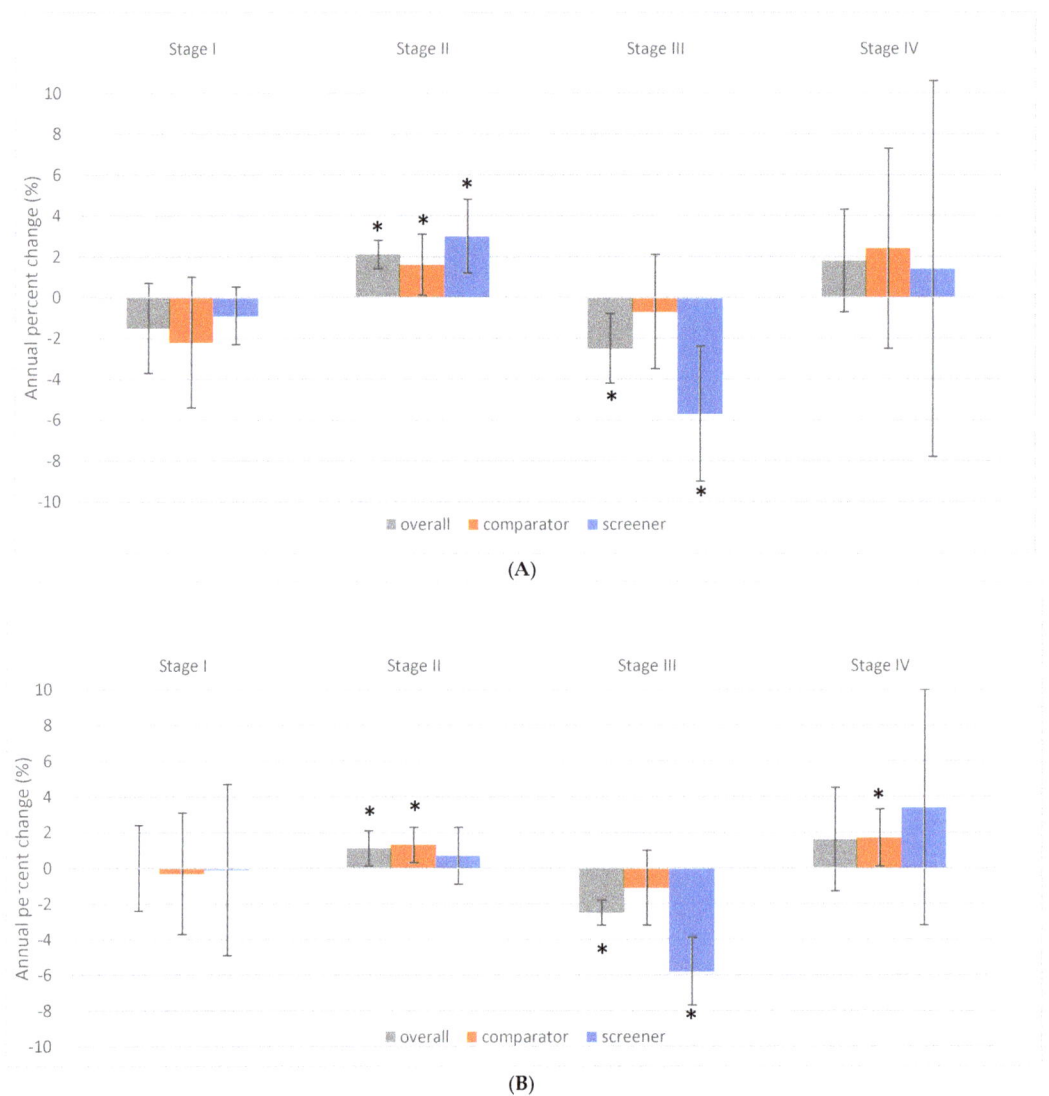

Figure 5. (**A**). Stage–specific female breast cancer incidence rate trends by jurisdictional screening status, ages 40 to 49 years, Canada excluding Quebec, 2011 to 2017. (**B**). Stage-specific female breast cancer incidence rate trends by jurisdictional screening status, ages 50 to 59 years, Canada excluding Quebec, 2011 to 2017. Note: Quebec is excluded because cases diagnosed in Quebec from 2011 onward had not been submitted to the Canadian Cancer Registry. Screeners: Alberta, British Columbia, Nova Scotia, Northwest Territories, and Prince Edward Island; Comparators: Manitoba, New Brunswick, Newfoundland and Labrador, Nunavut, Ontario, Saskatchewan, Yukon. The vertical error bars indicate 95% confidence intervals. Asterisks indicate the trend is significant at the $p < 0.05$ level. Source: Canadian Cancer Registry (1992 to 2018) at Statistics Canada [42]; provincial and territorial screening practices [49,50].

3.3. Stage Distribution of BC in Women 50–59 Related to Screening Guidelines for Women 40–49 Years Old

The incidence of stage I BC remained stable in women aged 50–59 over the same time period from 2011 to 2017 (Figures 4B and 5B). A significant average annual increase of 1.1% in the rate of diagnosis of stage II BC was observed ($p = 0.047$). Among stage III BC cases, there was a significant average decline of 2.5% per year ($p < 0.001$) which was mainly influenced by an annual reduction of 5.8% per year in the screener jurisdictions ($p = 0.001$). The overall trend for stage IV was not significant, but there was a significant average annual increase of 1.7% in metastatic disease among comparator women 50–59 ($p = 0.025$). This corresponded to a 10.3% increase in stage IV BC in these women over the six years.

3.4. Impact of Provincial/Territorial Screening Status on BC Stage at Diagnosis in Women Aged 40–49

BC stage distribution at diagnosis in women aged 40–49 was significantly different in screener versus comparator jurisdictions (Figure 6A). Higher proportions of stage I BC were diagnosed among screener jurisdictions (33.3% vs. 39.9%, $p < 0.001$), while comparators had proportionately more BC diagnosed at stage II (43.7% vs. 40.7%, $p < 0.001$), III (18.3% vs. 15.6%, $p < 0.001$) and IV (4.6% vs. 3.9%, $p = 0.001$). Among the BC cases that were coded as unstaged, 96.9% were diagnosed in the comparator province of Ontario (data not shown). As a consequence, there were significantly more unstaged BC cases among comparators than screeners, with an incidence rate ratio of 2.4 (data not shown).

Regression of provincial and territorial screening participation with an incidence of the stage at diagnosis revealed a significant relationship between screening and stage I BC ($p = 0.010$). An increase of 10 percentage points in the screening participation of women aged 40–49 was linearly associated with a 6.6 per 100,000 increase in the stage I incidence rate (Figure 7A) and with a non-significant 1.2 per 100,000 decrease in the rate of stage IV or metastatic disease ($p = 0.186$) (Figure 7B).

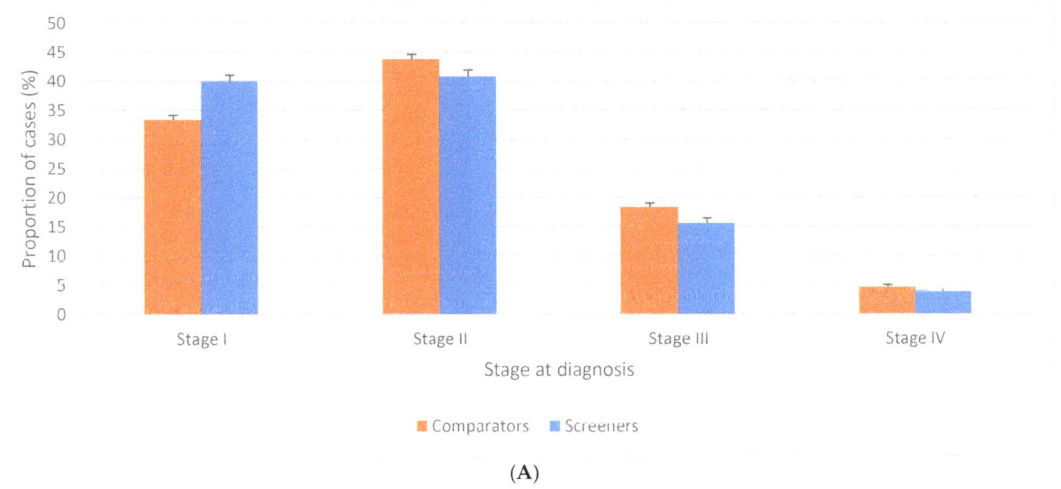

(A)

Figure 6. *Cont.*

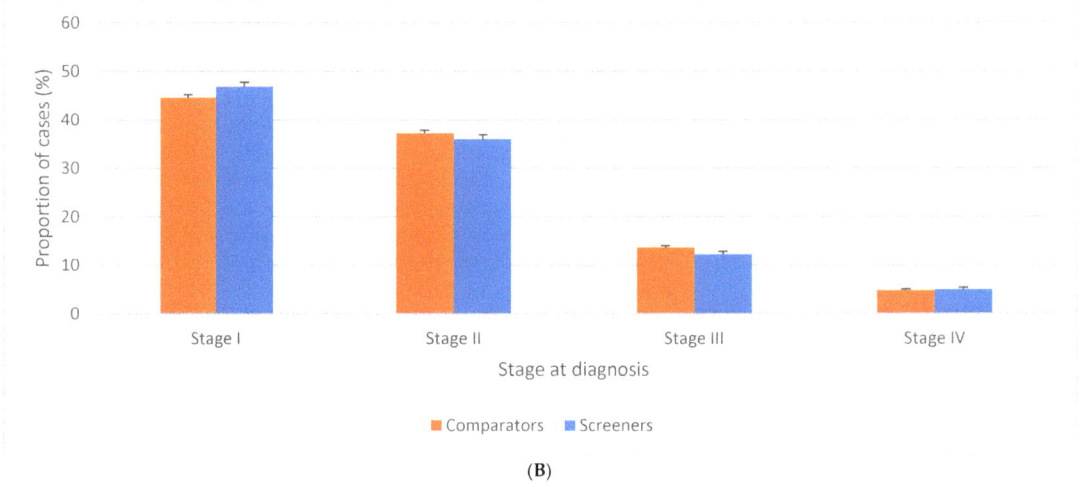

(B)

Figure 6. (**A**). Stage-specific distribution of female breast cancer cases by jurisdictional screening status, ages 40 to 49 years, Canada excluding Quebec, 2010 to 2017. (**B**). Stage-specific distribution of female breast cancer cases, ages 50–59 years, by jurisdictional screening status for women 40–49 years, Canada excluding Quebec, 2010 to 2017. Note: Quebec is excluded because cases diagnosed in Quebec from 2011 onward had not been submitted to the Canadian Cancer Registry. Screeners: Alberta, British Columbia, Nova Scotia, Northwest Territories, and Prince Edward Island; Comparators: Manitoba, New Brunswick, Newfoundland and Labrador, Nunavut, Ontario, Saskatchewan, Yukon. Source: Canadian Cancer Registry (1992 to 2018) at Statistics Canada [42,44]; provincial and territorial screening practices [49,50].

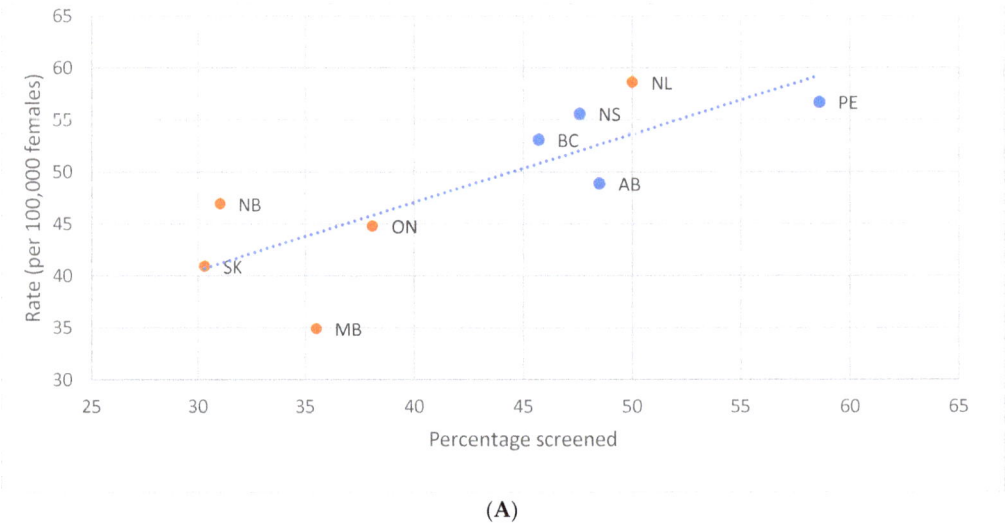

(A)

Figure 7. *Cont.*

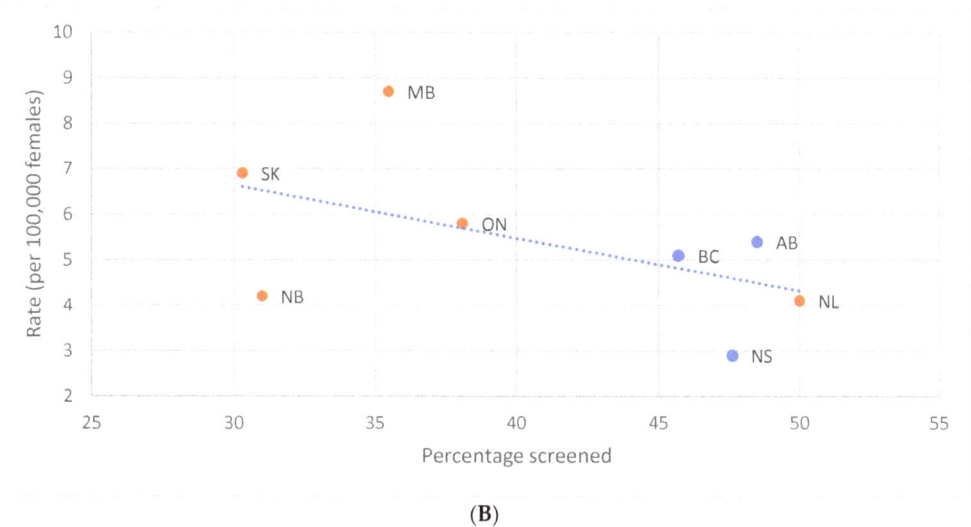

(**B**)

Figure 7. (**A**). Incidence rate of stage I female breast cancer during the 2011 to 2013 period by provincial screening participation rate in 2012, ages 40 to 49 years, selected provinces. (**B**). Incidence rate of stage IV female breast cancer during the 2011 to 2013 period by provincial screening participation rate in 2012, ages 40 to 49 years, selected provinces. Note: Orange dots denote comparators and blue dots denote screeners. Quebec is excluded because cases diagnosed in Quebec from 2011 onward had not been submitted to the Canadian Cancer Registry. The three Canadian territories (Yukon, Northwest Territories, and Nunavut) were excluded from the stage I and IV analyses, and Prince Edward Island from the stage IV analysis, because the number of incident cases was too small to be reliably compared against other jurisdictions. Source: Canadian Cancer Registry (1992 to 2018) and Canadian Community Health Survey [42,44]: Annual Component (2012) at Statistics Canada; provincial and territorial screening practices [49,50].

3.5. Impact of Provincial/Territorial Screening Status for Women Aged 40–49 on BC Stage at Diagnosis in Women Aged 50–59

The stage distribution of BC cases diagnosed among women aged 50–59 differed according to the screening practices—screener or comparator—used in their jurisdiction for 40–49 year-olds (Figure 6B). There was a lower proportion of stage I in women aged 50–59 at diagnosis (44.5% vs. 46.8%, $p < 0.001$), and higher proportions of stage II (37.2% vs. 36.0%, $p = 0.003$) and stage III (13.6% vs. 12.3%, $p < 0.001$) in the comparator than in the screener jurisdictions. No significant difference was observed between comparator and screener jurisdictions in terms of the proportion of cases diagnosed at stage IV.

4. Discussion

This study leveraged differences in provincial and territorial screening practices and used robust Canadian BC data to investigate the impact of mammography screening programs on women aged 40–49 and 50–59. Even with suboptimal screening participation, a stage shift was noted in jurisdictions without organised screening programs. A significant relationship between the degree of jurisdictional screening participation and the incidence rate of stage I BC at diagnosis was observed. On a proportionate basis, women aged 40–49 in comparator provinces were significantly more likely to be diagnosed with stages II, III, or IV BC than their screened peers. For the first time, it was observed that Canadian screening programs that included women in their 40s were associated with earlier stage migration in women aged 50–59. In jurisdictions where women in their 40s were not included in the screening programs, there were significantly higher rates of stages II and III BC in women aged 50–59, and a significant increase in the incidence of metastatic BC over time. The stage profile of BC was observed to have changed since 2011 when the CTFPHC recommended against screening women aged 40–49. Changes appeared more evident among women aged 40–49 than among women aged 50–59 for whom screening continued to be recommended. The ongoing screening activity, albeit lessened, for women aged 40–49 may have mitigated the extent of this shift.

These findings have implications for outcomes for these women, as stage III and IV BC have an overall five-year net survival of only 74.0% and 23.2% compared to 91.9% and 99.8% for stage II and I, respectively [54]. The profile of BC in women in their 40s is often of later stage (II, III, and IV) disease at diagnosis, compared to their screened peers in their fifties. This late-stage disease, along with the increased proportion of stage III BC in women aged 50–59, results in higher mortality and life years lost, given the young age at diagnosis and lower stage-specific survival [38]. In addition to the inherently increased mortality risk with later-stage disease, these women must also undergo treatments that are far more extensive than those for early BC. A diagnosis with late-stage BC often means more invasive surgeries such as mastectomy and axillary dissection, and more intensive and longer duration of therapy with chemotherapy and radiation, causing morbidity with potential long-term toxicities such as lymphedema, secondary malignancies, and cardiotoxicity [55].

The cost of annual mammography screening for women aged 40 to 49 has been estimated at CAD 2355 per woman [56]. However, these new costs would only be applicable to those women not already undergoing screening. They could also be partially offset by the reduction in the incremental costs of otherwise having to treat more stage II, III, and IV BC with increasingly complex and expensive therapies. In Ontario in 2014, the two-year treatment costs for stage I through IV BC were CAD 29,938; CAD 46,893; CAD 65,369, and CAD 66,627, respectively [57]. The treatment of hormone receptor-positive (HR+)/human epidermal growth factor 2 negative (HER2-) metastatic disease in Ontario from 2012 to 2017 cost more than CAD 1.2 billion [58]. These costs likely underestimate the current financial impacts of treating advanced BC. A two-year time frame does not capture all costs of stage III treatment, including recurrence and ongoing survivorship care, nor the full duration of treatment for metastatic disease. As well, these costs predate the introduction of cyclin-dependent kinase (CDK) inhibitors in metastatic BC, drugs which cost more than CAD 5000 per month [59] and can be continued for more than five years [60]. These costs also do not account for the loss of productivity from time away from the workforce, due to the lengthier treatment of more advanced cancers. The high costs of implementing a population-based screening program for all Canadian women 40–49 might be offset by a risk-stratified approach; research underway may provide greater insights into the best screening approach [61].

Several reasons for not screening women in their 40s have been cited: overdiagnosis, lead time bias, and the presence of more aggressive molecular subtypes which present with more advanced disease and have a higher risk of recurrence and death [62,63]. A recent analysis, after adjusting for tumour subtype and detection method (screening or diagnostic) showed no difference in survival for women aged 40–50 compared to women aged 51–60 [64]. This finding supports diagnosing breast cancers at an early stage in women aged 40–49, perhaps even more so if the cancers are aggressive. Overdiagnosis is more likely to be a concern in older populations who have higher rates of co-morbidities and is less likely to impact younger women with few underlying medical issues [38]. Overdiagnosis has been estimated to be <0.1% in women aged 40–49 [4]. Our study supports that cancers diagnosed in women in their 40s are not overdiagnosed, as higher proportions of stage III and metastatic disease in unscreened women suggest progression of the earlier stage BC diagnosed in screened women. An additional downside of breast cancer screening is that many women who are screened are never found to have breast cancer. Because 80% of women who develop breast cancer have no identifiable risk factors, a risk-based approach to limiting screening to only those at high risk has not been beneficial. Active research on strategies to evaluate a personalised approach to screening may include more intensive supplemental screening for some and reduced screening intensity for others [61].

Just as the absence of ethnicity in Canadian cancer data does not allow us to analyse BC outcomes related to race, current screening guidelines may not account for our racially diverse society. Screening guidelines are largely based on eight randomised controlled trials performed 30–60 years ago in Sweden, Scotland, the USA, and Canada [19]. Ethnicity was not recorded but given each country's population, it is likely that white women were mainly studied. The biology of BC differs based on ethnicity. The incidence of BC in White women peaks in their 60s, while the highest incidence for Black, Hispanic, and Asian women is in their 40s [65,66]. Higher mortality rates in Black women are independent of socioeconomic factors and are driven by higher rates of triple-negative BC, an aggressive cancer that is associated with later stage presentation and resultant lower survival [67–69]. Current screening guidelines amplify disparities, as the requirement for self-referral, or need for primary care referral for screening, decreases screening uptake, and skews participation to those patients who are health-literate and of a higher socioeconomic background [36]. Initiating breast screening at the age of 40 has been shown to reduce the mortality disparities between Black and White women and create a more equitable screening strategy [70].

This study has several limitations. It is a retrospective analysis of the impact of jurisdictional screening program policies. Quebec, the second largest jurisdiction in Canada, had to be excluded as their BC cases had not been submitted to the CCR for diagnosis years 2011 onward. None of the screener jurisdictions had optimal participation of >70%, and many of the comparator provinces had some screening activity, including greater than 50% in Newfoundland and Labrador. As such, our analysis likely underestimates the impact of organised screening programs. Among women aged 40–49, the five-year net survival estimates for unstaged and unknown stage BC cases are intermediate to that of stage II and III cases, and a few percentage points below stage I to IV combined [54]. Definitively staging these cases likely would have led to slightly higher proportions of late-stage disease in both screener and comparator groups, but more so in the comparator group given the higher rate of unstaged cases in this group. Although the CCHS survey questions attempt to measure screening mammograms only, we cannot definitively determine if the mammograms reported were diagnostic or for screening purposes. The inclusion of diagnostic mammograms in this study could overestimate late-stage or symptomatic, palpable cancers in the screener jurisdictions, thereby further attenuating the impacts of screening. Although the aim of screening is to detect cancers at an early stage, we did not have information about how the BC was diagnosed, and some cancers may have been detected symptomatically or as interval cancers. The power to detect trends in women in their 40s and 50s, especially with sub-analyses by screening status, was limited by the fact that we only have seven years of stage data. Because this study only evaluated invasive carcinomas, the impact on in situ disease was not assessed. Risk factors could not be assessed in this study and it is possible that 40–49-year-old women had more risk factors in the comparator than in the screening groups. However, given that we measured the stages of breast cancer at diagnosis this was unlikely to have significantly impacted the outcomes. In addition, the Canadian database did not record race or ethnicity, or breast tissue density, and we could not assess the impact of screening guidelines on the groups who would most likely be affected, such as Black and Asian women whose incidence of breast cancer peaks in the 40s, or those at higher risk. While the use of national registry data stands out as one of the main strengths of this study, the absence of statistical information on cancer recurrence and longer-term outcomes after an initial BC diagnosis narrows the scope of our conclusions to primary tumour cases. We were unable to evaluate breast cancer mortality outcomes using 10-year follow-ups for cases diagnosed from 2010–2017 as follow-up was restricted to the end of 2017.

This study presents important new information regarding the impact on Canadian women in their 40s and 50s of current BC mammography screening guidelines. The results can be used to reassess the optimum lower age for BC screening in Canada. Although women aged 40–49 have a lower incidence of breast cancer than those 50–59, women in both these age groups may have been negatively impacted by the exclusion of women younger than 50 from organised breast screening programs. This study supports two large observational trials [20,21], showing the benefit of breast cancer mortality reduction among women 40 years and older. Future research into the best method of including women 40–49 years old in population-based screening programs is needed. The thousands of Canadian women in their 40s who are diagnosed with BC each year have proportionally more stage III and metastatic cancers than women involved in organised screening, and there may be downstream stage migration with its associated decreased stage-specific survival in women aged 50–59. Identifying these cancers through screening at an early stage, where associated treatment costs are reduced relative to late-stage disease, could result in substantial savings for the Canadian health care system. The current screening guidelines are inequitable because they necessitate self-referral, selecting for health-literate women of higher socioeconomic status, and creating barriers for women who are required to have a primary care provider who will agree to the referral. These same guidelines preferentially benefit White women while disadvantaging ethnic groups with differing BC biology with an earlier peak incidence. Our guidelines may lead to increased treatment morbidity, and most importantly increased mortality. It is time to focus not on the harms of screening, but on the harms of not screening women aged 40–49.

5. Conclusions

Between 2010 and 2017, using national database registries, Canadian women 40–49 years old were diagnosed with significantly fewer stage I and more stages II and III breast cancers than women 50–59 years old. In the same period, women 40–49 years old in screening jurisdictions were diagnosed with significantly fewer stages II, III, and IV BC than those living in the comparator provinces. Screening policies for women 40–49 also had an impact on women 50–59 years old who had significantly lower rates of stages II and III BC in the screening vs. the comparator jurisdictions.

Author Contributions: Conceptualisation, A.N.W., J.M.S., L.F.E. and J.-M.B.; methodology, J.-M.B., L.F.E., A.N.W. and J.M.S.; software, J.-M.B., L.F.E. and A.N.W.; validation, A.N.W., J.M.S., L.F.E. and J.-M.B.; formal analysis, J.-M.B. and L.F.E.; investigation, J.-M.B., L.F.E., A.N.W., J.M.S., N.I. and M.A.K.; resources, J.M-.B., L.F.E., A.N.W., J.M.S., N.I. and M.A.K.; data curation, A.N.W., L.F.E., J.-M.B. and J.M.S.; writing—original draft preparation, A.N.W. and J.M.S.; writing—review and editing, J.-M.B., L.F.E., A.N.W., J.M.S., N.I. and M.A.K.; visualisation, A.N.W., J.M.S., L.F.E. and J. M.B.; supervision, J.-M.B., L.F.E., A.N.W. and J.M.S.; project administration, L.F.E. and J.-M.B. All authors have read and agreed to the published version of the manuscript.

Funding: This research received no external funding.

Institutional Review Board Statement: This study was a secondary analysis of nationally de-identified data collected by Statistics Canada, and as such, ethics approval was not required.

Informed Consent Statement: Patient consent was waived this study was a secondary analysis of nationally de-identified data collected by Statistics Canada.

Data Availability Statement: Aggregate data on cancer incidence counts and rates by stage are publicly available from Tables 13-10-0761-01 and 13-10-0762-01, patient- and tumor-level microdata files are confidential and can only be accessed through Statistics Canada's Research Data Centre Program.

Conflicts of Interest: The authors declare no conflict of interest.

References

1. Ellison, L.F. The cancer survival index: Measuring progress in cancer survival to help evaluate cancer control efforts in Canada. *Health Rep.* **2021**, *32*, 14–26. [CrossRef] [PubMed]
2. Statistics Canada 2022. The Daily—Cancer Incidence and Mortality Trends, 1984 to 2020. Available online: https://www150.statcan.gc.ca/n1/daily-quotidien/220204/dq220204b-eng.htm (accessed on 22 July 2022).
3. Brenner, D.R.; Poirier, A.; Woods, R.R.; Ellison, L.F.; Billette, J.M.; Demers, A.A.; Zhang, S.X.; Yao, C.; Finley, C.; Fitzgerald, N.; et al. Projected estimates of cancer in Canada in 2022. *CMAJ* **2022**, *194*, E601–E607. [CrossRef] [PubMed]
4. Grimm, L.J.; Avery, C.S.; Hendrick, E.; Baker, J.A. Benefits and Risks of Mammography Screening in Women Ages 40 to 49 Years. *J. Prim. Care Community Health* **2022**, *13*, 21501327211058322. [CrossRef]

5. Canadian Task Force on Preventive Health Care. Recommendations on screening for breast cancer in average-risk women aged 40–74 years. *CMAJ* **2011**, *183*, 1991–2001. [CrossRef] [PubMed]
6. Klarenbach, S.; Sims-Jones, N.; Lewin, G.; Singh, H.; Thériault, G.; Tonelli, M.; Doull, M.; Courage, S.; Garcia, A.J.; Thombs, B.D. Recommendations on screening for breast cancer in women aged 40–74 years who are not at increased risk for breast cancer. *CMAJ* **2018**, *190*, E1441–E1451. [CrossRef]
7. Shapiro, S.; Strax, P.; Venet, L. Periodic breast cancer screening in reducing mortality from breast cancer. *JAMA* **1971**, *215*, 1777–1785. [CrossRef]
8. Andersson, I.; Aspegren, K.; Janzon, L.; Landberg, T.; Lindholm, K.; Linell, F.; Ljungberg, O.; Ranstam, J.; Sigfusson, B. Mammographic screening and mortality from breast cancer: The Malmö mammographic screening trial. *Br. Med. J.* **1988**, *297*, 943–948. [CrossRef]
9. Tabár, L.; Gad, A.; Holmberg, L.; Ljungquist, U.; Group, K.C.P.; Fagerberg, C.; Baldetorp, L.; Gröntoft, O.; Lundström, B.; Månson, J.; et al. Reduction in mortality from breast cancer after mass screening with mammography: Randomised trial from the Breast Cancer Screening Working Group of the Swedish National Board of Health and Welfare. *Lancet* **1985**, *325*, 829–832. [CrossRef]
10. Huggins, A.; Muir, B.; Donnan, P.; Hepburn, W.; Prescott, R.; Anderson, T.; Lamb, J.; Alexander, F.; Chetty, U.; Forrest, P.; et al. Edinburgh trial of screening for breast cancer: Mortality at seven years. *Lancet* **1990**, *335*, 241–246. [CrossRef]
11. Frisell, J.; Lidbrink, E.; Hellström, L.; Rutqvist, L.E. Followup after 11 years–update of mortality results in the Stockholm mammographic screening trial. *Breast Cancer Res. Treat.* **1997**, *45*, 263–270. [CrossRef]
12. Miller, A.B.; Baines, C.J.; To, T.; Wall, C. Canadian National Breast Screening Study: 1. Breast cancer detection and death rates among women aged 40 to 49 years. *CMAJ* **1992**, *147*, 1459–1476, Erratum in *Can. Med. Assoc. J.* **1993**, *148*, 718.
13. Miller, A.B.; Baines, C.J.; To, T.; Wall, C. Canadian National Breast Screening Study: 2. Breast cancer detection and death rates among women aged 50 to 59 years. *CMAJ* **1992**, *147*, 1477–1488, Erratum in *Can. Med. Assoc. J.* **1993**, *148*, 718.
14. Bjurstam, N.; Björneld, L.; Duffy, S.W.; Smith, T.C.; Cahlin, E.; Eriksson, O.; Hafström, L.O.; Lingaas, H.; Mattsson, J.; Persson, S.; et al. The Gothenburg breast screening trial: First results on mortality, incidence, and mode of detection for women ages 39–49 years at randomization. *Cancer Interdiscip. Int. J. Am. Cancer Soc.* **1997**, *80*, 2091–2099. [CrossRef]
15. Hendrick, R.E.; Smith, R.A.; Rutledge, J.H., III; Smart, C.R. Benefit of screening mammography in women aged 40–49: A new meta-analysis of randomized controlled trials. *JNCI Monogr.* **1997**, *1997*, 87–92. [CrossRef] [PubMed]
16. Miller, A.B.; Wall, C.; Baines, C.J.; Sun, P.; To, T.; Narod, S.A. Twenty five year follow-up for BC incidence and mortality of the Canadian National Breast Screening Study: Randomised screening trial. *Bmj* **2014**, *348*, g366. [CrossRef] [PubMed]
17. Yaffe, M.J.; Seely, J.M.; Gordon, P.B.; Appavoo, S.; Kopans, D.B. The randomized trial of mammography screening that was not-A cautionary tale. *J. Med. Screen* **2022**, *29*, 7–11. [CrossRef] [PubMed]
18. Seely, J.M.; Eby, P.R.; Gordon, P.B.; Appavoo, S.; Yaffe, M.J. Errors in conduct of the CNBSS trials of breast cancer screening observed by research personnel. *J. Breast Imaging* **2022**, *4*, 135–143. [CrossRef]
19. Smart, C.R.; Hendrick, R.E.; Rutledge, J.H., III; Smith, R.A. Benefit of mammography screening in women ages 40 to 49 years. Current evidence from randomized controlled trials. *Cancer* **1995**, *75*, 1619–1626. [CrossRef]
20. Coldman, A.; Phillips, N.; Wilson, C.; Decker, K.; Chiarelli, A.M.; Brisson, J.; Zhang, B.; Payne, J.; Doyle, G.; Ahmad, R. Pan-Canadian study of mammography screening and mortality from breast cancer. *JNCI J. Natl. Cancer Inst.* **2014**, *106*, dju261. [CrossRef]
21. Duffy, S.W.; Tabár, L.; Yen, A.M.F.; Dean, P.B.; Smith, R.A.; Jonsson, H.; Törnberg, S.; Chen, S.L.S.; Chiu, S.Y.H.; Fann, J.C.Y.; et al. Mammography screening reduces rates of advanced and fatal breast cancers: Results in 549,091 women. *Cancer* **2020**, *126*, 2971–2979. [CrossRef]
22. Tabár, L.; Dean, P.B.; Chen, T.H.H.; Yen, A.M.F.; Chen, S.L.S.; Fann, J.C.Y.; Lin, A.T.-Y.; Smith, R.A.; Duffy, S.W. The incidence of fatal BC measures the increased effectiveness of therapy in women participating in mammography screening. *Cancer* **2019**, *125*, 515–523. [CrossRef] [PubMed]
23. Heller, D.R.; Chiu, A.S.; Farrell, K.; Killelea, B.K.; Lannin, D.R. Why Has Breast Cancer Screening Failed to Decrease the Incidence of de Novo Stage IV Disease? *Cancers* **2019**, *11*, 500. [CrossRef] [PubMed]
24. Bleyer, A.; Welch, H.G. Effect of three decades of screening mammography on breast-cancer incidence. *N. Engl. J. Med.* **2012**, *367*, 1998–2005. [CrossRef] [PubMed]
25. Autier, P.; Boniol, M.; Middleton, R.; Doré, J.F.; Héry, C.; Zheng, T.; Gavin, A. Advanced breast cancer incidence following population-based mammographic screening. *Ann. Oncol.* **2011**, *22*, 1726–1735. [CrossRef]
26. Kopans, D.B. Point: The New England Journal of Medicine article suggesting overdiagnosis from mammography screening is scientifically incorrect and should be withdrawn. *J. Am. Coll. Radiol.* **2013**, *10*, 317–319. [CrossRef]
27. Garfinkel, L.; Boring, C.C.; Heath, C.W., Jr. Changing trends. An overview of breast cancer incidence and mortality. *Cancer* **1994**, *74*, 222–227. [CrossRef]
28. Gaudette, L.A.; Silberberger, C.; Altmayer, C.A.; Gao, R.N. Trends in breast cancer incidence and mortality. *Health Rep.* **1996**, *8*, 29–37.
29. Taplin, S.H.; Ichikawa, L.; Buist, D.S.; Seger, D.; White, E. Evaluating organized BC screening implementation: The prevention of late-stage disease? *Cancer Epidemiol. Prev. Biomark.* **2004**, *13*, 225–234. [CrossRef]
30. Blumen, H.; Fitch, K.; Polkus, V. Comparison of treatment costs for breast cancer, by tumor stage and type of service. *Am. Health Drug Benefits* **2016**, *9*, 23–32.

31. Shen, Y.; Yang, Y.; Inoue, L.Y.; Munsell, M.F.; Miller, A.B.; Berry, D.A. Role of detection method in predicting BC survival: Analysis of randomized screening trials. *J. Natl. Cancer Inst.* **2005**, *97*, 1195–1203. [CrossRef]
32. Ugnat, A.M.; Xie, L.; Morriss, J.; Semenciw, R.; Mao, Y. Survival of women with breast cancer in Ottawa, Canada: Variation with age, stage, histology, grade and treatment. *Br. J. Cancer* **2004**, *90*, 1138–1143. [CrossRef] [PubMed]
33. Christiansen, S.R.; Autier, P.; Støvring, H. Change in effectiveness of mammography screening with decreasing breast cancer mortality: A population-based study. *Eur. J. Public Health* **2022**, *32*, 630–635. [CrossRef]
34. Yaffe, M.J.; Mainprize, J.G. Overdetection of Breast Cancer. *Curr. Oncol.* **2022**, *29*, 3894–3910. [CrossRef] [PubMed]
35. Ding, L.; Poelhekken, K.; Greuter, M.J.; Truyen, I.; De Schutter, H.; Goossens, M.; Houssami, N.; Van Hal, G.; de Bock, G.H. Overdiagnosis of invasive breast cancer in population-based breast cancer screening: A short-and long-term perspective. *Eur. J. Cancer* **2022**, *173*, 1–9. [CrossRef] [PubMed]
36. Giordano, L.; Stefanini, V.; Senore, C.; Frigerio, A.; Castagno, R.; Marra, V.; Dalmasso, M.; del Turco, M.R.; Paci, E.; Segnan, N. The impact of different communication and organizational strategies on mammography screening uptake in women aged 40–45 years. *Eur. J. Public Health* **2012**, *22*, 413–418. [CrossRef]
37. Loy, E.Y.; Molinar, D.; Chow, K.Y.; Fock, C. National Breast Cancer Screening Programme, Singapore: Evaluation of participation and performance indicators. *J. Med. Screen.* **2015**, *22*, 194–200. [CrossRef]
38. Ray, K.M.; Joe, B.N.; Freimanis, R.I.; Sickles, E.A.; Hendrick, R.E. Screening mammography in women 40–49 years old: Current evidence. *Am. J. Roentgenol.* **2018**, *210*, 264–270. [CrossRef]
39. Sprague, B.L.; Gangnon, R.E.; Burt, V.; Trentham-Dietz, A.; Hampton, J.M.; Wellman, R.D.; Kerlikowske, K.; Miglioretti, D.L. Prevalence of mammographically dense breasts in the United States. *JNCI J. Natl. Cancer Inst.* **2014**, *106*, dju255. [CrossRef]
40. Boyd, N.F.; Guo, H.; Martin, L.J.; Sun, L.; Stone, J.; Fishell, E.; Jong, R.A.; Hislop, G.; Chiarelli, A.; Minkin, S.; et al. Mammographic density and the risk and detection of breast cancer. *N. Engl. J. Med.* **2007**, *356*, 227–236. [CrossRef]
41. Seely, J.M.; Peddle, S.E.; Yang, H.; Chiarelli, A.M.; McCallum, M.; Narasimhan, G.; Zakaria, D.; Earle, C.C.; Fung, S.; Bryant, H.; et al. Breast Density and Risk of Interval Cancers: The Effect of Annual Versus Biennial Screening Mammography Policies in Canada. *Can. Assoc. Radiol. J.* **2022**, *73*, 90–100. [CrossRef]
42. Statistics Canada. Canadian Cancer Registry. Available online: http://www23.statcan.gc.ca/imdb/p2SV.pl?Function=getSurvey&SDDS=3207 (accessed on 6 June 2022).
43. Public Health Agency of Canada. Organized Breast Cancer Screening Programs in Canada. *Report on Program Performance in 2003 and 2004*. 2008. Available online: https://www.canada.ca/content/dam/phac-aspc/migration/phac-aspc/publicat/2008/obcsp-podcs-03-04/pdf/obcsp-podcs-03-04-eng.pdf (accessed on 22 June 2022).
44. Government of Canada SC. Canadian Community Health Survey: Public Use Microdata File. 2020. Available online: http://www150.statcan.gc.ca/n1/en/catalogue/82M0013X (accessed on 6 June 2022).
45. Cronin, K.A.; Miglioretti, D.L.; Krapcho, M.; Yu, B.; Geller, B.M.; Carney, P.A.; Onega, T.; Feuer, E.J.; Breen, N.; Ballard-Barbash, R. Bias associated with self-report of prior screening mammography. *Cancer Epidemiol. Biomark. Prev.* **2009**, *18*, 1699–1705. [CrossRef] [PubMed]
46. Statistics Canada. 2021. Available online: https://www150.statcan.gc.ca/n1/daily-quotidien/210519/dq210519b-eng.htm (accessed on 6 June 2022).
47. International Agency for Research on Cancer; World Health Organization; International Association of Cancer Registries; European Network of Cancer Registries. *International Rules for Multiple Primary Cancers (ICD-O Third Edition)*; IARC: Lyon, France, 2004. Available online: http://www.iacr.com.fr/images/doc/MPrules_july2004.pdf (accessed on 22 June 2022).
48. Byrd, D.R.; Carducci, M.A.; Compton, C.C.; Fritz, A.G.; Greene, F. *AJCC Cancer Staging Manual*; Edge, S.B., Ed.; Springer: New York, NY, USA, 2010; Volume 7, pp. 97–100.
49. Organized Breast Cancer Screening Programs in Canada. Available online: https://s22457.pcdn.co/wp-content/uploads/2019/01/Breast-Cancer-Screen-Perform-2008-EN.pdf (accessed on 22 June 2022).
50. Breast Cancer Screening in Canada; Monitoring & Evaluation of Quality Indicators–Results Report, January 2011 to December 2012. Available online: https://s22457.pcdn.co/wp-content/uploads/2019/01/Breast-Cancer-Screen-Quality-Indicators-Report-2012-EN.pdf (accessed on 22 June 2022).
51. Statistics Canada. Canadian Community Health Survey (CCHS)—Annual Component—2020 Microdata File. *User Guide*. 2021. Available online: https://www23.statcan.gc.ca/imdb/p2SV.pl?Function=getSurvey&SDDS=3226 (accessed on 6 June 2022).
52. *JoinPoint Regression Program*, Version 4.9.0.0; Statistical Methodology and Applications Branch, Surveillance Research Program, National Cancer Institute: Bethesda, MD, USA, 2020.
53. Agresti, A.; Coull, B.A. Approximate is better than 'exact' for interval estimation of binomial proportions. *Am. Stat.* **1998**, *52*, 119–126.
54. Ellison, L.F.; Saint-Jacques, N. *Five-Year Cancer Survival by Stage at Diagnosis in Canada*. [Manuscript Submitted for Publication]; Centre for Population Health Data, Statistics Canada: Ottawa, ON, Canada, 2022.
55. Wilkinson, A.N.; Boutet, C.E. Breast Cancer Survivorship Tool: Facilitating breast cancer survivorship care for family physicians and patients. *Can. Fam. Physician* **2020**, *66*, 321–326. [PubMed]
56. Mittmann, N.; Stout, N.K.; Tosteson, A.N.; Trentham-Dietz, A.; Alagoz, O.; Yaffe, M.J. Cost-effectiveness of mammography from a publicly funded health care system perspective. *Can. Med. Assoc. Open Access J.* **2018**, *6*, E77–E86. [CrossRef] [PubMed]

57. Mittmann, N.; Porter, J.; Rangrej, J.; Seung, S.; Liu, N.; Saskin, R.; Cheung, M.; Leighl, N.; Hoch, J.S.; Trudeau, M.; et al. Health system costs for stage-specific breast cancer: A population-based approach. *Curr. Oncol.* **2014**, *21*, 281–293. [CrossRef]
58. Brezden-Masley, C.; Fathers, K.E.; Coombes, M.E.; Pourmirza, B.; Xue, C.; Jerzak, K.J. A population-based comparison of treatment patterns, resource utilization, and costs by cancer stage for Ontario patients with hormone receptor-positive/HER2-negative breast cancer. *Breast Cancer Res. Treat.* **2021**, *185*, 507–515. [CrossRef]
59. pCODR Expert Review Committee (pERC) Final Recommendation. Available online: https://www.cadth.ca/sites/default/files/pcodr/Reviews2020/10195RibociclibFulvestrantMBC_fnRec_pERC%20Chair%20Approved_22April2020_final.pdf (accessed on 22 June 2022).
60. Slamon, D.J.; Neven, P.; Chia, S.; Jerusalem, G.; De Laurentiis, M.; Im, S.; Petrakova, K.; Bianchi, G.V.; Martín, M.; Nusch, A.; et al. Ribociclib plus fulvestrant for postmenopausal women with hormone receptor-positive, human epidermal growth factor receptor 2-negative advanced breast cancer in the phase III randomized MONALEESA-3 trial: Updated overall survival. *Ann. Oncol.* **2021**, *32*, 1015–1024. [CrossRef]
61. Gagnon, J.; Lévesque, E.; Borduas, F.; Chiquette, J.; Diorio, C.; Duchesne, N.; Dumais, M.; Eloy, L.; Foulkes, W.; Gervais, N.; et al. Recommendations on breast cancer screening and prevention in the context of implementing risk stratification: Impending changes to current policies. *Curr. Oncol.* **2016**, *23*, 615–625. [CrossRef]
62. Puliti, D.; Duffy, S.W.; Miccinesi, G.; De Koning, H.; Lynge, E.; Zappa, M.; Paci, E. Overdiagnosis in mammographic screening for breast cancer in Europe: A literature review. *J. Med. Screen.* **2012**, *19* (Suppl. S1), 42–56. [CrossRef]
63. Anders, C.K.; Johnson, R.; Litton, J.; Phillips, M.; Bleyer, A. Breast cancer before age 40 years. *Semin. Oncol.* **2009**, *36*, 237–249. [CrossRef]
64. Partridge, A.H.; Hughes, M.E.; Warner, E.T.; Ottesen, R.A.; Wong, Y.-N.; Edge, S.B.; Theriault, R.L.; Blayney, D.W.; Niland, J.C.; Winer, E.P.; et al. Subtype-dependent relationship between young age at diagnosis and breast cancer survival. *J. Clin. Oncol.* **2016**, *34*, 3308–3314. [CrossRef] [PubMed]
65. Stapleton, S.M.; Oseni, T.O.; Bababekov, Y.J.; Hung, Y.C.; Chang, D.C. Race/ethnicity and age distribution of breast cancer diagnosis in the United States. *JAMA Surg.* **2018**, *153*, 594–595. [CrossRef] [PubMed]
66. Oppong, B.A.; Obeng-Gyasi, S.; Relation, T.; Adams-Campbell, L. Call to action: Breast cancer screening recommendations for Black women. *Breast Cancer Res. Treat.* **2021**, *187*, 295–297. [CrossRef] [PubMed]
67. Rebner, M.; Pai, V.R. Breast cancer screening recommendations: African American women are at a disadvantage. *J. Breast Imaging* **2020**, *2*, 416–421. [CrossRef]
68. Kohler, B.A.; Sherman, R.L.; Howlader, N.; Jemal, A.; Ryerson, A.B.; Henry, K.A.; Boscoe, F.P.; Cronin, K.A.; Lake, A.; Noone, A.M.; et al. Annual Report to the Nation on the Status of Cancer, 1975–2011, Featuring Incidence of Breast Cancer Subtypes by Race/Ethnicity, Poverty, and State. *J. Natl. Cancer Inst.* **2015**, *107*, djv048, Erratum in *J. Natl. Cancer Inst.* **2015**, *107*, djv121. [CrossRef] [PubMed]
69. Monticciolo, D.L. Current guidelines and gaps in breast cancer screening. *J. Am. Coll. Radiol.* **2020**, *17*, 1269–1275. [CrossRef]
70. Chapman, C.H.; Schechter, C.B.; Cadham, C.J.; Trentham-Dietz, A.; Gangnon, R.E.; Jagsi, R.; Mandelblatt, J.S. Identifying Equitable Screening Mammography Strategies for Black Women in the United States Using Simulation Modeling. *Ann. Intern. Med.* **2021**, *174*, 1637–1646. [CrossRef]

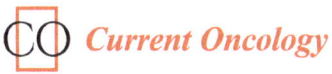

Article

Reducing Unnecessary Biopsies Using Digital Breast Tomosynthesis and Ultrasound in Dense and Nondense Breasts

Ibrahim Hadadi [1,2,*], Jillian Clarke [1], William Rae [1,3], Mark McEntee [1,4], Wendy Vincent [5] and Ernest Ekpo [1,6]

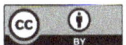

Citation: Hadadi, I.; Clarke, J.; Rae, W.; McEntee, M.; Vincent, W.; Ekpo, E. Reducing Unnecessary Biopsies Using Digital Breast Tomosynthesis and Ultrasound in Dense and Nondense Breasts. *Curr. Oncol.* 2022, 29, 5508–5516. https://doi.org/10.3390/curroncol29080435

Received: 21 June 2022
Accepted: 2 August 2022
Published: 4 August 2022

Publisher's Note: MDPI stays neutral with regard to jurisdictional claims in published maps and institutional affiliations.

Copyright: © 2022 by the authors. Licensee MDPI, Basel, Switzerland. This article is an open access article distributed under the terms and conditions of the Creative Commons Attribution (CC BY) license (https://creativecommons.org/licenses/by/4.0/).

[1] Medical Image Optimisation and Perception Group, Discipline of Medical Imaging Science, Faculty of Medicine and Health, The University of Sydney, Camperdown, NSW 2006, Australia
[2] Department of Radiological Sciences, Faculty of Applied Medical Sciences, King Khalid University, Abha 62529, Saudi Arabia
[3] Medical Imaging Department, Prince of Wales Hospital, Sydney, NSW 2031, Australia
[4] Discipline of Diagnostic Radiography, UGF 12 ASSERT, Brookfield Health Sciences, University College Cork, College Road, T12 AK54 Cork, Ireland
[5] Royal Prince Alfred Hospital, Sydney Local Health District, Camperdown, NSW 2050, Australia
[6] Orange Radiology, Laboratories and Research Centre, Calabar 540281, Nigeria
* Correspondence: ihad5571@uni.sydney.edu.au

Abstract: Aim: To compare digital breast tomosynthesis (DBT) and ultrasound in women recalled for assessment after a positive screening mammogram and assess the potential for each of these tools to reduce unnecessary biopsies. Methods: This data linkage study included 538 women recalled for assessment from January 2017 to December 2019. The association between the recalled mammographic abnormalities and breast density was analysed using the chi-square independence test. Relative risks and the number of recalled cases requiring DBT and ultrasound assessment to prevent one unnecessary biopsy were compared using the McNemar test. Results: Breast density significantly influenced recall decisions ($p < 0.001$). Ultrasound showed greater potential to decrease unnecessary biopsies than DBT: in entirely fatty (21% vs. 5%; $p = 0.04$); scattered fibroglandular (23% vs. 10%; $p = 0.003$); heterogeneously dense (34% vs. 7%; $p < 0.001$) and extremely dense (39% vs. 9%; $p < 0.001$) breasts. The number of benign cases needing assessment to prevent one unnecessary biopsy was significantly lower with ultrasound than DBT in heterogeneously dense (1.8 vs. 7; $p < 0.001$) and extremely dense (1.9 vs. 5.1; $p = 0.03$) breasts. Conclusion: Women with dense breasts are more likely to be recalled for assessment and have a false-positive biopsy. Women with dense breasts benefit more from ultrasound assessment than from DBT.

Keywords: DBT; ultrasound; benign biopsy; breast density; breast cancer

1. Introduction

Early detection of breast cancer is crucial to reducing mortality from the disease [1]. Population screening using mammography is the standard approach to early detection. The principal criterion for screening recommendation is patient age, although a family history of breast cancer is also a well-established risk factor for breast cancer. In the last two decades, high mammographic breast density as a risk factor has also gained significant attention in the literature due to the associated increase in breast cancer risk and the resultant reduced sensitivity of screening mammography [2]. Technological advances and the transition from film-screen to digital mammography (DM) reduced the masking effect of breast density and enhanced cancer detection [3]. However, there are still difficulties reading DM images of women with dense breasts [4]. Mammographically dense tissue has been demonstrated to increase radiologists' suspicion during the interpretation of screening mammograms, leading to higher recall rates for women with mammographically dense breasts [5].

Most women with dense breasts recalled for assessment have demonstrated negative or benign outcomes, with false positives ranging between 73% and 97% [6–10]. Unnecessary recalls increase the cost of screening, may cause psychosocial harm due to false-positive alarms, and can deter women from rescreening [11,12]. Digital breast tomosynthesis (DBT) and ultrasound can mitigate the limitations associated with DM, allowing for a more detailed evaluation of breast tissue and suspicious lesions by minimising superimposition of parenchymal densities [13–15]. In the United Kingdom National Health Service Breast Screening Programme, DBT assessment of women recalled at DM screening led to a 33% reduction in the benign biopsy rate [16], with lower false positives across mammographic features such as mass lesions and asymmetric densities. Some studies have also shown that using ultrasound is accurate in distinguishing between benign and malignant lesions and decreases the number of benign biopsies by 34% to 60% [17,18]. However, it is unclear how DBT and ultrasound compare when assessing women recalled and whether they reduce false-positive biopsies across different breast compositions.

Studies comparing DBT and ultrasound [19,20] have focused on incremental breast cancer detection in mammography-negative dense breasts. In one study [21], the effectiveness of ultrasound screening after the combination of DM and DBT was examined. Despite the widespread concurrent use of DBT and ultrasound in many clinical settings, no study has directly compared their diagnostic efficacy in mammography-recalled women to establish optimised assessment pathways. Importantly, no published work has compared the impact of these tools in reducing unnecessary biopsies of benign lesions, across various breast densities. We hypothesised that DBT and ultrasound result in equal numbers of unnecessary biopsies. Therefore, this study aims to compare the performance of DBT and ultrasound in women recalled for assessment after a positive screening mammogram and to compare the number of unnecessary biopsies in dense and nondense breasts.

2. Materials and Methods

2.1. Study Design and Patient Selection

This is a data linkage study of women recalled for assessment following a suspicious finding on their screening mammogram. Patients were included if they were recalled for assessment after a screening mammogram, had both DBT and ultrasound assessment, and underwent breast biopsy procedures. All screening mammograms of the recalled women were read by two radiologists who interpreted the images independently from each other. Any discrepancies between these two readers were resolved by a third radiologist.

A five-tier grading system was used to describe the findings on screening mammograms based on BreastScreen Australia's RANZCR breast imaging lesion classification system: grade 1 (normal or no abnormality); grade 2 (benign); grade 3 (indeterminate/equivocal); grade 4 (suspicious); grade 5 (malignant). Each breast was examined using two different mammographic views: the craniocaudal (CC) and the mediolateral oblique (MLO). If more mammography spot views were required, they were obtained. Women whose images were rated 3, 4, or 5 were recalled for assessment using DBT and ultrasound to confirm or rule out breast cancer. A needle biopsy was performed on breast lesions graded 3, 4, or 5 after these imaging assessment tools were assessed. Table 1 shows the baseline characteristics of women recalled for assessment.

Breast density was reported according to the Breast Imaging Reporting and Data System (BI-RADS 5th edition): BI-RADS A: "the breasts are almost entirely fatty"; BI-RADS B: "there are scattered areas of fibroglandular density"; BI-RADS C: "the breasts are heterogeneously dense, which may obscure small masses"; BI-RADS D: "the breasts are extremely dense, which lowers the sensitivity of mammography".

All DBT images used in this study were acquired using Selenia Dimensions (Hologic Inc.). Real time B-mode and colour doppler were performed using an ACUSON S2000 Ultrasound System (HELX Evolution with Touch Control, Siemens Medical Solutions), equipped with a 12L4 linear array transducer (12–4 MHz). Both DBT and ultrasound assessment results were evaluated according to the RANZCR breast imaging lesion classification scale.

Table 1. Characteristics of women recalled for assessment following a suspicious mammography finding.

Characteristic	No. (%)
Age (years)	
40–49	69 (12.8)
50–59	222 (41.2)
60–69	163 (30.3)
≥70	84 (15.7)
Breast Density	
Almost entirely fatty	64 (12)
Scattered areas of fibroglandular density	152 (28.2)
Heterogeneously dense	238 (44.2)
Extremely dense	84 (15.6)
Risk Factor of Breast Cancer (Personal/Family History)	
Yes	98 (18.2)
No	440 (81.8)

2.2. Statistical Analysis

We compared the performance of DBT and ultrasound in women recalled for assessment after a positive screening mammogram to test the hypothesis that there is no difference between DBT and ultrasound in reducing unnecessary benign biopsies. The comparisons were performed according to breast density (BI-RADS A, B, C, and D). Relative risks at a 95% confidence interval were calculated to establish how DBT and ultrasound decreased the likelihood of an unnecessary biopsy following screening mammography. Using needle biopsy results as the reference standard, the number of cases requiring DBT and ultrasound assessment to prevent one unnecessary biopsy was estimated to determine the likelihood of benefit. The number needed to be assessed is inversely proportional to the risk reduction [1/(absolute risk reduction)]. The ideal screening number would be 1, in which all the women recalled for assessment with benign lesions have benefited. The association between the recalled mammographic abnormalities and breast density was analysed using the chi-square independence test (χ^2 continuity correction). The McNemar test (χ^2 continuity correction) was used to determine the statistical significance between DBT and ultrasound. A p-value ≤ 0.05 was considered statistically significant. These statistical analyses were conducted via the open-source Jamovi software (2.3.0).

3. Results

The study included 550 mammographic lesions from 538 women, aged 40 to 94 years (mean age: 58.9, SD: ±8.94), recalled at breast cancer screening mammography between 2017 and 2019. Among the 550 lesions recalled, 60.4% were in dense breasts, and 39.6% were in nondense breasts. Breast density was found to influence recall decisions significantly. Mammographic abnormalities were more likely to be recalled when seen in dense breasts than in non-dense breasts ($p < 0.001$). The distribution of lesion types across dense and nondense breasts is shown in Table 2.

Table 2. Association between recall and breast density based on lesion features.

Radiologic Feature	Breast Density		Total	p-Value
	Nondense Breasts (Number of Benign Lesions)	Dense Breasts (Number of Benign Lesions)		
NSD	26 (16)	23 (10)	49	
Stellate	51 (5)	75 (7)	126	
Calcification	39 (18)	128 (53)	167	**<0.001**
Discrete mass	99 (32)	82 (44)	181	
Architectural distortion	3 (2)	24 (10)	27	
Total	218 (73)	332 (124)	550	

NSD: Nonspecific density; Nondense Breasts: almost entirely fatty & scattered areas of fibroglandular density; Dense Breasts: heterogeneously dense & extremely dense; Bold values indicate statistical significance at the p-value ≤ 0.05 level.

Table 3 shows that there is no difference in true negative proportions between DBT and ultrasound in nondense breasts (32.8% vs. 22%, respectively; $p = 0.2$). Conversely, in dense breasts, ultrasound showed a significantly higher proportion of true negatives than DBT (54.8% vs. 16.1%, respectively; $p < 0.001$).

Table 3. True negative proportions of DBT and ultrasound across dense and nondense breasts.

Assessment Tools	NO. of True Negative (%)	Negative Outcome (Biopsy)	p-Value	NO. of True Negative (%)	Negative Outcome (Biopsy)	p-Value
	Breast Density					
	Nondense Breasts			Dense Breasts		
DBT	16 (22)	73	0.2	20 (16.1)	124	**<0.001**
US	24 (32.8)	73		68 (54.8)	124	

Nondense Breasts: almost entirely fatty & scattered areas of fibroglandular density; Dense Breasts: heterogeneously dense & extremely dense; DBT: digital breast tomosynthesis; US: ultrasound; Bold values indicate statistical significance at the p-value ≤ 0.05 level.

Table 4 shows the potential reduction of unnecessary biopsies for DBT and ultrasound stratified according to breast density. Differences between DBT and ultrasound in terms of preventing one unnecessary biopsy are also presented. Among all recalled mammographic abnormalities, ultrasound showed greater potential to decrease unnecessary biopsies than DBT: entirely fatty (21% vs. 5%, respectively; $p = 0.04$); scattered fibroglandular (23% vs. 10%, respectively; $p = 0.003$); heterogeneously dense (34% vs. 7%, respectively; $p < 0.001$); extremely dense (39% vs. 9%, respectively; $p < 0.001$) breasts. The number of cases needing assessment to prevent one unnecessary biopsy was significantly lower with ultrasound than with DBT in heterogeneously dense breasts (1.8 vs. 7, respectively; $p < 0.001$) and extremely dense breasts (1.9 vs. 5.1, respectively; $p = 0.03$), but there were no significant differences in entirely fatty breasts (3.2 vs. 4.3, respectively; $p = 0.65$) and scattered fibroglandular densities (2.6 vs. 4.6, respectively; $p = 0.21$).

Table 4. The potential reduction of DBT and ultrasound to decrease unnecessary biopsies following screening mammography and the number of DBT and ultrasound examinations required to be assessed to prevent one unnecessary biopsy.

Parameter	Potential Reduction of DBT and Ultrasound to Decrease Unnecessary Biopsies after DM			Estimation Number of Benign Cases that Required Assessment by DBT and Ultrasound to Prevent One Unnecessary Biopsy		
	Relative Risk (95% CI)			NO. of Cases (ARR%)		
Breast Density	DBT	US	p-Value	DBT	US	p-Value
BI-RADS A	0.95 (0.89 to 1)	0.79 (0.70 to 0.90)	**0.04**	4.3 (23)	3.2 (30.7)	0.65
BI-RADS B	0.9 (0.85 to 0.95)	0.77 (0.70 to 0.84)	**0.003**	4.6 (21.7)	2.6 (66.7)	0.21
BI-RADS C	0.93 (0.89 to 0.96)	0.66 (0.60 to 0.73)	**<0.001**	7 (14.1)	1.8 (55.4)	**<0.001**
BI-RADS D	0.91 (0.85 to 0.97)	0.61 (0.51 to 0.72)	**<0.001**	5.1 (18.8)	1.9 (50)	**0.03**

BI-RADS A: almost entirely fatty; BI-RADS B: scattered areas of fibroglandular density; BI-RADS C: heterogeneously dense; BI-RADS D: extremely dense; DM: digital mammography; DBT: digital breast tomosynthesis; US: ultrasound; ARR: absolute risk reduction. Bold values indicate statistical significance at the p-value $\leq$ 0.05 level.

4. Discussion

We found strong evidence that the density of a woman's breast significantly influences recall decisions in a population-based screening program. Mammographic abnormalities were more likely to be recalled when seen in dense breasts than in nondense breasts. We also found that a significant number of the lesions found in women with dense breasts recalled for assessment were benign, and almost double the number of benign lesions recalled in women with nondense breasts. These findings suggest that around 1 in 3 women with dense breasts recalled for assessment had an unnecessary biopsy.

Several factors affect the interpretation of two-dimensional images and may be responsible for the high number of recalls, particularly in women with dense breasts. Summation artefacts caused by the superimposition of dense tissue on benign lesions may mimic breast cancer, which may have resulted in the high rate of unnecessary recalls [15,22]. False-positive or negative recall at screening may be due to perceptual or cognitive errors caused by factors such as poor lesion visibility and subtle or atypical cancer appearances [23]. It has been shown that breast density is more likely to cause perceptual errors such as false positives and negatives due to its ability to obscure subtle lesions or create difficulty in distinguishing lesions in distracting background breast tissue [14,24,25]. Such perceptual errors and the higher of cancer incidence in dense breasts may have contributed to the high recall of women with high breast density.

Mammographic abnormalities such as calcifications, masses with indistinct, spiculated or circumscribed margins, and asymmetries are frequent features of breast cancer [15,22,25]. Mammographic features such as calcifications and discrete masses constituted the largest proportion of benign biopsies. These two mammographic features are common findings in screening programs [26–28]. The high false-positive biopsies of these lesion types underscore the need for studies to establish the features of these lesions associated with malignancy to inform criteria for reducing unnecessary recall. Such studies may provide reasonable thresholds for identifying true positive lesions and reduce overtesting and unnecessary biopsies of benign lesions. Another factor that may have been responsible for the higher recall of benign lesions is lesion size. Screening quality can be judged by the detection of small cancers, defined as those with a diameter of $\leq$15 mm. Small-sized calcifications ($\leq$15 mm) and calcifications that cover a larger region of breast are more likely to be malignant [29–31]. However, the diameters of calcifications varied widely in our data. Malignancy may be established by a complex combination of lesion features including size, morphology, and shape. Studies that combine these features to predict malignancy may better inform criteria for recall and biopsy.

A major focus of our study was to examine the potential role of DBT and ultrasound in reducing unnecessary biopsies. Previous pieces of work that compared DBT and ultrasound focused on women with mammographically negative dense breasts [19,20] and showed that ultrasound has a higher false-positive rate than DBT. Our study focuses on women with mammographically suspicious findings recalled for assessment and shows that ultrasound has significantly greater potential to decrease unnecessary biopsies than DBT in all breast compositions. We found no significant difference in true negative proportions between ultrasound and DBT in nondense breasts. In dense breasts, ultrasound showed a significantly higher proportion of true negatives than DBT. We also found that the number of cases that required assessment to prevent one unnecessary biopsy was significantly lower with ultrasound than DBT in heterogeneously dense and extremely dense breasts. These findings suggest that every benign lesion in heterogeneously and extremely dense breasts being unnecessarily recalled has approximately a 50% (1 out of 2 benign lesions) chance of receiving benefit from ultrasound.

In women with nondense breasts, we found no significant difference between DBT and ultrasound in terms of the number of cases that required assessment to prevent one unnecessary biopsy. To the best of our knowledge, the current study was the first to compare DBT and ultrasound assessments of recalled lesions across dense and nondense breasts. Previous studies [15,25] that focused on ultrasound showed that mimickers of breast cancer with benign morphologic ultrasound features could be safely managed with ultrasound follow-up to establish stability and confirm benign status. In dense breasts, ultrasound was found to be a satisfactory alternative to biopsy for solid lesions with benign morphological ultrasound features because of the high negative predictive value (99.8%) [32]; this may reduce anxiety for women recalled for assessment.

Previous studies that sought to reduce unnecessary biopsies were based on DBT. In one of these studies [16] incorporating DBT into the diagnostic workup of mammographic abnormalities would have resulted in a reduction in the number of benign biopsies conducted during screening assessment. The authors reported that DBT enhances reader accuracy and confidence in judging whether mammographic abnormalities are cancerous or not, resulting in a decrease in biopsies from 69% to 36%. However, this study did not adjust for breast density and lesion characteristics. A study from the USA [33] showed that DBT has the potential to decrease unnecessary biopsies for all breast densities, with substantial reductions for women with heterogeneously dense breasts (21.3%) and extremely dense breasts (27.5%). Our study, based on an Australian population and radiologists, showed only modest potential of DBT to reduce unnecessary biopsies for women of all breast compositions: entirely fatty (5%), scattered fibroglandular (10%), heterogeneously dense (7%), and extremely dense breasts (9%). These differences may be due to the differences in study designs and recall classification criteria. Unlike the USA study, we included women recalled for assessment following a suspicious finding on their screening mammograms that were read by two radiologists who worked independently. Additionally, the RANZCR grade 3 used by BreastScreen Australia is classified as a positive finding that combines the BI-RADS 3 and BI-RADS 4A categories in the American College of Radiologists BI-RADS Atlas. These differences may have influenced the impact of DBT during assessment for recalled women.

Although ultrasound is an effective assessment tool to differentiate between benign and malignant lesions that appear suspicious on mammography, it is limited in accurately classifying calcifications. Therefore, mammography-recalled calcifications should not be wholly ruled out based on ultrasound findings. This is supported by a previous study [17] that suggested that women should be recalled for biopsy even if suspicious calcifications are considered normal during an ultrasound. This previous work also showed a decrease in the false-positive rate in screening mammography by incorporating ultrasound into the diagnostic work-up of suspicious findings. However, further studies are needed to estimate the benefit-to-harm ratio and costs of ultrasound and DBT as assessment tools.

Our study is not without limitations. First, it is a single-centre study. Second, the sample size is relatively small, and 60.4% of recalled lesions in our study were in dense breasts, representing a large proportion of recalled mammograms. Thus, a greater understanding of work-up for dense breasts might help screening programs better manage their assessment procedures and resources.

5. Conclusions

The mammographic breast density increases recall rates and biopsy recommendations, and women with dense breasts recalled for assessment are more likely to have a false-positive biopsy compared to those with fatty breasts. In dense breasts, ultrasound showed greater potential to decrease unnecessary biopsies than DBT, with every benign lesion in dense breasts being unnecessarily recalled having approximately a 50% chance of benefiting from ultrasound. DBT and ultrasound perform comparatively similar in reducing unnecessary benign biopsies in fatty breasts. Therefore, tailoring assessment pathways according to breast density may reduce unnecessary biopsies and anxiety in women recalled for assessment.

Author Contributions: Conceptualization, I.H., M.M. and E.E.; methodology, I.H. and E.E.; validation, I.H., E.E., M.M., J.C., W.R. and W.V.; analysis, I.H.; investigation, I.H. and E.E.; data collection, I.H.; writing—original draft preparation, I.H.; writing—review and editing, I.H., E.E., M.M., J.C., W.R. and W.V.; supervision, E.E. All authors have read and agreed to the published version of the manuscript.

Funding: This research received no external funding.

Institutional Review Board Statement: The study was conducted in accordance with the Declaration of Helsinki, and received ethics approval from the New South Wales health department (IRB: X19-0495) and local approval from Sydney Local Health District (2019/ETH13792), date of approval: 11 February 2020.

Informed Consent Statement: The Committee granted a waiver of the usual requirement for the consent of the individual for the use of their health information in a research project, in accordance with the Health Records and Information Privacy Act 2002 (NSW) and the NSW Privacy Commissioner's Statutory guidelines on research and the NHMRC Guidelines approved under Section 95A of the Privacy Act 1988.

Data Availability Statement: Data are available from the authors with the permission of BreastScreen NSW, Sydney Local Health District.

Acknowledgments: We want to thank Beby Thung Winata for assisting with data collection.

Conflicts of Interest: The authors declare no conflict of interest.

References

1. Nelson, H.D.; Tyne, K.; Naik, A.; Bougatsos, C.; Chan, B.K.; Humphrey, L.; U.S. Preventive Services Task Force. Screening for breast cancer: An update for the U.S. Preventive Services Task Force. *Ann. Intern Med.* **2009**, *151*, 727–737. [CrossRef] [PubMed]
2. Bond-Smith, D.; Stone, J. Methodological Challenges and Updated Findings from a Meta-analysis of the Association between Mammographic Density and Breast Cancer. *Cancer Epidemiol. Biomark. Prev.* **2019**, *28*, 22–31. [CrossRef] [PubMed]
3. Kerlikowske, K.; Hubbard, R.A.; Miglioretti, D.L.; Geller, B.M.; Yankaskas, B.C.; Lehman, C.D.; Taplin, S.H.; Sickles, E.A.; Breast Cancer Surveillance Consortium. Comparative effectiveness of digital versus film-screen mammography in community practice in the United States: A cohort study. *Ann. Intern Med.* **2011**, *155*, 493–502. [CrossRef]
4. Posso, M.; Louro, J.; Sánchez, M.; Román, M.; Vidal, C.; Sala, M.; Baré, M.; Castells, X. Mammographic breast density: How it affects performance indicators in screening programmes? *Eur. J. Radiol.* **2019**, *110*, 81–87. [CrossRef]
5. Ekpo, E.U.B.; Egbe, N.O.P.; Egom, A.E.B.; McEntee, M.F.P. Mammographic Breast Density: Comparison Across Women with Conclusive and Inconclusive Mammography Reports. *J. Med. Imaging Radiat. Sci.* **2015**, *47*, 55–59. [CrossRef] [PubMed]
6. Hong, S.; Song, S.Y.; Park, B.; Suh, M.; Choi, K.S.; Jung, S.E.; Kim, M.J.; Lee, E.H.; Lee, C.W.; Jun, J.K. Effect of Digital Mammography for Breast Cancer Screening: A Comparative Study of More than 8 Million Korean Women. *Radiology* **2020**, *294*, 247–255. [CrossRef] [PubMed]
7. Berg, W.A.; Zhang, Z.; Lehrer, D.; Jong, R.A.; Pisano, E.D.; Barr, R.G.; Böhm-Vélez, M.; Mahoney, M.C.; Evans, W.P.; Larsen, L.H. Detection of breast cancer with addition of annual screening ultrasound or a single screening MRI to mammography in women with elevated breast cancer risk. *JAMA* **2012**, *307*, 1394–1404.

8. Pisano, E.D.; Hendrick, R.E.; Yaffe, M.J.; Baum, J.K.; Acharyya, S.; Cormack, J.B.; Hanna, L.A.; Conant, E.F.; Fajardo, L.L.; Bassett, L.W.; et al. Diagnostic Accuracy of Digital versus Film Mammography: Exploratory Analysis of Selected Population Subgroups in DMIST. *Radiology* **2008**, *246*, 376–383. [CrossRef]
9. McDonald, E.S.; McCarthy, A.M.; Akhtar, A.L.; Synnestvedt, M.B.; Schnall, M.; Conant, E.F. Baseline screening mammography: Performance of full-field digital mammography versus digital breast tomosynthesis. *Am. J. Roentgenol.* **2015**, *205*, 1143–1148. [CrossRef]
10. Gilbert, F.J.; Tucker, L.; Gillan, M.G.C.; Willsher, P.; Cooke, J.; Duncan, K.A.; Michell, M.J.; Dobson, H.M.; Lim, Y.Y.; Suaris, T.; et al. Accuracy of Digital Breast Tomosynthesis for Depicting Breast Cancer Subgroups in a UK Retrospective Reading Study (TOMMY Trial). *Radiology* **2015**, *277*, 697–706. [CrossRef]
11. Brewer, N.T.; Salz, T.; Lillie, S.E. Systematic review: The long-term effects of false-positive mammograms. *Ann. Intern Med.* **2007**, *146*, 502–510. [CrossRef]
12. Zappa, M.; Spagnolo, G.; Ciatto, S.; Giorgi, D.; Paci, E.; Rosseli del Turco, M. Measurement of the costs in two mammographic screening programmes in the province of Florence, Italy. *J. Med. Screen* **1995**, *2*, 191–194. [CrossRef] [PubMed]
13. Peppard, H.R.; Nicholson, B.E.; Rochman, C.M.; Merchant, J.K.; Mayo, R.C., III; Harvey, J.A. Digital Breast Tomosynthesis in the Diagnostic Setting: Indications and Clinical Applications. *RadioGraphics* **2015**, *35*, 975–990. [CrossRef] [PubMed]
14. Rafferty, E.A. Digital Mammography: Novel Applications. *Radiol. Clin. N. Am.* **2007**, *45*, 831–843. [CrossRef] [PubMed]
15. Guirguis, M.S.; Adrada, B.; Santiago, L.; Candelaria, R.; Arribas, E. Mimickers of breast malignancy: Imaging findings, pathologic concordance and clinical management. *Insights Imaging* **2021**, *12*, 53. [CrossRef]
16. Sharma, N.; McMahon, M.; Haigh, I.; Chen, Y.; Dall, B.J.G. The Potential Impact of Digital Breast Tomosynthesis on the Benign Biopsy Rate in Women Recalled within the UK Breast Screening Programme. *Radiology* **2019**, *291*, 310–317. [CrossRef] [PubMed]
17. Tohno, E.; Umemoto, T.; Sasaki, K.; Morishima, I.; Ueno, E. Effect of adding screening ultrasonography to screening mammography on patient recall and cancer detection rates: A retrospective study in Japan. *Eur. J. Radiol.* **2013**, *82*, 1227–1230. [CrossRef]
18. Stavros, A.T.; Thickman, D.; Rapp, C.L.; Dennis, M.A.; Parker, S.H.; Sisney, G.A. Solid breast nodules: Use of sonography to distinguish between benign and malignant lesions. *Radiology* **1995**, *196*, 123–134. [CrossRef] [PubMed]
19. Tagliafico, A.S.; Calabrese, M.; Mariscotti, G.; Durando, M.; Tosto, S.; Monetti, F.; Airaldi, S.; Bignotti, B.; Nori, J.; Bagni, A.; et al. Adjunct Screening With Tomosynthesis or Ultrasound in Women With Mammography-Negative Dense Breasts: Interim Report of a Prospective Comparative Trial. *J. Clin. Oncol.* **2016**, *34*, 1882–1888. [CrossRef]
20. Tagliafico, A.S.; Mariscotti, G.; Valdora, F.; Durando, M.; Nori, J.; La Forgia, D.; Rosenberg, I.; Caumo, F.; Gandolfo, N.; Sormani, M.P. A prospective comparative trial of adjunct screening with tomosynthesis or ultrasound in women with mammography-negative dense breasts (ASTOUND-2). *Eur. J. Cancer* **2018**, *104*, 39–46. [CrossRef]
21. Yi, A.; Jang, M.J.; Yim, D.; Kwon, B.R.; Shin, S.U.; Chang, J.M. Addition of Screening Breast US to Digital Mammography and Digital Breast Tomosynthesis for Breast Cancer Screening in Women at Average Risk. *Radiology* **2021**, *298*, 568–575. [CrossRef] [PubMed]
22. Castells, X.; Torá-Rocamora, I.; Posso, M.; Román, M.; Vernet-Tomas, M.; Rodríguez-Arana, A.; Domingo, L.; Vidal, C.; Baré, M.; Ferrer, J.; et al. Risk of Breast Cancer in Women with False-Positive Results according to Mammographic Features. *Radiology* **2016**, *280*, 379–386. [CrossRef] [PubMed]
23. Ekpo, E.U.; Alakhras, M.; Brennan, P. Errors in Mammography Cannot be Solved Through Technology Alone. *Asian Pac. J. Cancer Prev.* **2018**, *19*, 291–301. [CrossRef]
24. Corsetti, V.; Houssami, N.; Ghirardi, M.; Ferrari, A.; Speziani, M.; Bellarosa, S.; Remida, G.; Gasparotti, C.; Galligioni, E.; Ciatto, S. Evidence of the effect of adjunct ultrasound screening in women with mammography-negative dense breasts: Interval breast cancers at 1year follow-up. *Eur. J. Cancer* **2011**, *47*, 1021–1026. [CrossRef]
25. Nassar, L.; Baassiri, A.; Salah, F.; Barakat, M.; Najem, E.; Boulos, F.; Berjawi, G. Stromal Fibrosis of the Breast: A Spectrum of Benign to Malignant Imaging Appearances. *Radiol. Res. Pract.* **2019**, *2019*, 5045908. [CrossRef] [PubMed]
26. Farshid, G.; Sullivan, T.; Downey, P.; Gill, P.G.; Pieterse, S. Independent predictors of breast malignancy in screen-detected microcalcifications: Biopsy results in 2545 cases. *Br. J. Cancer* **2011**, *105*, 1669–1675. [CrossRef]
27. Stomper, P.C. The prevalence and distribution of well circumscribed nodules on screening mammography: Analysis of 1500 mammograms. *Breast Dis.* **1991**, *4*, 197–203.
28. Farshid, G.; Walker, A.; Battersby, G.; Sullivan, T.; Gill, P.G.; Pieterse, S.; Downey, P. Predictors of malignancy in screen-detected breast masses with indeterminate/equivocal (grade 3) imaging features. *Breast* **2011**, *20*, 56–61. [CrossRef]
29. Fondrinier, E.; Lorimier, G.; Guerin-Boblet, V.; Bertrand, A.-F.; Mayras, C.; Dauver, N. Breast Microcalcifications: Multivariate Analysis of Radiological and Clinical Factors for Carcinoma. *World J. Surg.* **2002**, *26*, 290–296. [CrossRef] [PubMed]
30. James, J.J.; Evans, A.J.; Pinder, S.E.; Macmillan, R.D.; Wilson, A.R.M.; Ellis, I.O. Is the Presence of Mammographic Comedo Calcification Really a Prognostic Factor for Small Screen-detected Invasive Breast Cancers? *Clin. Radiol.* **2003**, *58*, 54–62. [CrossRef]
31. Nyante, S.J.; Lee, S.S.; Benefield, T.S.; Hoots, T.N.; Henderson, L.M. The association between mammographic calcifications and breast cancer prognostic factors in a population-based registry cohort. *Cancer* **2017**, *123*, 219–227. [CrossRef] [PubMed]

32. Graf, O.; Helbich, T.H.; Hopf, G.; Graf, C.; Sickles, E.A. Probably Benign Breast Masses at US: Is Follow-up an Acceptable Alternative to Biopsy? *Radiology* **2007**, *244*, 87–93. [CrossRef] [PubMed]
33. Richard, E.; Sharpe, J.; Venkataraman, S.; Phillips, J.; Dialani, V.; Fein-Zachary, V.J.; Prakash, S.; Slanetz, P.J.; Mehta, T.S. Increased Cancer Detection Rate and Variations in the Recall Rate Resulting from Implementation of 3D Digital Breast Tomosynthesis into a Population-based Screening Program. *Radiology* **2016**, *278*, 698–706. [CrossRef]

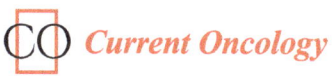

Article

Female Healthcare Workers' Knowledge, Attitude towards Breast Cancer, and Perceived Barriers towards Mammogram Screening: A Multicenter Study in North Saudi Arabia

Anfal Mohammed Alenezi [1,*], Ashokkumar Thirunavukkarasu [2], Farooq Ahmed Wani [3], Hadil Alenezi [4], Muhannad Faleh Alanazi [5], Abdulaziz Saud Alruwaili [6], Rasha Harbi Alashjaee [6], Faisal Harbi Alashjaee [6], Abdulaziz Khalid Alrasheed [7] and Bandar Dhaher Alshrari [6]

[1] Department of Surgery, College of Medicine, Jouf University, Sakaka 72388, Saudi Arabia
[2] Department of Community and Family Medicine, College of Medicine, Jouf University, Sakaka 72388, Saudi Arabia; ashokkumar@ju.edu.sa
[3] Department of Pathology, College of Medicine, Jouf University, Sakaka 72388, Saudi Arabia; fawani@ju.edu.sa
[4] Department of Radiology and Nuclear Medicine, Security Forces Hospital, Riyadh 11481, Saudi Arabia; hmaalenezi@sfh.med.sa
[5] Division of Radiology, Department of Internal Medicine, College of Medicine, Jouf University, Sakaka 72388, Saudi Arabia; mfalanazi@ju.edu.sa
[6] College of Medicine, Jouf University, Sakaka 72388, Saudi Arabia; alnosairy.9@gmail.com (A.S.A.); rashaintj@gmail.com (R.H.A.); f65aisal@gmail.com (F.H.A.); drbanderalsharari@gmail.com (B.D.A.)
[7] Department of General Surgery, King Saud Medical City, Riyadh 12745, Saudi Arabia; a.alrasheed@ksmc.med.sa
* Correspondence: amaalenezi@ju.edu.sa; Tel.: +966-599739619

Citation: Alenezi, A.M.; Thirunavukkarasu, A.; Wani, F.A.; Alenezi, H.; Alanazi, M.F.; Alruwaili, A.S.; Alashjaee, R.H.; Alashjaee, F.H.; Alrasheed, A.K.; Alshrari, B.D. Female Healthcare Workers' Knowledge, Attitude towards Breast Cancer, and Perceived Barriers towards Mammogram Screening: A Multicenter Study in North Saudi Arabia. *Curr. Oncol.* **2022**, *29*, 4300–4314. https://doi.org/10.3390/curroncol29060344

Received: 15 May 2022
Accepted: 14 June 2022
Published: 15 June 2022

Publisher's Note: MDPI stays neutral with regard to jurisdictional claims in published maps and institutional affiliations.

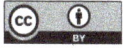

Copyright: © 2022 by the authors. Licensee MDPI, Basel, Switzerland. This article is an open access article distributed under the terms and conditions of the Creative Commons Attribution (CC BY) license (https://creativecommons.org/licenses/by/4.0/).

Abstract: Breast cancer is the most commonly diagnosed cancer among women in the Kingdom of Saudi Arabia and other Middle East countries. This analytical cross-sectional study assessed knowledge, attitude towards breast cancer, and barriers to mammogram screening among 414 randomly selected female healthcare workers from multiple healthcare facilities in northern Saudi Arabia. Of the studied population, 48.6% had low knowledge, and 16.1% had a low attitude towards breast cancer risk factors and symptoms. The common barriers to mammogram screening were fear to discover cancer (57.2%) and apprehension regarding radiation exposure (57%). Logistic regression analysis found that lack of awareness regarding mammogram was significantly associated with age ($p = 0.030$) and healthcare workers category (ref: physicians: $p = 0.016$). In addition, we found a significant negative correlation between knowledge and barrier scores (Spearman's rho: -0.315, $p < 0.001$). It is recommended to develop target-oriented educational programs for the healthcare workers, which would empower them to educate the community regarding the risk factors and the importance of mammogram screening. Furthermore, a prospective study is warranted in other regions of the Kingdom of Saudi Arabia to understand the region-specific training needs for the healthcare workers.

Keywords: breast cancer; risk factors; screening mammography; knowledge assessment; barriers; questionnaire examination

1. Introduction

Breast cancer is one of the significant public health issues worldwide affecting women after puberty, as stated by the World Health Organization (WHO). In 2020, there were 2.3 million cases and 685,000 deaths worldwide due to breast cancer [1]. Several international surveys reported that breast cancer causes more disability-adjusted life years among women than any other cancer in the world [2,3]. Even though the etiology for breast cancer has not been completely understood, certain risk factors, including older age, genetic predisposition, family history, early menarche, late menopause, exogenous hormone usage, and obesity, play a significant role in the breast cancer development [4,5]. In the Kingdom of Saudi Arabia (KSA), breast cancer ranks as the number one reported cancer (14.2%), and cancer-related deaths among women have an increasing annual incidence of 3.01% and a mortality of 0.93% [6,7].

Various screening methods are available for detecting breast cancer at an earlier stage, including breast self-examination, clinical breast examination, and ultrasound; however, mammography remains the primary screening modality used worldwide. In the KSA, the mammography screening technique is used for early detection of breast cancer, and it uses low-frequency X-rays to detect the features of microcalcification or mass in the breast [8,9]. As per the American Cancer Society's guidelines, breast cancer screening to be started at 40 years of age and annual screening to be done from 45 years of age. Considering the higher incidence of breast cancer in the KSA, the Ministry of Health has recommended breast cancer screening through mammogram for all women aged from 40 to 50 years for every two years and women aged 51 to 69 years should have regular mammograms for every one to two years [10]. In the KSA, Breast Cancer Early Detection (BCED) program aims to increase early-detected cases and reduce breast cancer mortality. As per the BCED, mammogram screening is available free of cost in hospitals, selected primary health centers, and mobile clinics for Saudi nationals and public sector workers. Women are enrolled in mammogram screening programs by raising awareness through different modalities [11].

Recent epidemiological studies reported that women with inadequate knowledge regarding risk factors and susceptibility to breast cancer were less likely to accept breast cancer screening methods. Other factors associated with the low uptake of mammogram screening programs were low income, low education, and lack of information regarding available screening methods [12,13].

Healthcare workers (HCWs) play a critical role in imparting knowledge regarding available health services improving access and screening services provided by the concerned authorities. They also help in changing the behavior of an individual, families, and communities through different health-promotion activities [14,15]. Hence, it is essential to improve the knowledge and skills of the HCWs. These factors can be achieved among the HCWs by continuously assessing the current awareness, perception, and barriers towards breast cancer screening programs.

Hence, the present study assessed the knowledge and attitude towards breast cancer among the female HCWs and identified the correlation between knowledge and attitude. This study also aimed to identify the barriers to breast cancer screening programs among them.

2. Materials and Methods

2.1. Study Design and Setting

The current analytical cross-sectional survey was conducted in the Aljouf region from December 2021 to April 2022. This region is situated in the northern part of the KSA, with a total population of about 500,000. Healthcare in the Aljouf region is delivered by the ministry of health (MOH), private sectors, and other ministries through four levels: primary, secondary, specialty hospitals, and medical cities. There are 62 primary health centers, 13 general hospitals, and 2 specialty hospitals in this region under the MOH, KSA.

2.2. Inclusion and Exclusion Criteria

We included all the female HCW categories working in the MOH sector for a minimum duration of one year, namely doctors, nurses, pharmacists, lab technicians, and other categories. We excluded the HCWs on vacation, in different sectors (other than MOH), and those unwilling to give informed consent to participate in the present survey.

2.3. Sample Size Estimation

By using Cochran's formula ($n = z^2 pq/e^2$), we estimated the minimum required female participants needed for this research. The following values were considered while calculating sample size, namely n = minimum size of the necessary sample, z = 1.96 at the confidence level of 95%, p = expected proportion (we took 50% as the p-value to get the maximum sample size), and $q = 1 - p$ and e = margin of error at 5%. Considering all the above-specified values, the estimated minimum required sample size was 384. Finally, we adjusted the sample size to 480, with the expected 20% non-response rate.

2.4. Sampling Method

A multistage probability sampling method was performed to select the required study participants. In the first stage, we chose one general hospital, one tertiary care hospital, and all the PHCs from the Aljouf region. The research team used the lot technique to choose one general hospital and one specialty hospital from the available facilities. In the second stage, the required number of participants from each type of healthcare facility was selected based on the probability proportional to size in the following steps. Finally, we applied a systematic sampling method to select the female HCWs based on the allotted number.

2.5. Ethical Consideration

After obtaining ethical clearance from the Aljouf regional research ethics committee, Qurayat health affairs, MOH (approval number 126), the data collectors began the survey. The following considerations were made to avoid ethical issues:

1. Informed consent—The study participants were briefed about this study, and their willingness to participate (informed consent) was obtained.
2. Risk to the participants: There was no risk for the participants, as it was questionnaire-based research.
3. Respect for anonymity, privacy, and confidentiality: The collected details did not have any identification details of the study participants, and only the overall results of the participants were reported after the completion of the study. Hence, we maintained the anonymity of the respondents.

2.6. Data Collection Tool

The present study used a standardized self-administered questionnaire prepared by a team of experts from general surgery, radiology, and public health departments based on existing pieces of literature [16–18]. The structured questionnaire was tested for required validity and reliability. The independent experts examined the face and content validity of the data collection tool. Furthermore, we conducted a pilot study among the 30 different HCWs categories to understand the cultural adaptability and reliability in the local settings. All the pilot study participants agreed that the data collection tool was simple and easy to understand, and there were no missing data found in the completed data collection forms. The pilot study's test score reliability coefficient (Cronbach's alpha) for knowledge, attitude, and barrier scores were 0.78, 0.81, and 0.83, respectively, which showed good reliability in the present form of the survey questionnaire. Hence, the research team collected the data with the same data collection tool. The survey tool consisted of four sections; the first part inquired about socio-demographic details of the HCWs, including age (years), nationality, marital status, highest education qualification, current working healthcare facility, work experience duration, and HCW category. The second part consisted of sixteen questions. Of the sixteen questions, the first ten questions are related to the common risk factors (such as early puberty, late menopause, and family history), and the following six questions were related to common breast cancer symptoms. The participants were asked to choose "yes", "no", or "do not know". We gave a score of one for correct answers (response as yes) and zero for wrong answers (response as no or do not know). The third part consisted of ten questions related to the attitude of the HCWs towards breast cancer and patients diagnosed with breast cancer. The participants responded on a 5-point Likert scale ranging from strongly agree to strongly disagree, and scores were given from 5 (strongly agreed) to 1 (strongly disagree). The final part included ten questions about the barriers to uptake of the mammogram screening program, including fear of the procedure, embarrassment due to breast-related tests, apprehension regarding radiation exposure, and fear of discovering cancer. The presence of a barrier was scored as one, and the absence of a barrier was scored as zero. Furthermore, the research team categorized knowledge, attitude, and barriers into high (80% and above of total scores), medium (60–79% of total scores), and low (less than 60% of total scores). Our categorization is as per the original Bloom's cut-off point and is supported by previous studies conducted among the HCWs in the KSA and other parts of the world. In Saudi Arabia, the HCWs are expected to have high knowledge ($\geq$80%) of common public health problems, as they play a crucial role in preventing diseases by health education and delivering healthcare services implemented by the concerned authorities [19,20]. Hence, we combined low and good scores as a single category for logistic regression analysis, and previously conducted surveys among the HCWs strongly support and justify our categorization.

2.7. Data Collection Procedure

After necessary administrative approvals from the concerned healthcare facilities, the data collectors initiated the survey. We used an electronic shareable document (Google form) with the IRB-approved questionnaire for data collection. After briefing about the research rationale and objectives and obtaining informed consent, the selected HCWs were requested to fill the google form on the personal electronic device of the data collectors. For data security, the research team decided to give authorization only to the principal investigator to access, download, and export the survey's spreadsheet. In addition, the research team made three attempts in two weeks to communicate with the selected participants. The HCWs who were unwilling to participate and those who could not be communicated with despite three attempts were recorded as non-respondents.

2.8. Statistical Analysis

We used the statistical package for social sciences, version 21, to export data from spreadsheets, coding, recoding, and analysis (SPSS Statistics for Windows, Armonk, NY, USA: IBM Corp.). The categorical and other descriptive results are presented as numbers (frequencies) and proportions (%), while the continuous data are presented as mean and standard deviation (SD). Initially, we performed the Shapiro–Wilk normality assumption test for the knowledge, attitude, and barriers scores. We found that all three types of scores did not meet the normality assumption ($p < 0.001$). Hence, we executed the Spearman's correlation coefficient rank test was also used to find the strength and direction of correlation between knowledge, attitude, and barriers scores. Finally, we performed a multivariable analysis using the binomial logistic regression method to find the significantly associated socio-demographic factors with the knowledge, attitude, barriers, and awareness of the MOH, Saudi Arabia's recommendation for mammogram screening for breast cancer. All the statistical analysis used in this research is two-tailed, and the p-value less than 0.05 was set as statistically significant.

3. Results

Of the 480 selected participants, 414 completed the survey with a response rate of 86.3%. Table 1 depicts the background characteristics of the study participants. Of the 414 responses, the majority (68.6%) are Saudi nationals, married (58.0%), bachelor's degree holders (68.8%), nurses, and midwives (45.2%). The mean $\pm$ SD age of the studied population was 31.17 $\pm$ 6.04 years. Regarding work settings, 23.4%, 43.0%, and 33.6% of the participants worked at PHCs, general hospitals (secondary care), and tertiary care centers, respectively.

Table 2 presents the participants' knowledge regarding breast cancer risk factors and symptoms. Regarding breast cancer risk factors, the highest proportion of correct answers was observed regarding family history of breast cancer (79.0%) and smoking (66.2%). In comparison, the lowest proportion of correct answers was seen with regards to early puberty (26.8%) and late first pregnancy (31.2%). More than three-fourths of the HCW's correctly responded regarding change in size or shape of the breast (80.9%), non-painful lumps in the breast (75.1%), and nipple discharge (74.2%) being the risk factors of breast cancer.

Table 1. Background characteristics of the female healthcare workers (HCWs) (n = 414).

Variables	Frequency	%
Age in years (mean ± SD)	31.17 ± 6.04	
Nationality		
Saudi	284	68.6
Non-Saudi	130	31.4
Marital status		
Married	240	58.0
Single	145	35.0
Divorced/Widowed	29	7.0
Education		
Diploma	73	17.6
Bachelors	285	68.8
Masters and above	56	15.5
Work setting		
Primary health centers (PHC)	97	23.4
General hospital	178	43.0
Tertiary care hospital	139	33.6
HCWs category		
Physicians	83	20.0
Nurse and midwifes	187	45.2
Pharmacist	43	10.5
Lab technicians	35	9.1
Other categories	66	17.2
Work experience in healthcare settings (mean ± SD)	5.91 ± 4.7	
Currently suffering from breast-related symptoms like breast pain, nipple discharge, etc.		
No	397	95.9
Yes	17	4.1
Family history of breast cancer		
No	358	86.5
Yes	56	13.5

We found that more than one-third of the participants had barriers in all ten categories. Barriers were commonly found as fear of discovering cancer (57.2%) and apprehension regarding radiation exposure (57%). Nearly half (48.6%) of the HCWs responded that embarrassment due to breast-related tests was their primary barrier to mammogram screening uptake (Table 3).

Of the 414 respondents, 93 (22.5%), 106 (25.6%), and 69 (16.7%) had high scores in the knowledge, attitude, and barriers categories, respectively. In comparison, 201 (79.1%), 79 (19.1%), and 254 (61.4%) had low scores in the knowledge, attitude, and barriers categories, respectively (Figure 1).

Table 2. Participants knowledge regarding breast cancer risk factors and symptoms (*n* = 414).

No/Do Not Know	Yes	No/Do Not Know
	n (%)	*n* (%)
Risk factors		
Age—Women with age 35 years or older	249 (60.1)	165 (39.9)
First pregnancy after 30 years	129 (31.2)	285 (68.8)
Early puberty	111 (26.8)	303 (73.2)
Late menopause	151 (36.5)	263 (63.5)
Women who do not breastfeed	216 (52.2)	198 (47.8)
Obesity	202 (48.8)	212 (51.2)
Family history of breast cancer	327 (79.0)	87 (21.0)
Lack of physical activity	170 (41.1)	244 (58.9)
Smoking	274 (66.2)	140 (33.8)
Hormone therapy	271 (65.5)	143 (34.5)
Symptoms		
Non-painful lumps in the breast	311 (75.1)	103 (24.9)
Breast redness or change in color	283 (68.4)	131 (31.6)
Nipple discharge	307 (74.2)	107 (25.8)
Severe weight loss	213 (51.4)	201 (48.6)
Axillary lymph node enlargement	323 (78.0)	91 (22.0)
Change in size or shape of the breast	335 (80.9)	79 (19.1)

Table 3. Barriers towards uptake of mammogram screening among the participants (*n* = 414).

Barriers	Yes *n* (%)	No *n* (%)
Screening for breast cancer is not worthwhile	142 (34.3)	272 (65.7)
Apprehension regarding radiation exposure	236 (57.0)	178 (43.0)
Fear of pain related to clinical examination	231 (55.8)	183 (44.2)
Mammogram is not important	133 (32.1)	282 (67.9)
Embarrassment due to breast-related tests	201 (48.6)	213 (51.4)
Fear to discover cancer	237 (57.2)	177 (42.8)
Cancer has no cure	136 (32.9)	278 (67.1)
The test may be rejected by the family	148 (35.7)	266 (64.3)
No family history of breast cancer	154 (37.2)	260 (62.8)
Fear of not knowing the procedure	203 (49.0)	211 (51.0)

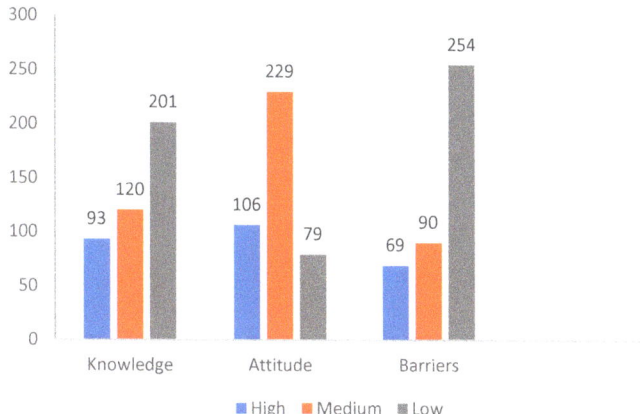

Figure 1. Knowledge, attitude, and barrier categories.

Table 4 shows the association between the knowledge subcategories and sociodemographic characteristics of the participating HCWs. Firstly, the univariate analysis was performed to compare each exposure (independent) variable with the knowledge subscales, and then, binomial logistic (multivariate analysis) were performed after adjusted with other covariables. In the univariate analysis, the characteristics that were significantly associated with the knowledge subcategories were age group (ref: up to 30 years: OR = 1.68, 95% CI = 1.06–2.67, p = 0.038), nationality (ref: Saudi: OR = 2.60, 95% CI = 1.62–4.19, p = 0.001), education (ref: diploma holders: OR = 2.96, 95% CI = 1.53–4.10, p = 0.001), HCWs category (ref: other categories: OR = 6.31, 95% CI = 4.91–8.10, p = 0.001), and family history of breast cancer (ref: no: OR = 1.93, 95% CI = 1.07–3.34, p = 0.037). The binomial logistic regression revealed only the following two characteristics were significantly associated with knowledge subscales, namely education status (ref: diploma holders: Adjusted OR (AOR) = 2.47, 95% CI = 1.54–4.53, p = 0.001) and HCW category (ref: other categories: AOR = 4.11, 95% CI = 2.86–5.76, p = 0.017).

Attitude subcategories and their association with sociodemographic characteristics are depicted in Table 5. The univariate analysis found that attitude subcategories were significantly associated with nationality (ref: Saudi: AOR = 1.34, 95% CI = 1.02–1.63, p = 0.017) and family history of breast cancer (ref: no: AOR = 2.73, 95% CI = 1.89–6.14, p = 0.001). However, logistic regression analysis did not reveal any significant association between independent variables and attitude subcategories.

Table 6 shows the association between barriers subcategories and sociodemographic characteristics of the participated HCWs. The binomial logistic regression revealed that only the following two characteristics were significantly associated with barriers subcategories: nationality (ref: Saudi: AOR = 1.66, 95% CI = 1.14–2.3, p = 0.015) and marital status (ref: married: AOR = 0.47, 95% CI = 0.28–0.69, p = 0.037).

Of the studied population, 66.2% were aware about the MOH, Saudi Arabia's recommendation for mammogram screening for breast cancer In the binomial logistic regression analysis, after adjusting with other covariables of the study, we found only age (ref: up to 30 years: OR = 0.91, 95% CI = 0.83–0.97, p = 0.030) and HCWs categories (ref: other categories: OR = 1.83, 95% CI = 1.12–2.98, p = 0.001 for nurses and OR = 4.08, 95% CI = 3.01–5.79, p = 0.001 for physicians) were significantly associated with the awareness regarding MOH, Saudi Arabia's recommendation for mammogram screening for breast cancer (Table 7).

The spearman's rank correlation test revealed a significant positive correlation between knowledge and attitude scores (rho = 0.195, p = 0.001). In addition, we found a negative correlation between knowledge of the breast cancer risk factors and symptoms with the barriers towards uptake of mammogram screening (rho = −0.315, p = 0.001) (Table 8).

Table 4. Binomial regression analysis between participants' socio-demographic characteristics and knowledge towards breast cancer (n = 414).

Characteristics	Total HCWs (n = 414)	Knowledge Low/Medium (n = 321) n (%)	Knowledge High (n = 93) n (%)	Univariate Analysis Low/Medium vs. High Unadjusted or (95% CI)	p-Value **	Multivariate Analysis * Low/Medium vs. High Adjusted or (95% CI)	p-Value **
Age (years)							
Up to 30	237	193 (81.4)	44 (18.6)	Ref		Ref	
Above 30	177	128 (72.3)	49 (27.7)	1.68 (1.06–2.67)	0.038	0.82 (0.37–1.82)	0.622
Nationality							
Saudi	284	236 (83.1)	48 (16.9)	Ref		Ref	
Non-Saudi	130	85 (65.3)	45 (34.6)	2.60 (1.62–4.19)	0.001	1.61 (0.83–3.11)	0.159
Marital status							
Married	240	179 (74.6)	51 (25.4)	Ref		Ref	
Single	145	118 (81.4)	27 (18.6)	0.67 (0.40–1.13)	0.181	0.75 (0.38–1.49)	0.408
Divorced/Widowed	29	24 (82.8)	5 (17.2)	1.01 (0.85–1.34)	0.071	0.86 (0.24–3.01)	0.809
Education							
Diploma	73	68 (93.2)	5 (6.8)	Ref		Ref	
Bachelors	285	234 (82.1)	51 (17.9)	1.85 (1.12–2.91)	0.028	2.48 (0.844–4.22)	0.099
Masters and above	56	19 (33.9)	37 (66.1)	2.96 (1.53–4.12)	0.001	2.47 (1.54–4.53)	0.001
Work setting							
PHC	97	68 (70.1)	29 (29.9)	Ref		Ref	
General hospital	178	146 (82.0)	32 (18.0)	1.34 (0.85–1.67)	0.384	0.56 (0.37–1.16)	0.117
Tertiary care hospital	139	107 (77.0)	32 (23.0)	0.87 (0.63–1.82)	0.165	0.59 (0.27–1.26)	0.173
HCWs category							
Other categories	144	130 (90.3)	14 (9.7)	Ref		Ref	
Nurse and midwifes	187	161 (86.1)	26 (13.9)	1.51 (0.75–2.99)	0.251	1.45 (0.68–3.01)	0.334
Physicians	83	30 (36.1)	53 (63.9)	6.31 (4.91–8.10)	0.001	4.11 (2.86–5.76)	0.017
Work experience in healthcare setting		5.91 ± 4.7		1.054 (1.01–1.10)	0.022	0.92 (0.72–1.66)	0.083
Family history of breast cancer							
No	358	284 (78.2)	74 (21.8)	Ref		Ref	
Yes	56	37 (73.2)	19 (26.8)	1.93 (1.07–3.34)	0.037	1.17 (0.87–2.24)	0.071

* Variables adjusted for logistic regression (enter method): Age category, nationality, marital status, education, work setting, HCWs category, work experience, and family history of breast cancer. ** Significant value less than 0.05 (two-tailed test).

Table 5. Binomial regression analysis between participants' socio-demographic characteristics and attitude towards breast cancer (n = 414).

Characteristics	Total HCWs (n = 414)	Attitude		Univariate Analysis Low/Medium vs. High		Multivariate Analysis * Low/Medium vs. High	
		Low/Medium (n = 308) n (%)	High (n = 106) n (%)	Unadjusted or (95% CI)	p-Value **	Adjusted or (95% CI)	p-Value **
Age (years)							
Up to 30	237	181 (76.4)	56 (23.6)	Ref		Ref	
Above 30	177	127 (71.8)	50 (28.2)	1.29 (0.82–1.98)	0.294	1.29 (0.66–2.53)	0.452
Nationality							
Saudi	284	215 (75.7)	69 (24.3)	Ref		Ref	
Non-Saudi	130	93 (71.5)	37 (28.5)	1.34 (1.02–1.63)	0.037	1.31 (0.75–2.28)	0.348
Marital status							
Married	240	179 (74.6)	61 (25.4)	Ref		Ref	
Single	145	110 (110)	35 (24.1)	0.93 (0.68–1.51)	0.783	0.96 (0.54–1.72)	0.469
Divorced/Widowed	29	19 (65.5)	10 (34.5)	1.54 (0.58–2.68)	0.188	1.57 (0.65–3.57)	0.340
Education							
Diploma	73	56 (76.7)	17 (23.3)	Ref		Ref	
Bachelors	285	215 (75.4)	70 (24.6)	1.07 (0.79–1.67)	0.092	1.03 (0.52–2.06)	0.359
Masters and above	56	37 (66.1)	19 (33.9)	1.69 (0.78–3.68)	0.187	1.21 (3.23)	0.699
Work setting							
PHC	97	70 (72.2)	27 (27.8)	Ref		Ref	
General hospital	178	125 (70.2)	53 (29.8)	1.10 (0.64–1.90)	0.531	1.94 (0.67–2.13)	0.547
Tertiary care hospital	139	113 (81.3)	26 (18.7)	0.59 (0.42–1.43)	0.103	0.58 (0.38–1.12)	0.104
HCWs category							
Other categories	144	106 (73.6)	38 (26.4)	Ref		Ref	
Nurse and midwifes	187	148 (79.1)	39 (20.9)	0.74 (0.44–1.23)	0.245	0.71 (0.41–1.24)	0.227
Physicians	83	54 (65.1)	29 (34.9)	1.49 (0.84–2.69)	0.184	1.36 (0.65–2.86)	0.421
Work experience in healthcare setting		5.91 ± 4.7		1.01 (0.96–1.12)	0.967	0.96 (0.86–1.03)	0.092
Family history of breast cancer							
No	358	281 (78.5)	77 (21.5)	Ref		Ref	
Yes	56	27 (48.2)	29 (51.8)	3.73 (1.89–6.14)	0.001	1.28 (0.42–2.88)	0.661

* Variables adjusted for logistic regression (enter method): Age category, nationality, marital status, education, work setting, HCWs category, work experience, and family history of breast cancer. ** Significant value less than 0.05 (two-tailed test).

Table 6. Binomial regression analysis between participants' socio-demographic characteristics and barriers to uptake mammogram screening (n = 414).

Characteristics	Total HCWs (n = 414)	Barriers High (n = 160) n (%)	Barriers Low/Medium (n = 254) n (%)	Univariate Analysis Low/Medium vs. High Unadjusted or (95% CI)	p-Value **	Multivariate Analysis * Low/Medium vs. High Adjusted or (95% CI)	p-Value **
Age (years)							
Up to 30	237	94 (39.7)	143 (60.3)	Ref		Ref	
Above 30	177	66 (37.3)	111 (62.7)	1.12 (0.74–1.65)	0.624	0.79 (0.53–1.39)	0.969
Nationality							
Saudi	284	121 (42.6)	163 (57.4)	Ref		Ref	
Non-Saudi	130	39 (30.0)	91 (70.0)	2.73 (2.11–3.68)	0.005	1.66 (1.14–2.32)	0.015
Marital status							
Married	240	79 (32.9)	161 (67.1)	Ref		Ref	
Single	145	66 (45.5)	79 (54.5)	0.59 (0.39–0.76)	0.014	0.47 (0.28–0.69)	0.037
Divorced/Widowed	29	15 (51.7)	14 (48.3)	0.46 (0.31–0.59)	0.049	0.48 (0.21–1.08)	0.076
Education							
Diploma	73	33 (45.2)	40 (54.8)	Ref		Ref	
Bachelors	285	114 (40.0)	171 (60.0)	1.24 (0.74–2.01)	0.420	1.01 (0.56–1.85)	0.969
Masters and above	56	13 (23.2)	43 (66.8)	2.73 (1.27–4.91)	0.011	1.55 (0.59–3.05)	0.369
Work setting							
PHC	97	39 (40.2)	58 (59.8)	Ref		Ref	
General hospital	178	71 (39.9)	107 (60.1)	(0.61–1.68)	0.959	1.07 (0.63–1.83)	0.808
Tertiary care hospital	139	50 (36.0)	89 (64.0)	1.20 (0.70–2.04)	0.509	1.16 (0.64–2.09)	0.625
HCWs category							
Other categories	144	64 (44.4)	80 (55.6)	Ref		Ref	
Nurse and midwifes	187	75 (40.1)	112 (59.9)	1.20 (0.77–1.86)	0.428	0.58 (0.28–1.19)	0.139
Physicians	83	21 (25.3)	62 (74.7)	2.36 (1.30–4.28)	0.015	0.58 (0.28–1.21)	0.148
Work experience in healthcare setting		5.91 ± 4.7		0.99 (0.95–1.03)	0.675	0.94 (0.89–1.01)	0.068
Family history of breast cancer							
No	358	139 (38.8)	219 (61.2)	Ref		Ref	
Yes	56	21 (37.5)	35 (62.5)	1.06 (0.59–1.89)	0.850	1.04 (0.57–1.92)	0.898

* Variables adjusted for logistic regression (enter method): Age category, nationality, marital status, education, work setting, HCWs category, work experience, and family history of breast cancer. ** Significant value less than 0.05 (two-tailed test).

Table 7. Binomial regression analysis between participants' socio-demographic characteristics and awareness on the MOH, Saudi Arabia's recommendation for mammogram screening for breast cancer (n = 414).

Characteristics	Total HCWs (n = 414)	Awareness Status No (n = 140) n (%)	Awareness Status Yes (n = 274) n (%)	Univariate Analysis No vs. Yes Unadjusted or (95% CI)	p-Value **	Multivariate Analysis * No vs. Yes Adjusted or (95% CI)	p-Value **
Age (years)							
Up to 30	237	93 (39.2)	144 (60.8)	Ref		Ref	
Above 30	177	47 (26.6)	130 (73.4)	1.99 (1.32–3.01)	0.001	0.81 (0.66–0.94)	0.039
Nationality							
Saudi	284	111 (39.1)	173 (60.9)	Ref		Ref	
Non-Saudi	130	29 (22.3)	101 (77.7)	1.26 (0.82–1.95)	0.292	0.85 (0.51–1.44)	0.553
Marital status							
Married	240	66 (27.5)	174 (72.5)	Ref		Ref	
Single	145	60 (41.4)	85 (58.6)	0.72 (0.47–1.12)	0.148	1.13 (0.66–1.84)	0.665
Divorced/Widowed	29	14 (48.3)	15 (51.7)	0.87 (0.75–0.98)	0.010	0.75 (0.52–1.46)	0.061
Education							
Diploma	73	23 (31.5)	50 (68.5)	Ref		Ref	
Bachelors	285	110 (38.6)	175 (61.4)	0.79 (0.46–1.37)	0.404	0.95 (0.61–1.69)	0.133
Masters and above	56	7 (12.5)	49 (87.5)	1.81 (0.89–3.68)	0.102	1.30 (0.71–2.77)	0.076
Work setting							
PHC	97	25 (25.8)	72 (74.2)	Ref		Ref	
General hospital	178	62 (34.8)	116 (65.2)	0.81 (0.49–1.35)	0.418	1.03 (0.60–1.78)	0.521
Tertiary care hospital	139	53 (38.1)	86 (61.9)	0.67 (0.39–1.16)	0.153	0.88 (0.48–1.61)	0.682
HCWs category							
Other categories	144	73 (50.7)	71 (49.3)	Ref		Ref	
Nurse and midwifes	187	56 (29.9)	131 (70.1)	1.19 (0.74–1.91)	0.479	1.01 (0.62–1.69)	0.972
Physicians	83	11 (13.3)	72 (86.7)	2.38 (1.33–4.10)	0.003	2.12 (1.35–3.18)	0.017
Work experience in healthcare setting		5.91 ± 4.7		1.06 (1.02–1.12)	0.005	1.02 (0.96–1.09)	0.487
Family history of breast cancer							
No	358	120 (33.5)	238 (66.5)	Ref		Ref	
Yes	56	20 (35.7)	36 (64.3)	1.12 (0.72–2.91)		1.46 (0.79–2.68)	0.223

* Variables adjusted for logistic regression (enter method): Age category, nationality, marital status, education, work setting, HCWs category, work experience, and family history of breast cancer. ** Significant value less than 0.05 (two-tailed test).

Table 8. Correlation between knowledge, attitude, and barriers scores (Spearman's rank correlation).

Variable	Rho */p-Value **
Knowledge–Attitude	0.195/0.001
Knowledge–Barrier	−0.315/0.001
Attitude–Barrier	0.060/0.226

* Spearman's rank correlation coefficient, ** significant at 0.05 level (two-tailed).

4. Discussion

In spite of the availability of these programs, a low-level mammogram screening uptake was prevalent in all sectors of the population living in all provinces of the KSA. A study conducted in the KSA reported that among 1135 women aged 50 years and above, 92% never had mammogram screening [21].

We conducted the current study among the 414 randomly selected different categories of HCWs. The present study found that a high proportion of the HCWs recognized family history and smoking as risk factors for developing breast cancer. In contrast, the lowest proportion of the participants reported early puberty, late menopause, and physical inactivity as risk factors. Similar to the current study findings, a study done by in Jordan found that female participants were highly aware of family history as a risk factor. However, only one-third recognized early puberty as a risk factor [12]. A recently conducted survey in the KSA found results in contrast to the present study. Another study done in 2020 found a lower proportion of their study participants was aware of these risk factors. The possible reason for this variation could be the difference in study settings and inclusion and exclusion criteria [16,22]. Our study revealed that nearly half of the female HCWs had low knowledge of breast cancer risk factors and symptoms regarding overall knowledge categories. A study conducted in the Riyadh region of KSA among the healthcare professionals from a tertiary care center and another study conducted in a Nigerian urban city also found similar findings [22,23].

The binomial logistic regression analysis of the current study found that knowledge scores were significantly associated with age group, nationality, level of education, and HCWs categories. Similar to the current study findings, a survey conducted among the female primary HCWs found a significant association between knowledge with the HCWs' profession and education status [24]. The present study results revealed that only 25.2% of the HCWs had a high attitude towards breast cancer, and the attitude score was lower among the Saudi nationals than the expatriates. We could not find any other sociodemographic characteristic that was significantly associated with the attitude. Interestingly, in a Vietnam study, a higher proportion of females had a positive attitude towards breast cancer and related procedures [17]. The dissimilarities between our study and the later study are attributed to the variations in study settings, cultural characteristics, and the applied survey tools. A qualitative survey conducted in Australia reported that most of the participants had a positive perception of personalized mammogram screening, and more than 90% of them had undergone mammogram screening. The contrasting results could be due to differences in the screening model. In the KSA, the breast cancer early-detection program aims to enhance the awareness of mammogram screening through a mass approach. There is no personalized screening model available, as explored by an Australian study [25]. Even though the latter study was done in Australia, a personalized breast cancer screening model could be implemented in the KSA, where a well-established healthcare system is available as per the international standards.

Healthcare services utilization, including mammogram screening utilization by the public, is influenced by numerous barriers [16,26–28]. Our study revealed that more than one-third of the HCWs working in the MOH were not aware of the MOH, Saudi Arabia's recommendation for mammogram screening for breast cancer. Moreover, the present study demonstrated that fear of discovering cancer, apprehension regarding radiation exposure, and embarrassment due to breast-related tests were the common barriers to mammogram screening uptake. Similar to the present study, some other studies conducted in the KSA and other Arab countries also reported that embarrassment due to breast examination, fear of discovering cancer, and fear of radiation were the common barriers faced by the women [16,18]. In contrast, a survey conducted in 2022 among Spanish health professionals reported that workload and financial limitations were the common barriers they faced [29]. Another study reported that being busy and lack of perceived susceptibility were the significant barriers perceived by the female HCWs [27]. The possible differences in the results might be due to the conservative nature of societies in the KSA and other Arab countries. The current study found that the barriers to mammogram screening were significantly higher among Saudi nationals, divorced/widowers, diploma holders, and other HCWs categories such as pharmacists, lab technicians, and physiotherapists. Similar to our study findings, some other authors also found that lower education is one of the predictors of barriers to mammogram screening [16,30].

Health literacy is an individual's competence and knowledge to understand and make a proper decision on the health-related needs of them and others. A high level of health literacy and knowledge is critical for making a proper health-related decision [31,32]. The research team attempted to find the correlation between the knowledge and attitude of the HCWs to the barriers to uptake of mammogram screening. The present study results suggest that HCWs' knowledge is negatively correlated with the barriers to uptake mammogram screening. The present study results are supported by a survey conducted in 2020 among Jordanian women [18]. In their study, more participants with a good knowledge of breast cancer reported having a mammogram than the participants with insufficient knowledge. In the KSA, the healthcare sciences curriculum is developed based on rapid change in the demography, pattern of disease, and health care needs. The healthcare students are taught about major public health problems relevant to global and local health needs. The traditional classroom learning is supplemented through additional programs such as community health activities and health promotion activities in the field. To keep up with the changing demands, the curriculum is constantly updated and incorporated into the healthcare sciences colleges' study plan [33]. Improvements to the current training program for the HCWs and curriculum that stresses the importance of the breast cancer prevention program might facilitate them to work with greater effectiveness and improve the uptake of screening mammography by the eligible women in the community [34,35].

The WHO Global Breast Cancer Initiatives is an essential collaboration formed in 2021 to empower women and reduce breast-cancer-related deaths by 2.5% and save 25 million lives by 2040. This aim can be achieved by raising awareness of breast cancer and the importance of early detection to the HCWs, as they play a central role in strengthening the existing healthcare system [36,37].

Based on the above-mentioned findings, it is recommended to develop evidence-based and target-oriented educational programs for the HCWs, which would empower them to educate the community regarding the risk factors of breast cancer and the importance of early detection. Additionally, concerned authorities may consider changing their strategies from a mass approach to a personalized risk assessment and screening method. Furthermore, a prospective study is warranted in other regions of the KSA to understand the region-specific training needs for the HCWs.

The research team conducted the current survey using the validated tool with an adequate sample size using the standard methodology. At the same time, certain constraints need to be considered during the interpretation of this survey's results. Firstly, this study design is cross-sectional and can find only the association, not the causation. Secondly, there is a possibility of bias due to self-reported studies present in this study. Thirdly, the present study assessed female HCWs' knowledge, attitude, and barriers, not the general population. Hence, the current study's findings may not be generalized to all sections of the KSA. Finally, we included only the HCWs working at the ministry of health, KSA. Nonetheless, the current research explored critical aspects of one of the significant global health issues to be addressed immediately.

5. Conclusions

The present study depicted that the knowledge was significantly associated with age group, nationality, level of education, and HCWs categories. However, attitude was significantly associated only with the nationality of the HCW's. Overall, the knowledge and attitude among the northern Saudi HCWs were found to be inadequate. There were several barriers reported by the HCWs to utilizing the free mammogram services provided by the MOH, KSA, and these barriers correlated negatively with the HCW's knowledge of breast cancer. The need of the hour is to develop evidence-based and target-oriented educational programs for the HCWs, who in turn can play a pivotal role in educating the community regarding the risk factors of breast cancer and the importance of its early detection.

Author Contributions: Conceptualization, A.M.A., A.T., H.A., R.H.A. and F.A.W.; methodology, A.T., A.K.A., M.F.A., F.H.A., B.D.A. and A.M.A.; software, A.T., M.F.A. and A.S.A.; validation, A.T., A.S.A., A.M.A. and A.K.A.; formal analysis, A.K.A., F.A.W. and A.M.A.; investigation, A.S.A., R.H.A., F.H.A. and M.F.A.; resources, A.M.A. and M.F.A.; data curation, H.A., A.T., M.F.A. and F.A.W.; writing—original draft preparation, A.M.A., A.K.A., A.T., F.A.W. and H.A.; writing—review and editing, M.F.A., A.S.A., R.H.A., F.H.A. and M.F.A.; visualization, H.A.; supervision, M.F.A.; project administration, A.M.A., A.T. and F.A.W.; funding acquisition, A.M.A. All authors have read and agreed to the published version of the manuscript.

Funding: This research received no external funding.

Institutional Review Board Statement: The study was conducted in accordance with the Declaration of Helsinki and approved by the Aljouf regional research ethics committee, Qurayat health affairs, Ministry of Health, Saudi Arabia (approval number 126).

Informed Consent Statement: Informed consent was obtained from all subjects involved in the study.

Data Availability Statement: The data presented in this study are available on request from the corresponding author.

Acknowledgments: The authors would like to thank the Ministry of Health, Jouf health affairs for their cooperation in completing research.

Conflicts of Interest: The authors declare no conflict of interest.

References

1. WHO. Breast Cancer. Available online: https://www.who.int/news-room/fact-sheets/detail/breast-cancer (accessed on 15 January 2021).
2. Ji, P.; Gong, Y.; Jin, M.L.; Hu, X.; Di, G.H.; Shao, Z.M. The Burden and Trends of Breast Cancer from 1990 to 2017 at the Global, Regional, and National Levels: Results From the Global Burden of Disease Study 2017. *Front. Oncol.* **2020**, *10*, 650. [CrossRef] [PubMed]
3. Global Burden of Disease 2019 Cancer Collaboration. Cancer Incidence, Mortality, Years of Life Lost, Years Lived With Disability, and Disability-Adjusted Life Years for 29 Cancer Groups From 2010 to 2019: A Systematic Analysis for the Global Burden of Disease Study 2019. *JAMA Oncol.* **2022**, *8*, 420–444. [CrossRef] [PubMed]
4. Alkabban, F.M.; Ferguson, T. Breast Cancer. In *StatPearls*; StatPearls Publishing: Treasure Island, FL, USA, 2022.
5. CDC. What Are the Risk Factors for Breast Cancer? Available online: https://www.cdc.gov/cancer/breast/basic_info/risk_factors.htm (accessed on 10 January 2022).
6. Albeshan, S.M.; Alashban, Y.I. Incidence trends of breast cancer in Saudi Arabia: A joinpoint regression analysis (2004–2016). *J. King Saud Univ.-Sci.* **2021**, *33*, 101578. [CrossRef]
7. Alqahtani, W.S.; Almufareh, N.A.; Domiaty, D.M.; Albasher, G.; Alduwish, M.A.; Alkhalaf, H.; Almuzzaini, B.; Al-Marshidy, S.S.; Alfraihi, R.; Elasbali, A.M.; et al. Epidemiology of cancer in Saudi Arabia thru 2010–2019: A systematic review with constrained meta-analysis. *AIMS Public Health* **2020**, *7*, 679–696. [CrossRef]
8. Reeves, R.A.; Kaufman, T. Mammography. In *StatPearls*; StatPearls Publishing: Treasure Island, FL, USA, 2022.
9. Ghodsi, Z.; Hojjatoleslami, S. Breast self examination and mammography in cancer screening: Women health protective behavior. *J. Prev. Med. Hyg.* **2014**, *55*, 46–49. [PubMed]
10. MOH. Breast Cancer Screening. Available online: https://www.moh.gov.sa/en/HealthAwareness/Campaigns/Breastcancer/Pages/ray.aspx (accessed on 21 January 2022).
11. MOH. Breast Cancer Early Detection (BCED). Available online: https://www.moh.gov.sa/en/Ministry/Projects/breast-cancer/Pages/default.aspx (accessed on 12 March 2022).

12. Ayoub, N.M.; Al-Taani, G.M.; Almomani, B.A.; Tahaineh, L.; Nuseir, K.; Othman, A.; Mensah, K.B. Knowledge and Practice of Breast Cancer Screening Methods among Female Community Pharmacists in Jordan: A Cross-Sectional Study. *Int. J. Breast Cancer 2021*, *2021*, 9292768. [CrossRef] [PubMed]
13. Abeje, S.; Seme, A.; Tibelt, A. Factors associated with breast cancer screening awareness and practices of women in Addis Ababa, Ethiopia. *BMC Women's Health* **2019**, *19*, 4. [CrossRef]
14. Hartzler, A.L.; Tuzzio, L.; Hsu, C.; Wagner, E.H. Roles and Functions of Community Health Workers in Primary Care. *Ann. Fam. Med.* **2018**, *16*, 240–245. [CrossRef]
15. WHO. Health Professions Network. Available online: https://www.who.int/teams/health-workforce/health-professions-networks/ (accessed on 13 February 2022).
16. Abdel-Salam, D.M.; Mohamed, R.A.; Alyousef, H.Y.; Almasoud, W.A.; Alanzi, M.B.; Mubarak, A.Z.; Osman, D.M. Perceived Barriers and Awareness of Mammography Screening Among Saudi Women Attending Primary Health Centers. *Risk Manag. Healthc. Policy* **2020**, *13*, 2553–2561. [CrossRef]
17. Toan, D.T.T.; Son, D.T.; Hung, L.X.; Minh, L.N.; Mai, D.L.; Hoat, L.N. Knowledge, Attitude, and Practice Regarding Breast Cancer Early Detection Among Women in a Mountainous Area in Northern Vietnam. *Cancer Control* **2019**, *26*, 107327481986377. [CrossRef]
18. Al-Mousa, D.S.; Alakhras, M.; Hossain, S.Z.; Al-Sa'Di, A.G.; Al Hasan, M.; Al-Hayek, Y.; Brennan, P.C. Knowledge, Attitude and Practice Around Breast Cancer and Mammography Screening Among Jordanian Women. *Breast Cancer Targets Ther.* **2020**, *12*, 231–242. [CrossRef] [PubMed]
19. Thirunavukkarasu, A.; Almulhim, A.K.; Albalawi, F.A.; Alruwaili, Z.M.; Almajed, O.A.; Alruwaili, S.H.; Almugharriq, M.M.; Alruwaili, A.S.; Alkuwaykibi, M.K. Knowledge, Attitudes, and Practices towards Diabetic Retinopathy among Primary Care Physicians of Saudi Arabia: A Multicenter Cross-Sectional Study. *Healthcare* **2021**, *9*, 1697. [CrossRef] [PubMed]
20. Ukwenya, V.O.; Fuwape, T.A.; Fadahunsi, T.I.; Ilesanmi, O.S. Disparities in knowledge, attitude, and practices of infection prevention and control of Lassa fever among health care workers at The Federal Medical Centre, Owo, Ondo State, Nigeria. *Pan. Afr. Med. J.* **2021**, *38*, 357. [CrossRef] [PubMed]
21. El Bcheraoui, C.; Basulaiman, M.; Wilson, S.; Daoud, F.; Tuffaha, M.; AlMazroa, M.A.; Memish, Z.A.; Al Saeedi, M.; Mokdad, A.H. Breast cancer screening in Saudi Arabia: Free but almost no takers. *PLoS ONE* **2015**, *10*, e0119051. [CrossRef] [PubMed]
22. Heena, H.; Durrani, S.; Riaz, M.; Alfayyad, I.; Tabasim, R.; Parvez, G.; Abu-Shaheen, A. Knowledge, attitudes, and practices related to breast cancer screening among female health care professionals: A cross sectional study. *BMC Women's Health* **2019**, *19*, 122. [CrossRef]
23. Akhigbe, A.O.; Omuemu, V.O. Knowledge, attitudes and practice of breast cancer screening among female health workers in a Nigerian urban city. *BMC Cancer* **2009**, *9*, 203. [CrossRef]
24. Erdem, Ö.; Toktaş, İ. Knowledge, Attitudes, and Behaviors about Breast Self-Examination and Mammography among Female Primary Healthcare Workers in Diyarbakır, Turkey. *BioMed Res. Int.* **2016**, *2016*, 6490156. [CrossRef]
25. Lippey, J.; Keogh, L.A.; Mann, G.B.; Campbell, I.G.; Forrest, L.E. "A Natural Progression": Australian Women's Attitudes about an Individualized Breast Screening Model. *Cancer Prev. Res.* **2019**, *12*, 383–390. [CrossRef]
26. Matranga, D.; Maniscalco, L. Inequality in Healthcare Utilization in Italy: How Important Are Barriers to Access? *Int. J. Environ. Res. Public Health* **2022**, *19*, 1697. [CrossRef]
27. Nazzal, Z.; Sholi, H.; Sholi, S.B.; Sholi, M.B.; Lahaseh, R. Motivators and barriers to mammography screening uptake by female health-care workers in primary health-care centres: A cross-sectional study. *Lancet* **2018**, *391*, S51. [CrossRef]
28. Al-Zalabani, A.H.; Alharbi, K.D.; Fallatah, N.I.; Alqabshawi, R.I.; Al-Zalabani, A.A.; Alghamdi, S.M. Breast Cancer Knowledge and Screening Practice and Barriers Among Women in Madinah, Saudi Arabia. *J. Cancer Educ.* **2018**, *33*, 201–207. [CrossRef] [PubMed]
29. Laza-Vásquez, C.; Hernández-Leal, M.J.; Carles-Lavila, M.; Pérez-Lacasta, M.J.; Cruz-Esteve, I.; Rué, M.; On Behalf of the Decido, G. Barriers and Facilitators to the Implementation of a Personalized Breast Cancer Screening Program: Views of Spanish Health Professionals. *Int. J. Environ. Res. Public Health* **2022**, *19*, 1406. [CrossRef]
30. Gan, Y.X.; Lao, C.K.; Chan, A. Breast cancer screening behavior, attitude, barriers among middle-aged Chinese women in Macao, China. *J. Public Health* **2018**, *40*, e560–e570. [CrossRef] [PubMed]
31. Rowlands, G. Health literacy. *Hum. Vaccines Immunother.* **2014**, *10*, 2130–2135. [CrossRef] [PubMed]
32. Ratzan, S.; Parker, R.; Selden, C.; Zorn, M. *National Library of Medicine Current Bibliographies in Medicine: Health Literacy*; National Institutes of Health, US Department of Health and Human Services: Bethesda, MD, USA, 2000.
33. Al-Mohaithef, M.; Javed, N.B.; Elkhalifa, A.M.; Tahash, M.; Chandramohan, S.; Hazazi, A.; Elhadi, F.E.M. Evaluation of Public Health Education and Workforce Needs in the Kingdom of Saudi Arabia. *J. Epidemiol. Glob. Health* **2020**, *10*, 96–106. [CrossRef]
34. Yeoh, K.G. The future of medical education. *Singap. Med. J.* **2019**, *60*, 3–8. [CrossRef]
35. Couper, I.; Ray, S.; Blaauw, D.; Ng'wena, G.; Muchiri, L.; Oyungu, E.; Omigbodun, A.; Morhason-Bello, I.; Ibingira, C.; Tumwine, J.; et al. Curriculum and training needs of mid-level health workers in Africa: A situational review from Kenya, Nigeria, South Africa and Uganda. *BMC Health Serv. Res.* **2018**, *18*, 553. [CrossRef]
36. Anderson, B.O.; Ilbawi, A.M.; Fidarova, E.; Weiderpass, E.; Stevens, L.; Abdel-Wahab, M.; Mikkelsen, B. The Global Breast Cancer Initiative: A strategic collaboration to strengthen health care for non-communicable diseases. *Lancet Oncol.* **2021**, *22*, 578–581. [CrossRef]
37. Duggan, C.; Trapani, D.; Ilbawi, A.M.; Fidarova, E.; Laversanne, M.; Curigliano, G.; Bray, F.; Anderson, B.O. National health system characteristics, breast cancer stage at diagnosis, and breast cancer mortality: A population-based analysis. *Lancet Oncol.* **2021**, *22*, 1632–1642. [CrossRef]

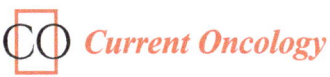

Article

Overdetection of Breast Cancer

Martin J. Yaffe * and James G. Mainprize

Physical Sciences Platform, Sunnybrook Research Institute, Toronto, ON M4N3M5, Canada; james.mainprize@sri.utoronto.ca
* Correspondence: martin.yaffe@sri.utoronto.ca; Tel.: +1-416-480-5715

Abstract: Overdetection (often referred to as overdiagnosis) of cancer is the detection of disease, such as through a screening program, that would otherwise remain occult through an individual's life. In the context of screening, this could occur for cancers that were slow growing or indolent, or simply because an unscreened individual would have died from some other cause before the cancer had surfaced clinically. The main harm associated with overdetection is the subsequent overdiagnosis and overtreatment of disease. In this article, the phenomenon is reviewed, the methods of estimation of overdetection are discussed and reasons for variability in such estimates are given, with emphasis on an analysis using Canadian data. Microsimulation modeling is used to illustrate the expected time course of cancer detection that gives rise to overdetection. While overdetection exists, the actual amount is likely to be much lower than the estimate used by the Canadian Task Force on Preventive Health Care. Furthermore, the issue is of greater significance in older rather than younger women due to competing causes of death. The particular challenge associated with in situ breast cancer is considered and possible approaches to avoiding overtreatment are suggested.

Keywords: breast cancer screening; breast cancer; overdetection; Canadian National Breast Screening Study; overdiagnosis; overtreatment; microsimulation

1. Introduction

The overdiagnosis of breast cancer has been suggested by some to be the largest harm associated with breast cancer screening [1–4]. Overdiagnosis refers to the diagnosis of breast cancers that normally would not have appeared in a woman's life, i.e., had not caused harm, before she had died of some other cause. In the case of breast screening, this would come about because of the smaller threshold in lesion size (and presumably development) provided by the screening modality. This provides lead time, and it is this lead time that contributes to the reduction in mortality and morbidity that has been demonstrated in women who participate in screening compared to those who do not [1,5]. If cancers detected earlier through screening would not have surfaced or done harm if they had remained undetected, then they can be considered to have been overdiagnosed, or more correctly, overdetected [6], a term that will be used throughout the remainder of this article when referring to detection by screening, while "overdiagnosis" will be used to refer to pathologic assessments.

Consider a cohort of women of the same age at a given time point. It would be expected that a certain number of breast cancers, illustrated schematically in Figure 1a as discs, would be initiated in the cohort each year. The cancers would vary in size and growth rate according to a variety of driving factors. At an early point, as illustrated on the left in the figure, they would not have yet reached the threshold for detectability; however, as time elapses, the cancers grow and at some point become large or noticeable enough to be detected by the women or by a clinician. Additionally, as shown in the figure, at a point that may occur before or after the threshold for clinical detectability is reached, they have become sufficiently advanced that they will be destined to become lethal (discs indicated with "x"s), or at least their treatment would impose considerable morbidity. The initiation

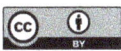

Citation: Yaffe, M.J.; Mainprize, J.G. Overdetection of Breast Cancer. *Curr. Oncol.* **2022**, *29*, 3894–3910. https://doi.org/10.3390/curroncol29060311

Received: 14 April 2022
Accepted: 17 May 2022
Published: 30 May 2022

Publisher's Note: MDPI stays neutral with regard to jurisdictional claims in published maps and institutional affiliations.

Copyright: © 2022 by the authors. Licensee MDPI, Basel, Switzerland. This article is an open access article distributed under the terms and conditions of the Creative Commons Attribution (CC BY) license (https://creativecommons.org/licenses/by/4.0/).

of cancer is a continuous process over time with a rate that is age-dependent, so that as time progresses new, earlier cancers are added to the population of previously undetected cancers that have grown larger.

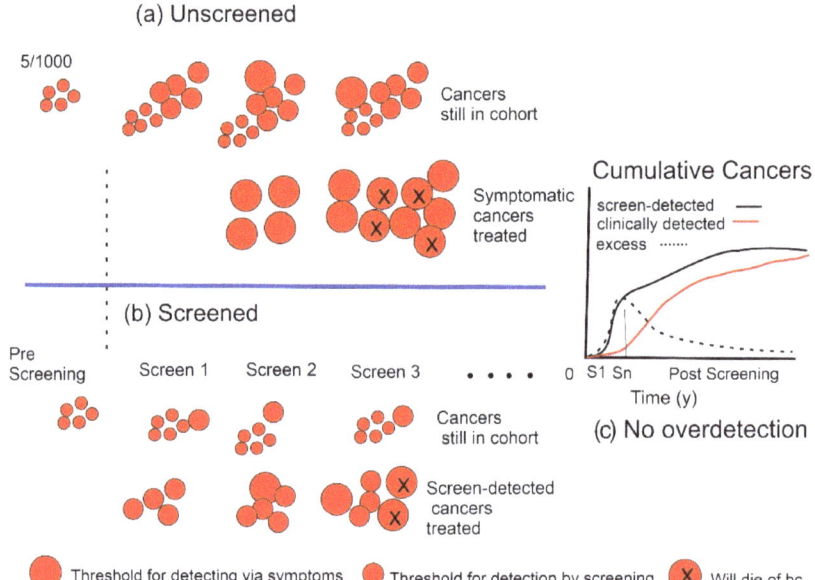

Figure 1. (**a**) Illustrates the initiation and growth of breast cancers in an unscreened population (e.g., 1000 women). Size of the lesion is represented by the diameter of the discs. X indicates cancers that will result in death. (**b**) The effect of screening. In (**a**,**b**), the lower rows indicate cancers that have been detected and treated, while upper rows show cancers in the cohort that have not yet been detected. (**c**) Difference (excess) in the cumulative number of cancers found in screened (black curve) versus unscreened (red curve) individuals, depicted in the graph as the dashed line, increases during the period of screening. In this example where there is no overdetection, cancers are found and treated earlier in the screened group; however, after screening ends at Sn, the number in the unscreened group will catch up over time, eliminating the excess.

The principle of screening is illustrated for an identical cohort of women in Figure 1b. If a suitable test is available to which the cohort is exposed at regular intervals and the threshold for lesion detectability is smaller than the clinical detection threshold, then cancers can be found and treated before they reach that clinical threshold. In this screened cohort, the cancers that are detected and treated are shown on the lower track, while those that remain undetected in those women are shown on the upper track. The time that it takes for cancers to grow from the size threshold of the screening test to the threshold for clinical detectability is the lead time afforded by screening. The term "size" is used loosely here as a surrogate for detectability because other factors that develop over time such as changes in morphology may also affect the detection threshold. The expectation is that there would have been less progression in size, a lower probability that metastasis has occurred and a greater chance of avoiding death from those earlier cancers. This paradigm has been demonstrated to be correct through multiple randomized trials, case–control and observational studies, e.g., [1,5,7].

Eventually, most of the equivalent cancers found earlier in the screened cohort would surface in the unscreened women due to symptoms or accidental detection. In the case of very slow growing (indolent) cancers (grey discs in Figure 2), however, these may not have the potential to progress beyond a certain point or to metastasize and, therefore, would not become lethal or at least not been clinically detectable in the absence of screening before the individual had died of some other cause. Under these conditions, the woman would never have been aware that she had cancer. This phenomenon of overdetection is illustrated in Figure 2b. More of these cancers with limited malignant potential will be detected in a screened population. To the extent that this occurs, the total numbers of cancers detected (and treated) in a cohort of women participating in screening will exceed the corresponding numbers in an unscreened cohort (Figure 2c).

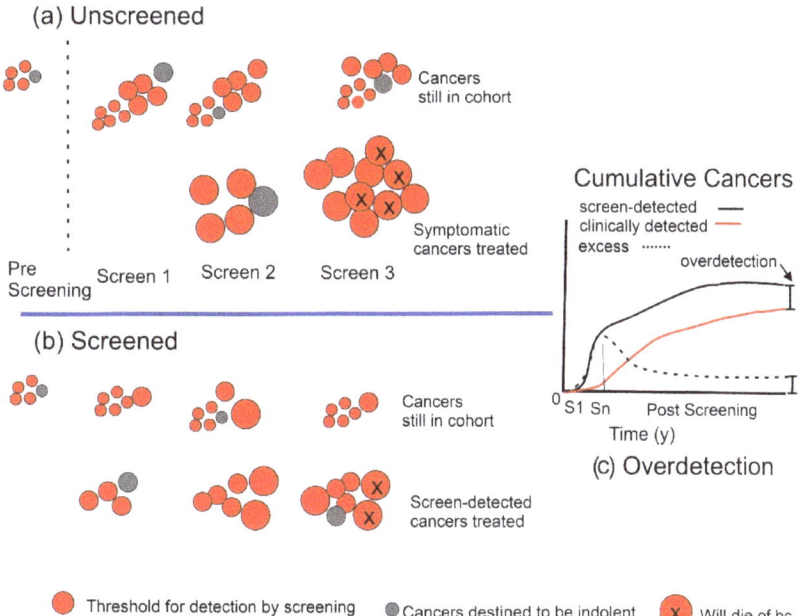

Figure 2. Initiation and growth of breast cancers in the presence of cancers with limited malignant potential. (**a**) An unscreened population. Grey discs indicate cancers that are destined not to be lethal. (**b**) The effect of screening. Lower row indicates cancers that have been detected and treated, while upper row indicates cancers in the cohort that have not yet been detected. (**c**) Overdetection. After screening ends at Sn, the initial excess of cancers in the screened grouped will not be completely eliminated over time.

The actual diagnosis of breast cancer is performed by a pathologist on biopsied tissue. A concern regarding overdetection is that a woman who otherwise would not have experienced the anxiety and other negative factors associated with having breast cancer would have become a breast cancer patient.

Overdetected cancers are real cancers and should not be confused with the so-called false positive results of screening, where further imaging or biopsy, triggered by an equivocal screening examination, demonstrates that suspicious results on screening are not cancer. The main point is that there is no direct benefit to the individual from finding overdetected cancers. They are currently an unavoidable collateral finding associated with the earlier detection and treatment of other cancers that would indeed otherwise likely become lethal.

Overdetection by screening can be considered as having two components: (1) detection of nonprogressive cancers and (2) detection of cancers that are progressive, but where the progression is sufficiently slow such that they would not have been detected in unscreened women before they would have died from a cause other than breast cancer. In a recent publication, for women in the age range 50–74 screened biennially who were monitored by the Breast Cancer Surveillance Consortium in the U.S., Ryser et al. estimated the rate of overdetection at 15% [8]. In their Bayesian inference study of 718 cancer diagnoses in 36,000 women, they estimated that one-third of overdetected cancers were indolent, while the other two-thirds were progressive but had not emerged before death had occurred due to another cause. Overdetection via the second mechanism is more likely to occur in older than younger women at time of screening because competing causes of death are higher in the former and, therefore, it is more likely that a cancer will not be detected in her unscreened counterpart before she dies.

Overdiagnosis, in its true sense, occurs when the pathology examination is not able to distinguish potentially aggressive from indolent cancers. The harms of overdiagnosis are the morbidities associated with overtreatment if this occurs. The same limitations can result in underdiagnosis and subsequent undertreatment, with a heightened probability of recurrence or death. Both of these are harms of the diagnostic process and the processes leading to therapeutic choices. It is worth mentioning that not all cancers that are overdetected are overdiagnosed. In some cases, the pathologist can identify disease at a very low risk for recurrence at biopsy. However, unlike the trend toward active surveillance in prostate cancer, where some men choose not to be treated for minimal disease, most women currently receive some level of treatment after a diagnosis of breast cancer. Some of these cancers are undoubtedly overtreated. It is, of course, also possible for cancers detected symptomatically to be over or underdiagnosed.

The main difference between screen-detected and symptomatically detected cancers is that the former tend to be smaller and earlier stage making the diagnostic procedure more challenging. This implies that overdiagnosis is more likely to occur in in situ than in invasive disease. The probability of detecting in situ cancer is greatly increased with screening and, therefore, these lesions require special consideration.

1.1. In Situ Cancers

In situ cancers are rarely detected in unscreened women, whereas in a cohort of women routinely screened with mammography, they constitute 20–30% of detected cancers. It has been argued that in situ cancer (which, here, will be loosely referred to as ductal carcinoma in situ or DCIS) should not be considered as a cancer in that, in itself, it does not have the potential to be lethal. If this were the case, then it could be considered that in situ cancer alone might be responsible for an overdetection rate of 20–30%. Certainly, of those cancers overdetected because they are nonprogressive, in situ cancers likely represent a large proportion. Glasiou et al. used Australian registry data to estimate overdetection for various cancers and concluded that for breast cancer there was an overall 22% overdetection of which 9% was for in situ cancers [9].

Nevertheless, in situ disease cannot simply be dismissed as being innocuous. It is well established that, if treated by breast conserving surgery alone, there will be ipsilateral recurrence in about 28% of cases and half of these will appear as invasive cancer [10–12]. The use of radiation therapy reduces local recurrence by a factor of two. More recent work by Solin et al. showed recurrence rates of 25% for high grade lesions 1 cm or smaller and 14% for larger (2.5 cm or larger) low or intermediate grade in situ cancer. Again, in each case, about half the recurrences were as invasive cancer [13]. The optimization of strategies of how to manage in situ cancers detected by screening is, therefore, a topic of great interest and some efforts in this direction will be described later in this article.

1.2. Estimating the Amount of Overdetection from Screening

There have been many attempts to estimate the amount of overdetection that would result from screening. All of these suffer from various limitations, and this is responsible for wide variation among estimates [5,8,14,15]. For example, Bleyer and Welch [16] extrapolated historical breast cancer incidence data before the onset of breast cancer screening from the SEER Registry to predict what incidence should be in the current era and compared with actual incidence to estimate the excess that they assumed was attributable to overdetection from screening. While conceptually this approach is sound, uncertainties in the year-to-year increase in background age-specific incidence rates, lack of information in SEER on the mode of cancer detection and other sources of variability made their calculation extremely unreliable. Small differences in the assumptions of the values of some of the extrapolation parameters could result in very high estimates of overdetection or even of underdetection [8,17,18].

Puliti et al. and Etzioni and Gulatti have identified several of the critical factors required in the estimation of overdetection [19,20] and these include accounting for effects of lead time from screening and differences in cancer risk between comparison groups [19]. Puliti et al. have suggested that when these effects have been appropriately accounted for, the fraction of cancers that have been overdetected is on the order of 1–10%.

Ideally, overdetection would be assessed through a randomized trial, where women in one arm receive screening and those in the other do not. This would eliminate possible differences between the two groups that could be responsible for differences in breast cancer incidence. Both arms would be followed for cancers detected during the period of the screening intervention and for a time period afterwards that is no less than the lead time provided by screening. To avoid bias, it is essential that the quality of the follow-up is identical for the two trial arms. During the post-intervention period, neither group would receive screening. The number of breast cancers occurring in each group would be carefully and thoroughly monitored and the difference would provide a measure of overdetection.

In such a trial, it would be expected that initially there would be an excess of cancers in the screened group due to their earlier detection. After a delay due to the screening lead time, the corresponding cancers would begin to appear in the control group and there would be a compensating decrease in the excess as illustrated in the graph in Figure 1c. If there was no overdetection occurring, then after the appropriate follow-up time, the excess would be neutralized.

Such an idealized trial is almost impossible to achieve. As in all randomized screening trials, there will be crossover effects due to the noncompliance of women assigned to screening as well as some women in the control group seeking screening outside the trial. If this occurs, it will cause an initial reduction in the measure of overdetection.

The screening behavior of women after the period of the intervention will also affect the estimated overdetection. The measure will be most accurate if neither group receives screening during the post-intervention follow up. Given human behavior this situation is unlikely to be achieved. If there is more post-intervention screening in the screening arm, overdetection will be overestimated and, if there is a greater degree of screening in the control group, the estimated overdetection fraction will be reduced.

1.3. Example–Canadian National Breast Screening Study

An example of the problems of estimating overdetection can be seen in the publication by Baines et al. of their revised estimates of overdetection of breast cancer using data from the two randomized controlled trials in the Canadian National Breast Screening Study (CNBSS) [21]. This analysis was an update from Miller et al., 2014, who had originally provided estimates based on the merged data from the two studies [22]. The revised estimates by Baines et al. were considerably larger than the previously published values.

The calculation used by Baines et al. was very simple. In each arm of the RCT, the total number of breast cancers found, which comprised screen-detected cancers or other cancers, were totaled over the period of observation. The estimated overdetection at a given point in time was obtained by dividing the difference in these totals between the study and control groups (the excess cancers) by the number of screen-detected breast cancers in the study group during the period of intervention.

Different authors have employed other denominators in this calculation [1]. Those who wish to accentuate the effect tend to choose the smallest number and vice versa. It is not clear that any particular choice is most correct, but the effect on the estimate of overdetection can be large and comparison of studies requires that the same denominator be used in all cases.

In CNBSS1, women in the age range 40–49 years in the intervention (MP) arm received annual mammography and physical examination, while the control group (UC) received a single physical examination at entry followed by "usual care" in the community, whose nature was undefined [23]. Women aged 50–59 at entry in the intervention (MP) arm of CNBSS2 received mammography plus clinical examination by a nurse (by a physician in Quebec) annually, while those in the control (PE) arm received annual clinical examination only [24].

The estimates of overdetection by Baines et al. are far higher than values published by other authors based on data from randomized trials or observational studies of service screening [19,21]. We, therefore, attempted to examine the results reported by Baines et al. to determine if these estimates were supported by their data. We also conducted microsimulation for the purpose of understanding mechanisms that could lead to the discrepancy in results.

2. Materials and Methods

For each of the two studies, CNBSS1 and CNBSS2, Baines et al. reported the cumulative number of invasive cancers and total (invasive and in situ) cancers that had accrued in each trial arm during the period that screening took place (denoted here as Years −4 to 0) and at 1, 2, 3, 4, 5, 10, 15 and 20 years after the study screening examinations terminated [21]. The differences between these two sets of numbers represented the in situ cancers. We observed the patterns in the accumulation of invasive, total and in situ cancers over time to assess if these patterns reflected those expected in a cohort of Canadian women.

Modelling

To predict the expected number of cancers in a randomized trial of screening, we utilized the OncoSim-Breast model, a microsimulation tool, based partially on the NCI CISNET Wisconsin-Harvard model that has been described previously [25,26]. OncoSim Breast has been validated by comparing its estimates with empirical breast cancer incidence both in an era prior to the implementation of screening programs and after programs were in place. There is no explicit modelling of a mechanism for overdetection in the algorithm; however, a range of cancer progression and growth rates are incorporated in the software. This would provide a distribution of cancers with varying levels of aggressiveness in the simulated population. Some of the slower-growing cancers "created" in the model should exhibit the phenomenon of overdetection. In particular, the model treats in situ and invasive cancers as parallel, partially independent processes. As in situ cancers develop over time, they have a probability of either transitioning into the invasive phenotype or remaining in situ and this can also give rise to overdetection.

The modeling represents a study even more rigorous than the conditions of a randomized trial in that the characteristics of the simulated participants are not only statistically similar, but rather they are perfectly matched; essentially, the simulation creates a study in which each woman in one cohort is matched with her identical twin in the other. For CNBSS1, we simulated a set of birth cohorts of women equally distributed over birth years, such that women would be in the age range of 40–49 at the beginning of the trial. The model inputs assume that prior to the beginning of the trial there is no screening in either arm. For half of the women (MP arm), the model was configured to estimate the number of in situ and invasive breast cancers that would be detected each year if the women received annual screening mammography and clinical examination. For the other half (UC), the model simulated a single screen by clinical examination in the year of entrance to the study and then followed the cohort without any screening intervention, again estimating the number of in situ and invasive cancers that would surface.

For CNBSS2, the same approach was taken; however, the interventions for the two study arms included a total of 40,000 women who would be in their 50s at the onset of the trial. The MP group received clinical examination and mammography annually, while the PE group received only annual clinical breast examination.

For both studies, for the purpose of modelling, it was assumed that no screening occurred in either trial arm after the intervention period. To reduce stochastic noise in modeling, 32 million histories were run and the results were scaled down to the 25,000 women in each arm for CNBSS1 and 20,000 for CNBSS2.

3. Results

3.1. CNBSS Findings

Figure 3 illustrates the excess in cancers found in the Study arm compared to the Control arm in each of the CNBSS trials. For invasive cancers, at the end of 5 years of the screening intervention (defined here as time 0), there was an excess of 59 and 79 cancers in the younger and older groups, respectively. When all cancers (invasive and in situ) were considered, the corresponding excesses were 92 and 115 cancers, respectively. It can then be inferred that there were 33 excess in situ cancers found in CNBSS1 and 36 in CNBSS2 over the period of screening. However, there is a dramatic difference between the trials in how the excesses varied as time elapsed after the screening intervention in the two trials.

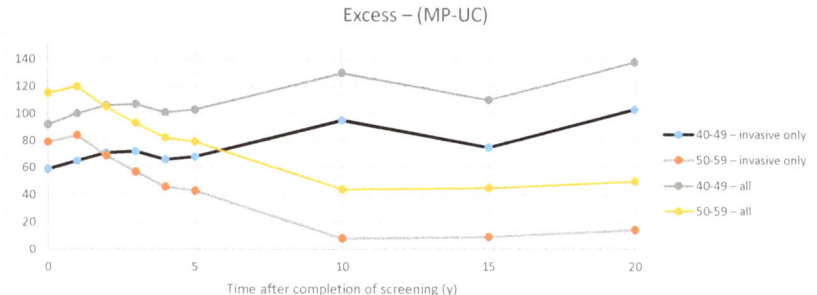

Figure 3. Excess invasive cancers in the study group compared to the controls in the two CNBSS trials.

Using the definition employed by Baines et al. for observation periods between t = 0 and 20 years after succession of screening (t = 20 y), for invasive cancers, the estimated overdetection fraction ranged from 28% to 48% at t = 0 and at t = 20 y, respectively, in the women in their 40s and between 29% and 5% for women in their 50s. Estimates were higher (36–53% in the younger group and 35% to 15% at t = 0 and 20 y, respectively, in the older group) when both all cancers (in situ and invasive) were considered.

In CNBSS2, for invasive cancers, the behavior over time is as would be expected with the excess gradually diminishing over the first 10 years after the period of screening as cancers gradually surface (without the benefit of screening lead time) in the control group. When the in situ cancers are included, the absolute excess that they represent at t = 0 appears to persist over time.

In CNBSS1, perplexingly, the excess of invasive cancers actually increases over the 20-year post-screening follow-up period. As in CNBSS2, the absolute contribution of in situ cancers to the excess appears to be essentially constant.

3.2. Modelling

For CNBSS1 the model breast cancer predictions are shown in Figure 4 for those in the mammography and usual care arms of the trial as well as for unscreened women. Here, annual screening begins at −4 years and Year 0 represents the point when screening ends. In Figure 5, the excess cancers (difference between MP and UC arms) are shown with separate curves for invasive cancers, all cancers and for DCIS only. Figures 6 and 7 show the corresponding predictions for cancer incidence and excess cancers for the older women in CNBSS2.

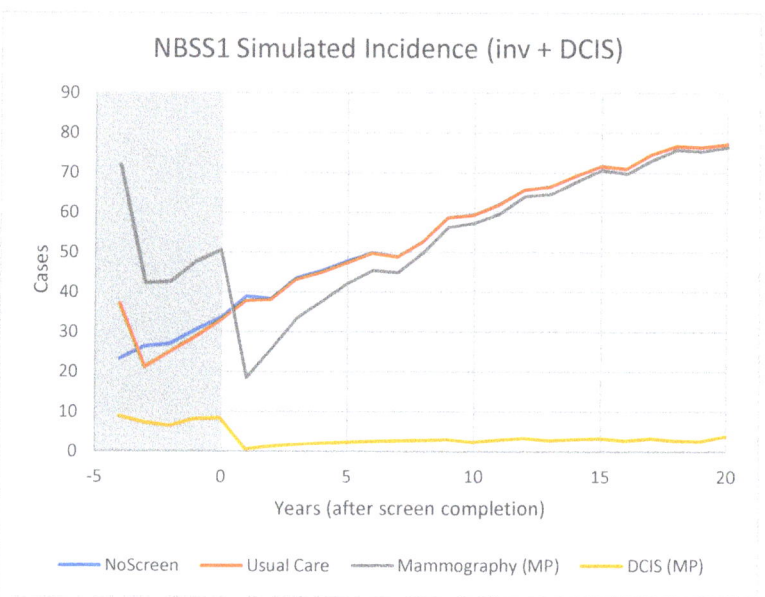

Figure 4. Predicted cases of breast cancer (OncoSim-Breast model) for women who are unscreened and in the Mammography or Usual Care arms of the CNBSS1 trial.

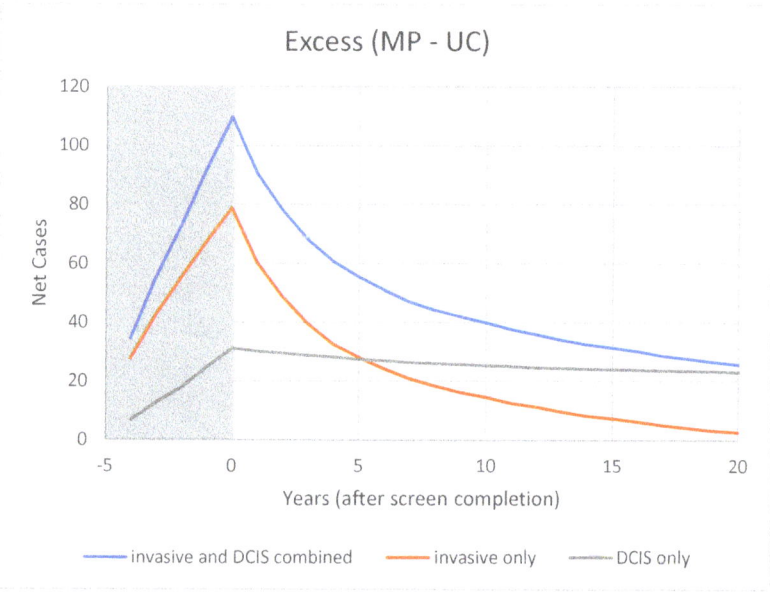

Figure 5. Modeled cumulative excess breast cancer detection in CNBSS1 from OncoSim-Breast. Shaded area represents screening period.

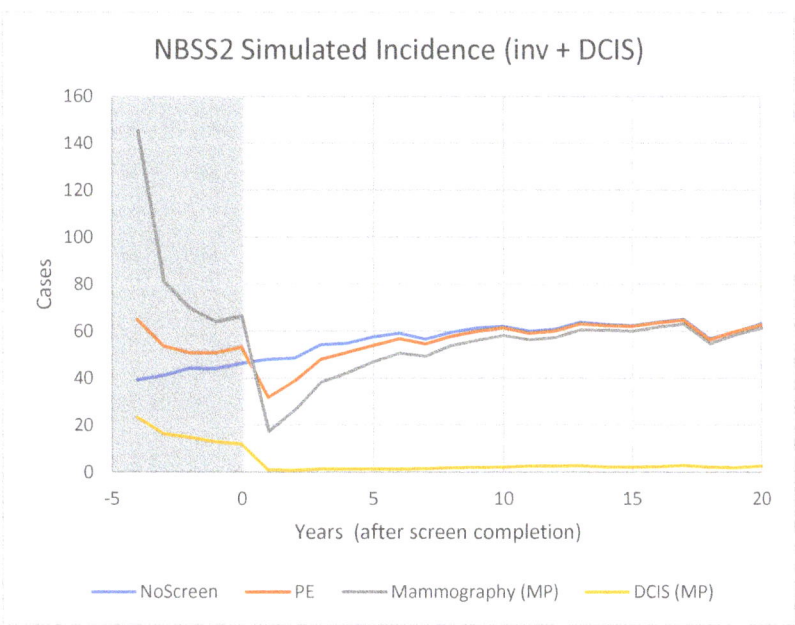

Figure 6. Predicted incidence of breast cancer (OncoSim-Breast model) for women who are unscreened and in the Mammography or Physical Examination arms of the CNBSS2 trial.

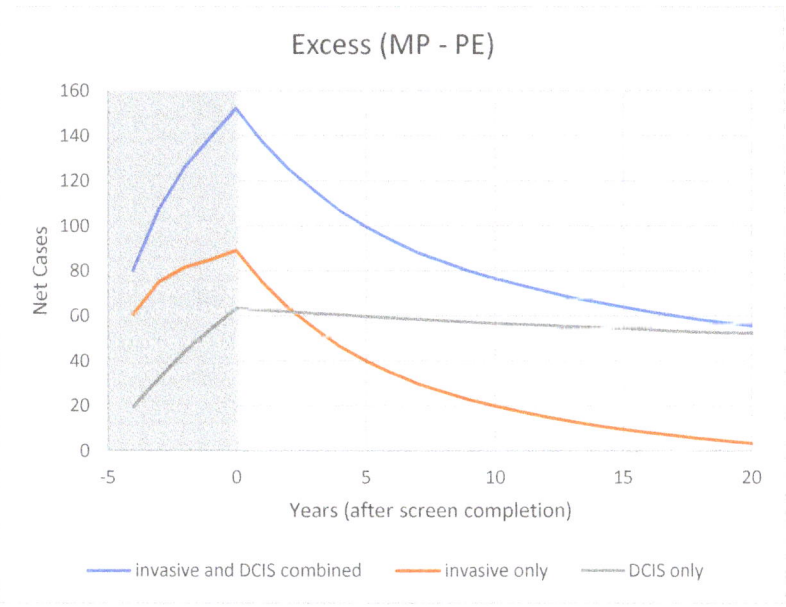

Figure 7. Modeled cumulative excess breast cancer detection in CNBSS2 from OncoSim-Breast.

4. Discussion

The rationale underlying effective breast cancer screening is that the screening intervention provides lead time; cancers will be found earlier in the screened group. In the CNBSS trials, this would cause an initial excess of cancers in the MP arms and that excess would persist (a) as long as women in one arm were screened, while in the other they were not, or (b) where the lead time in one trial arm was greater than in the other. Both of these conditions would be expected to occur in CNBSS1 because of the use of only one initial physical examination in the UC arm. The second condition would be in effect in CNBSS2 where less lead time would be expected in the PE arm at each screen as compared to that which received mammography plus clinical examination. At some point, however, it would be expected that the cancer incidence in the control arms would begin to catch up and the excess would diminish. As seen in Figure 3, this is exactly what was observed for invasive cancers in the older women in CNBSS2, but this was not seen in CNBSS1. If the excess cancers in the MP group were due to overdetection during the screening period, it would be expected that the absolute excess should remain constant after the intervention. From the continuing increase in the excess in CNBSS1 with time, we can deduce that factors other than overdetection are at play.

The most obvious explanation is that more women with breast cancer or who were more likely to develop breast cancer were recruited into the MP trial arms. The first factor would explain part of the initial excess in cancers in the MP arms in both trials; the second could contribute to the failure of the UC group in CNBSS1 to "catch up" in the number of invasive cancers over successive years.

Another explanation is there was some causal factors associated with screening in the MP arms that would contribute to more cancers. For example, it has been suggested that the additional radiation exposure from X-rays or the compression of the breast in the mammography might be responsible [27]; however, no credible evidence has emerged to support these hypotheses [28–30].

Finally, the thoroughness of cancer ascertainment during the post-screening follow up could be different between the MP and control arms. This possibility was suggested by Baines et al. as a possible contributor to the overestimation of overdetection [21]. This is plausible, especially in CNBSS1, because, by having only a single initial screen, women in the UC group were likely to have much less interaction with the Study than those in the MP arm.

4.1. Excess of In Situ Cancers

The CNBSS publications presented data on the number of invasive plus in situ cancers found by screening and otherwise, but did not separately indicate the number of in situ cancers found during the period of screening [23,24]. On the other hand, in their overdiagnosis publication, Baines et al. did present both the total number of invasive cancers and invasive plus in situ cancers in each study arm for CNBSS1 and CNBSS2 at the end of the screening period and for times out to 20 years beyond that [21]. The curves in Figure 3 demonstrate the excess in cancer detection in the MP group over the control group in each trial. The differences between the two curves are also plotted and at Year 0 indicate the excess number of in situ cancers detected in the MP arms during the screening period. This was 33 cancers in CNBSS1 (10% of cancers) and 42 in CNBSS2 (11.1% of cancers).

Following the period of screening intervention, if further screening does not occur, the detection of in situ cancers in both arms should fall dramatically. Under these conditions, it is unlikely that cancers in the control arm corresponding to those in the mammography arm that were detected as in situ cancers (and created that excess) will be detected when they are in situ. If the cancers progress, it is more likely that they will subsequently be detected as invasive cancers during the post-screening follow-up of the control group. If they do not progress to become invasive, it is likely that they will never be detected if the control group remains unscreened after $t = 0$. In this latter case, they contribute to overdetection.

This may explain why, as seen in Figure 3, the curves for total cancers and for invasive cancers remain essentially parallel; the initial excess in in situ cancers remains constant up to 20 years post-screening. All other factors being equal, this would suggest that many of the excess in situ cancers in the MP arms of CNBSS did not progress to become invasive and that much of the overdetection reported in that study is associated with in situ cancer. In situ cancer is not homogeneous [31] and it is possible that in CNBSS, particularly with concerns due to poor image quality, many of those detected were of the less aggressive phenotypes.

It is interesting that, from Baines et al., by subtracting the number of invasive cancers from the total number of cancers reported, it appears that over the 20 years after the screening intervention, only four and two additional in situ cancers were added in the MP and UC arms, respectively, to those detected during the screening period in CNBSS1. For CNBSS2, only a single in situ cancer was added in each arm over that period. This almost certainly implies that there was no effective post-intervention follow-up of in situ events, even though some degree of screening must have occurred in women in both arms during that time. Possibly cancer registries used for ascertaining cancers arising after $t = 0$ y simply did not record in situ cancers or possibly the overall ascertainment process had gaps.

4.2. Model Predictions

The model predictions for CNBSS1 (Figure 4) demonstrate the expected characteristics of the events in a screening regimen. In this case, the model was configured to simulate a screening intervention in the form of a randomized controlled trial with five annual examinations. The curve for unscreened women serves as a reference; there is a gradual monotonic rise of incidence corresponding mainly to increasing age.

For CNBSS1, at the onset of screening (-4 y), the model predicts a sharp increase in incidence in the arm screened with mammography corresponding to the detection of cancers whose state of development exceeded the threshold for screen detection, but had not yet reached that required to surface symptomatically. Once this "prevalence" screen has occurred, the predicted incidence rates are lower because many of the cancers that had accumulated prior to the onset of screening have been removed from the pool for detection. It might be expected that if there are slow growing or indolent cancers present these would largely be found in that initial prevalence screen along with newer, more aggressive cancers.

A sharp increase compared to no screening is also seen at the single screen of the control (UC) group, but in this case the increase is smaller, under the assumption that mammography was more sensitive than physical examination (higher threshold for detection). While the mammography screened group would include both invasive and in situ cancers, very few in situ cancers would be found in the controls. After the first examination at -4 y, the control group would no longer receive screening, so incidence would fall slightly below the level for unscreened women because some of the cancers had been found earlier due to the lead time provided by an expert clinical examination.

As shown in Figure 5 for CNBSS1, the lead time provided by mammography screening and the greater sensitivity for in situ cancer would be expected to cause an excess in the cumulative cancers detected in the screened group and this would build up gradually over the five screening examinations. After $t = 0$, the excess of invasive cancers in the MP arm is gradually compensated by a greater number in the control arm. Although half of the excess disappeared at 2.5 y and 75% by 7 y, the excess is not completely cancelled until 23 y, suggesting that there is a broad range of growth rates in these cancers detected by screening. At $t = 20$ y (25 years post entry), the predicted overdetection is 2% for invasive cancers and 13% for invasive plus in situ cancers. This provides a very different picture as to what happens to the excess cancers after the intervention period than that seen in Figure 3 in the data presented by Baines et al. [21] who estimated overdetection rates of 48% and 53%, respectively, at the same time point.

The predicted mortality reduction for five annual screens at $t = 10$y is 9% compared to the UC arm. This modest mortality reduction occurs because there were only five screens and the control group received an initial physical exam. Compared to no screening, the model predicts a 16.5% mortality reduction for five screens and 50% reduction for annual screening between ages 50 and 74 [32].

It may be worth making a comment about the effect of the choice of denominator in the calculation. If the number of cancers found in the MP arm (284) had been used rather than the number of screen-detected cancers (213), the overdetection estimate for invasive cancers would have dropped from 48% to 36%.

In CNBSS2 (Figure 6), there is a similar behavior at −4 y in both trial arms, again with a larger increase for the women receiving mammography. Screening continues for four more exams, again building up an excess in the mammography group (Figure 7) that is maximum at the cessation of screening (0 y). This predicted excess is greater than for CNBSS1 despite there being fewer women in the cohort; however, the timing of the decrease in excess cancers is similar to that for CNBSS1.

At $t = 20$ y (25 years post-entry), the predicted overdetection is 1% for invasive cancers and 16% for invasive plus in situ cancers compared to 5% and 16% from Baines et al. The predicted mortality reduction for five annual screens is 6% compared to the PE arm and 16.5% compared to no screening.

It should be mentioned that, although the model was calibrated against empirical incidence data, it is, of course, not perfect, and one should not overinterpret the numerical predictions. While it provides a mechanistic picture of the elements of screening, there are limited data available to describe the development of DCIS and the rate and degree of its transition to invasive cancer, so that there is considerable uncertainty in modeling the timing associated with the disappearance of the excess created by in situ cancers. Nevertheless, the modeling points to a similar behavior as seen both CNBSS trials in that the excess associated with in situ cancers persists for several decades, suggesting a significant sub-population of nonprogressive in situ cancers.

What are the most plausible explanations for the difference in behavior between the two trials and between the experimental and modeling results for CNBSS1? One possibility is that the women in the MP arm had a higher likelihood of having breast cancer. An anomaly of the CNBSS is that women received a clinical breast examination before they were entered in the register for the trial and, therefore, the suggestion has been put forward that non-randomness could have been introduced at this point, prompted by the findings of the nurse examiner [33]. There is now evidence that this did occur for some of the women, particularly those with advanced cancers at study entry, and this is a credible explanation for the fact that the CNBSS trials were the only RCTs that did not show a mortality benefit associated with routine mammography screening [5]. However, there is a suggestion that the imbalance was not limited to advanced cancers. Because in the prevalence (trial entry) episode of screening in both trials a physical examination of the breast was conducted on women in both trial arms, this provides a point in time where one can compare the number of cancers detectable by palpation between the arms. Although the differences did not reach statistical significance, the authors reported that there were approximately 10% more palpable cancers detected in the MP arm than in the usual care arm of CNBSS1 [23]. In CNBSS2, the excess was 13% [24]. Given that the procedure for detection of palpable cancers was the same in the two study arms and that the same nurses and physicians performed the examinations for both trial arms, such a difference is unexpected, whatever its cause, and would contribute in part to an apparent increase in overdetection.

Another possibility is suggested by the difference in the follow-up in the control groups between CNBSS1 and CNBSS2. In the former, after the initial clinical examination, women in the "Usual Care" arm reported on the incidence of breast cancer primarily through mailed, self-administered questionnaires, while women in the control arm of CNBSS2 received four more annual episodes of clinical examination during the screening epoch and presumably developed a closer relationship and commitment to communicating with study personnel during the subsequent follow-up. A similar situation existed in the study arms of both trials. It is possible that cancer arising after the single screening interaction in the Usual Care arm was under-reported and this would lead to an overestimate of overdetection. Supporting this finding is the observation in the publication by Baines et al. that virtually no DCIS was reported in the UC arm for the 20-year period following the screening intervention [21].

The CNBSS trials were heavily criticized due to the poor quality of the mammography. This is supported by the observation that the mean diameter of cancers in the screened group was only 2 mm smaller than that in the control group [22]. This suggests that the lead time afforded by mammography in CNBSS for actively growing cancers was relatively short. Additionally, while the mean diameter of cancers detected in CNBSS was about 2.1 cm, those cancers that were detected at the point where they were nonpalpable had a mean diameter of 1.4 cm. Therefore, most of the cancers detected by screening in the CNBSS were palpable and as mentioned above, there was a tendency for more of those cancers to be in the MP trial arms. In addition, the nonpalpable cancers most likely to be detected with poor quality mammography would be those that grew more slowly and, therefore, possibly would not reach the point of clinical detectability for many years, explaining the long tail in the curve for excess invasive cancers.

The observation that the excess invasive cancers increased over time after the period of screening intervention casts suspicion on the reliability of the use of data from the CNBSS1 trial for estimating overdetection. Documented problems with fair randomization and the tendency toward more palpable cancers in the MP arms of both trials adds to these concerns [23,24,33]. The one observation from these trials that does merit further consideration is the persistence of the excess that is associated with screen-detected in situ cancer.

4.3. Overtreatment

The main harm attributed to overdetection of breast cancer is overtreatment. Overtreatment can be considered to be any treatment whatsoever if the cancer is truly overdetected; however, it can also be unnecessarily harsh or aggressive treatment of slowly progressing cancers.

The greatest concerns regarding the overtreatment of breast cancer have been for in situ disease, which is most commonly treated with breast-conserving surgery and radiation therapy. There are now guidelines for acceptable margins (2 mm) for breast conserving surgery that will reduce re-excision rates [34]. For disease that has a low risk of recurring, the possibility of omitting radiotherapy can be considered [35].

However, it is also crucial that in situ disease not be undertreated. In a SEER review of over 144,000 women diagnosed with DCIS, Giannakeas et al. concluded: " ... the risk of dying of breast cancer was increased 3-fold after a diagnosis of DCIS" "(compared to women without a diagnosis of DCIS)" [36].

More recently, it has been shown that a multigene panel based on 12 genes associated with invasive cancer recurrence is predictive of local recurrence after DCIS. Combined with the categorical values of age at diagnosis and tumor diameter, low/medium/high DCIS score can predict a range of 10-year recurrence risks of 6.67 varying from 49% to 7% [37,38]. Further work by the same group in a cohort of 1362 women diagnosed with DCIS in Ontario, Canada, found that the application of the Oncotype DX 21 gene recurrence score was prognostic for invasive local recurrence and risk of breast cancer death [39]. These multigene assays help to predict an individual's risk of recurrence, which can improve treatment recommendations integrating individual-based risk assessment with individual preferences. Further research is underway to identify biomarkers that predict which women with DCIS would and would not benefit from radiation therapy, thereby reducing overtreatment associated with earlier detection of cancer.

5. Conclusions

Screening tends to detect breast cancers when they are smaller and at earlier stage and has a marked effect on the detection of in situ cancer [40]. The detection of some of these cancers, which are very slow growing or indolent, provides little or no benefit and should be considered as overdetection. In some cases, however, the degree of overdetection has been greatly overestimated [3,4,21], or at least the estimates are not on solid ground.

Currently, because there are no reliable and accepted in vivo tests to determine which cancers will be progressive and no way of determining which women will die of other causes before an undetected progressive cancer is found clinically, overdetection is a necessary tradeoff for the substantial mortality and morbidity reduction opportunities provided by screening. Nevertheless, overdetection, and more importantly, overtreatment remain issues that must be addressed, particularly for in situ disease.

At the same time, there are opportunities for the improvement of detecting aggressive cancers through screening methods that are preferentially sensitive to these cancers, such as contrast-enhanced imaging [41], or approaches such as breast tomosynthesis that are intended to make cancers more conspicuous by overcoming tissue superposition effects. In addition, the radiomic analysis of screening images could allow better in vivo characterization to more accurately determine which findings require biopsy [42,43] or are indicative of aggressive disease. For example, Tabar et al. have created subclassifications of mammographic findings previously generically referred to as "DCIS" to distinguish acinar findings, which tend to be lower risk from the more ominous presentations accompanied by linear calcifications in the major lactiferous ducts, likely indicating that neoductgenesis is already occurring [44].

Harms associated with overdetection can also be mitigated by reducing subsequent overdiagnosis, through more definitive pathology tools for analysis and characterization of samples from needle biopsy, thereby reducing the amount of over (and, in some cases, under) treatment [35,37–39,45–48].

While it is tempting to reduce overdetection by limiting screening to those who are perceived to be at greatest risk of developing cancer, often referred to as "personalized screening" [49–53], this does not really target the problem as it is the aggressiveness of the cancer or lack thereof, not the likelihood of incidence that is the main driving factor for overdetection. Personalized screening is an excellent concept and research in this area could be of great value, but until we have risk prediction tools whose negative predictive value is extremely high, this would be a dangerous path to follow as it would result in the missed opportunity for the earlier detection and effective treatment of many potentially lethal cancers.

Finally, women, the general public and health care providers must be clearly, accurately and appropriately informed of the benefits provided by screening as well as the limitations or harms associated with phenomena such as overdetection. This has often been conducted poorly or inaccurately and without any weighting related to quality of life, ascribing inappropriately high harms to false positive screens and overdetection [3]. Others have suggested more useful and positive approaches to communication [54]. To allow informed decision making, and as an indicator of respect for human life, it is critically important that this is performed more effectively in the future.

Author Contributions: Conceptualization, M.J.Y.; methodology, J.G.M. and M.J.Y.; software, J.G.M.; validation, J.G.M. and M.J.Y.; formal analysis, J.G.M. and M.J.Y.; writing—original draft preparation, M.J.Y.; writing—review and editing, M.J.Y. and J.G.M. All authors have read and agreed to the published version of the manuscript.

Funding: This research received no external funding.

Data Availability Statement: All data supporting the results reported in this article can be found in the published work listed in the references. Input parameters and results produced from use of the OncoSim-Breast model can be obtained upon reasonable requests to the authors.

Acknowledgments: The authors are grateful to Claude Nadeau at Statistics Canada and Jean Yong at The Canadian Partnership Against Cancer for their valuable assistance. Jean Seely (University of Ottawa) reviewed early drafts of the manuscript and provided helpful suggestions for improvement.

Eileen Rakovitch (Odette Cancer Centre) generously shared her insights on avoiding overtreatment of in situ breast cancer.

Conflicts of Interest: Yaffe holds shares in Volpara Health Technologies, a manufacturer of software for analyzing medical images and conducts some collaborative research in breast cancer imaging with GE Healthcare under an agreement with his institution. Neither organization was involved in any way with this project.

References

1. Marmot, M.G.; Altman, D.G.; Cameron, D.A.; Dewar, J.A.; Thompson, S.G.; Wilcox, M. The benefits and harms of breast cancer screening: An independent review. *Br. J. Cancer* **2013**, *108*, 2205–2240. [CrossRef] [PubMed]
2. Nelson, H.D.; Pappas, M.; Cantor, A.; Griffin, J.; Daeges, M.; Humphrey, L. Harms of breast cancer screening: Systematic review to update the 2009 U.S. Preventive Services Task Force recommendation. *Ann. Int. Med.* **2016**, *164*, 256–267. [CrossRef] [PubMed]
3. Klarenbach, S.; Sims-Jones, N.; Lewin, G.; Singh, H.; Thériault, G.; Tonelli, M.; Doull, M.; Courage, S.; Garcia, A.J.; Thombs, B.D. Recommendations on screening for breast cancer in women 40–74 years of age who are not at increased risk for breast cancer. *CMAJ* **2018**, *190*, E1441–E1451. [CrossRef]
4. Welch, H.G. Cancer Screening—The good, the bad, and the ugly. *JAMA Surg.* **2022**. [CrossRef]
5. International Agency for Research on Cancer. *Breast Cancer Screening IARC Handbook of Cancer Prevention*; International Agency for Research on Cancer: Lyon, France, 2016; Volume 15.
6. Brodersen, J.; Schwartz, L.M.; Heneghan, C.; O'Sullivan, J.W.; Aronson, J.K.; Woloshin, S. Overdiagnosis: What it is and what it isn't. *BMJ Evid. Based Med.* **2018**, *23*, 1–3. [CrossRef]
7. Coldman, A.; Phillips, N.; Wilson, C.; Decker, K.; Chiarelli, A.M.; Brisson, J.; Zhang, B.; Payne, J.; Doyle, G.; Ahmad, R. Pan-Canadian Study of Mammography Screening and Mortality from Breast Cancer. *JNCI J. Natl. Cancer Inst.* **2014**, *106*, dju261. [CrossRef] [PubMed]
8. Ryser, M.D.; Lange, J.; Inoue, L.Y.T.; O'Meara, E.S.; Gard, C.; Miglioretti, D.L.; Bulliard, J.L.; Brouwer, A.F.; Hwang, E.S.; Etzioni, R.B. Estimation of Breast Cancer Overdiagnosis in a U.S. Breast Screening Cohort. *Ann. Int. Med.* **2022**, *175*, 471–478. [CrossRef]
9. Glasziou, P.P.; Jones, M.A.; Pathirana, T.; Barratt, A.L.; Bell, K.J. Estimating the magnitude of cancer overdiagnosis in Australia. *Med. J. Aust.* **2020**, *212*, 163–168. [CrossRef]
10. Collins, L.C.; Achacoso, N.; Haque, R.; Nekhlyudov, L.; Fletcher, S.W.; Quesenberry, C.P.; Schnitt, S.J.; Habel, L.A. Risk factors for noninvasive and invasive local recurrence in patients with ductal carcinoma in situ. *Breast Cancer Res. Treat.* **2013**, *139*, 453–460. [CrossRef]
11. Early Breast Cancer Trialists' Collaborative Group (EBCTCG). Overview of the Randomized Trials of Radiotherapy in Ductal Carcinoma In Situ of the Breast. *J. Natl. Cancer Inst. Monogr.* **2010**, *41*, 162–177.
12. Rakovitch, E.; Nofech-Mozes, S.; Narod, S.A.; Hanna, W.; Thiruchelvam, D.; Saskin, R.; Taylor, C.; Tuck, A.; Sengupta, S.; Elavathil, L.; et al. Can we select individuals with low risk ductal carcinoma in situ (DCIS)? A population-based outcomes analysis. *Breast Cancer Res. Treat.* **2013**, *138*, 581–590. [CrossRef] [PubMed]
13. Solin, L.J.; Gray, R.; Hughes, L.L.; Wood, W.C.; Lowen, M.A.; Badve, S.S.; Baehner, F.L.; Ingle, J.N.; Perez, E.A.; Recht, A.; et al. Surgical excision without radiation for ductal carcinoma in situ of the breast: 12-year results from the ECOG-ACRIN E5194 Study. *J. Clin. Oncol.* **2015**, *33*, 3938–3944. [CrossRef] [PubMed]
14. Moss, S. Overdiagnosis and overtreatment of breast cancer: Overdiagnosis in randomised controlled trials of breast cancer screening. *Breast Cancer Res.* **2005**, *7*, 230–234. [CrossRef] [PubMed]
15. Zahl, P.H.; Jørgensen, K.J.; Gotzsche, P.C. Overestimated lead times in cancer screening has led to substantial underestimation of overdiagnosis. *Br. J. Cancer* **2013**, *109*, 2014–2019. [CrossRef] [PubMed]
16. Bleyer, A.; Welch, H.G. Effect of Three Decades of Screening Mammography on Breast-Cancer Incidence. *N. Engl. J. Med.* **2012**, *367*, 1998–2005. [CrossRef]
17. Kopans, D.B. Arguments against mammography screening continue to be based on faulty science. *Oncologist* **2014**, *19*, 107–112. [CrossRef]
18. Yaffe, M.J.; Pritchard, K.I. Commentary: Overdiagnosing Overdiagnosis. *Oncologist* **2014**, *19*, 103–106. [CrossRef]
19. Puliti, D.; Duffy, S.W.; Miccinesi, G.; de Koning, H.; Lynge, E.; Zappa, M.; Paci, M.; the EUROSCREEN WorkingGroup. Overdiagnosis in mammographic screening for breast cancer in Europe: A literature review. *J. Med. Screen.* **2012**, *19*, 42–56. [CrossRef]
20. Etzioni, R.; Gulati, R. Recognizing the limitations of cancer overdiagnosis studies: A first step towards overcoming them. *J. Natl. Cancer Inst.* **2016**, *108*, djv345. [CrossRef]
21. Baines, C.J.; To, T.; Miller, A.B. Revised estimates of overdiagnosis from the Canadian National Breast Screening Study. *Prev. Med.* **2016**, *90*, 66–71. [CrossRef]
22. Miller, A.B.; Wall, C.; Baines, C.J.; Sun, P.; To, T.; Narod, S.A. Twenty five year followup for breast cancer incidence and mortality of the Canadian National Breast Screening Study: Randomised screening trial. *BMJ* **2014**, *348*, g366. [CrossRef] [PubMed]

23. Miller, A.B.; Baines, C.J.; To, T.; Wall, C. Canadian National Breast Screening Study: 1. Breast cancer detection and death rates among women aged 40 to 49 years. *CMAJ* **1992**, *147*, 1459–1476. [PubMed]
24. Miller, A.B.; Baines, C.J.; To, T.; Wall, C. Canadian National Breast Screening Study: 2. Breast cancer detection and death rates among women aged 50 to 59 years. *CMAJ* **1992**, *147*, 1477–1488. [PubMed]
25. Yong, J.H.E.; Nadeau, C.; Flanagan, W.M.; Coldman, A.J.; Asakawa, K.; Garner, R.; Fitzgerald, N.; Yaffe, M.J.; Miller, A.B. The OncoSim-Breast cancer microsimulation model. *Curr. Oncol.* **2022**, *29*, 1619–1633. [CrossRef]
26. CISNET Wisconsin Model of Breast Cancer. 2013. Available online: https://cisnet.flexkb.net/mp/pub/CISNET_ModelProfile_BREAST_UWISC_001_07232013_58567.pdf (accessed on 27 May 2022).
27. Epstein, S.S.; Bertell, R.; Seaman, B. Dangers and unreliability of mammography: Breast examination is a safe, effective, and practical alternative. *Int. J. Health Serv.* **2001**, *31*, 605–615. [CrossRef]
28. Miglioretti, D.L.; Lange, J.; van den Broek, J.J.; Lee, C.I.; van Ravesteyn, N.T.; Ritley, D.; Kerlikowske, K.; Fenton, J.J.; Melnikow, J.; de Koning, H.J.; et al. Radiation-Induced Breast Cancer Incidence and Mortality From Digital Mammography Screening: A Modeling Study. *Ann. Int. Med.* **2016**, *164*, 205–214. [CrossRef]
29. Yaffe, M.J.; Mainprize, J.G. Risk of Radiation-induced Breast Cancer from Mammographic Screening. *Radiology* **2010**, *258*, 98–105. [CrossRef]
30. Hendrick, R.E. Radiation doses and cancer risks from breast imaging studies. *Radiology* **2010**, *257*, 246–253. [CrossRef]
31. Pinder, S.E. Ductal carcinoma in situ (DCIS): Pathological features, differential diagnosis, prognostic factors and specimen evaluation. *Mod. Pathol.* **2010**, *23*, S8–S13. [CrossRef]
32. Yaffe, M.J.; Mainprize, J.G. The Value of All-Cause Mortality as a Metric for Assessing Breast Cancer Screening. *J. Natl. Cancer Inst.* **2020**, djaa025. [CrossRef]
33. Yaffe, M.J.; Seely, J.E.; Gordon, P.B.; Appavoo, S.; Kopans, D.B. The Randomized trial of mammography screening that was not—A cautionary tale. *J. Med. Screen.* **2022**, *29*, 7–11. [CrossRef] [PubMed]
34. Morrow, M.; Van Zee, K.J.; Solin, L.J.; Houssami, N.; Chavez-MacGregor, M.; Harris, J.R.; Horton, J.; Hwang, S.; Johnson, P.L.; Marinovich, M.L.; et al. Society of Surgical Oncology-American Society for Radiation Oncology-American Society of Clinical Oncology Consensus Guideline on Margins for Breast-Conserving Surgery With Whole-Breast Irradiation in Ductal Carcinoma in Situ. *Pract Radiat Oncol.* **2016**, *6*, 287–295. [CrossRef] [PubMed]
35. Collins, L.C.; Laronga, C.; Wong, J.S. Ductal Carcinoma In Situ: Treatment and Prognosis. Available online: http://www.uptodate.com/contents/ductal-carcinoma-in-situ-treatment-and-prognosis (accessed on 27 May 2022).
36. Giannakeas, V.; Sopik, V.; Narod, S.A. Association of a Diagnosis of Ductal Carcinoma In Situ with Death from Breast Cancer. *JAMA Netw. Open.* **2020**, *3*, e2017124. [CrossRef] [PubMed]
37. Paszat, L.; Sutradhar, R.; Zhou, L.; Nofech-Mozes, S.; Rakovitch, E. Including the ductal carcinoma-in-situ (DCIS) score in the development of a multivariable prediction model for recurrence after excision of DCIS. *Clin. Breast Cancer* **2019**, *19*, 35–46. [CrossRef]
38. Rakovitch, E.; Gray, R.; Baehner, F.L.; Sutradhar, R.; Crager, M.; Gu, S.; Nofech-Mozes, S.; Badve, S.S.; Hanna, W.; Hughes, L.L.; et al. Refined estimates of local recurrence risks by DCIS score adjusting for clinicopathological features: A combined analysis of ECOG-ACRIN E5194 and Ontario DCIS cohort studies. *Breast Cancer Res. Treat.* **2018**, *169*, 359–369. [CrossRef]
39. Rakovitch, E.; Sutradhar, R.; Nofech-Mozes, S.; Gu, S.; Fong, C.; Hanna, W.; Paszat, L. 21-Gene Assay and Breast Cancer Mortality in Ductal Carcinoma In Situ. *JNCI J. Natl. Cancer Inst.* **2021**, *113*, djaa179. [CrossRef]
40. Ernster, V.L.; Ballard-Barbash, R.; Barlow, W.E.; Zheng, Y.; Weaver, D.L.; Cutter, G.; Yankaskas, B.C.; Rosenberg, R.; Carney, P.A.; Kerlikowske, K.; et al. Detection of ductal carcinoma in situ in women undergoing screening mammography. *J. Natl. Cancer Inst.* **2002**, *94*, 1546–1554. [CrossRef]
41. Kuhl, C. Abbreviated breast MRI for screening women with dense breast: The EA1141 trial. *Br. J. Radiol.* **2018**, *91*, 20170441. [CrossRef]
42. Pisano, E.D.; Yaffe, M.J. Breast cancer screening: Should tomosynthesis replace digital mammography? *JAMA* **2014**, *311*, 2488–2489. [CrossRef]
43. Rahbar, H.; McDonald, E.S.; Lee, J.G.M.; Partridge, S.C.; Lee, C.I. How Can Advanced Imaging Be Used to Mitigate Potential Breast Cancer Overdiagnosis? *Acad. Radiol.* **2016**, *23*, 768–773. [CrossRef]
44. Tabár, L.; Dean, P.B.; Lee Tucker, F.; Yen, A.M.; Chen, S.L.; Jen, G.H.H.; Wang, J.W.; Smith, R.A.; Duffy, S.W.; Chen, T.H. A new approach to breast cancer terminology based on the anatomic site of tumour origin: The importance of radiologic imaging biomarkers. *Eur. J. Radiol.* **2022**, *149*, 110189. [CrossRef] [PubMed]
45. Hwang, E.S.; Hyslop, T.; Lynch, T.; Frank, E.; Pinto, D.; Basila, D.; Collyar, D.; Bennett, A.; Kaplan, C.; Rosenberg, S.; et al. The COMET (Comparison of Operative versus Monitoring and Endocrine Therapy) trial: A phase III randomised controlled clinical trial for low-risk ductal carcinoma in situ (DCIS). *BMJ Open* **2019**, *9*, e026797. [CrossRef] [PubMed]
46. Sparano, J.A.; Gray, R.J.; Makower, D.F.; Pritchard, K.I.; Albain, K.S.; Hayes, D.F.; Geyer, C.E., Jr.; Dees, E.C.; Goetz, M.P.; Olson, J.A., Jr.; et al. Adjuvant Chemotherapy Guided by a 21-Gene Expression Assay in Breast Cancer. *N. Engl. J. Med.* **2018**, *379*, 111–121. [CrossRef] [PubMed]

47. Harris, L.N.; Ismaila, N.; McShane, L.M.; Andre, F.; Collyar, D.E.; Gonzalez-Angulo, A.M.; Hammond, E.H.; Kuderer, N.M.; Liu, M.C.; Mennel, R.G.; et al. Use of biomarkers to guide decisions on adjuvant systemic therapy for women with early-stage invasive breast cancer: American Society of Clinical Oncology Clinical Practice Guideline. *J. Clin. Oncol.* **2016**, *34*, 1134–1150. [CrossRef]
48. Katz, S.J.; Jagsi, R.; Morrow, M. Reducing Overtreatment of Cancer With Precision Medicine: Just What the Doctor Ordered. *JAMA* **2018**, *319*, 1091–1092. [CrossRef]
49. Allweis, T.M.; Hermann, N.; Berenstein-Molho, R.; Guindy, M. Personalized Screening for Breast Cancer: Rationale, Present Practices, and Future Directions. *Ann. Surg. Oncol.* **2021**, *28*, 4306–4317. [CrossRef]
50. Pashayan, N.; Antoniou, A.C.; Ivanus, U.; Esserman, L.J.; Easton, D.F.; French, D.; Sroczynski, G.; Hall, P.; Cuzick, J.; Evans, D.G.; et al. Personalized early detection and prevention of breast cancer: ENVISION consensus statement. *Nat. Rev. Clin. Oncol.* **2020**, *17*, 687–705. [CrossRef]
51. Román, M.; Sala, M.; Domingo, L.; Posso, M.; Louro, J.; Castells, X. Personalized breast cancer screening strategies: A systematic review and quality assessment. *PLoS ONE* **2019**, *14*, e0226352. [CrossRef]
52. Brooks, J.D.; Nabi, H.H.; Andrulis, I.L.; Antoniou, A.C.; Chiquette, J.; Després, P.; Devilee, P.; Dorval, M.; Droit, A.; Easton, D.F.; et al. Personalized Risk Assessment for Prevention and Early Detection of Breast Cancer: Integration and Implementation (PERSPECTIVE I&I). *J. Pers. Med.* **2021**, *11*, 511. [CrossRef]
53. Mukhtar, R.A.; Wong, J.G.M.; Esserman, L.J. Preventing overdiagnosis and overtreatment: Just the next step in the evolution of breast cancer care. *J. Natl. Compr. Cancer Netw.* **2015**, *13*, 737–743. [CrossRef]
54. Hersch, J.; Barratt, A.; McGeechan, K.; Jansen, J.; Houssami, N.; Dhillon, H.; Jacklyn, G.; Irwig, L.; McCaffery, K. Informing Women About Overdetection in Breast Cancer Screening: Two-Year Outcomes From a Randomized Trial. *J. Natl. Cancer Inst.* **2021**, *113*, 1523–1530. [CrossRef] [PubMed]

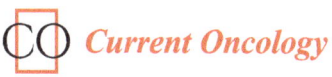

Article

Radiomic and Artificial Intelligence Analysis with Textural Metrics Extracted by Contrast-Enhanced Mammography and Dynamic Contrast Magnetic Resonance Imaging to Detect Breast Malignant Lesions

Roberta Fusco [1], Elio Di Bernardo [1], Adele Piccirillo [2], Maria Rosaria Rubulotta [3], Teresa Petrosino [3], Maria Luisa Barretta [3], Mauro Mattace Raso [3], Paolo Vallone [3], Concetta Raiano [3], Raimondo Di Giacomo [4], Claudio Siani [4], Franca Avino [4], Giosuè Scognamiglio [5], Maurizio Di Bonito [5], Vincenza Granata [3,*,†] and Antonella Petrillo [3,†]

[1] Medical Oncolody Division, Igea SpA, 80013 Naples, Italy; r.fusco@igeamedical.com (R.F.); e.dibernardo@igeamedical.com (E.D.B.)
[2] Department of Electrical Engineering and Information Technologies, Università degli Studi di Napoli Federico II, 80125 Naples, Italy; adelepiccirillo@gmail.com
[3] Radiology Division, Istituto Nazionale Tumori-IRCCS-Fondazione G. Pascale, 80131 Naples, Italy; m.rubulotta@istitutotumori.na.it (M.R.R.); t.petrosino@istitutotumori.na.it (T.P.); m.barretta@istitutotumori.na.it (M.L.B.); m.mattaceraso@istitutotumori.na.it (M.M.R.); p.vallone@istitutotumori.na.it (P.V.); c.raiano@istitutotumori.na.it (C.R.); a.petrillo@istitutotumori.na.it (A.P.)
[4] Senology Surgical Division, Istituto Nazionale Tumori-IRCCS-Fondazione G. Pascale, 80131 Naples, Italy; r.digiacomo@istitutotumori.na.it (R.D.G.); c.siani@istitutotumori.na.it (C.S.); f.avino@istitutotumori.na.it (F.A.)
[5] Pathology Division, Istituto Nazionale Tumori-IRCCS-Fondazione G. Pascale, 80131 Naples, Italy; g.scognamiglio@istitutotumori.na.it (G.S.); m.dibonito@istitutotumori.na.it (M.D.B.)
* Correspondence: v.granata@istitutotumori.na.it; Tel.: +39-081-590-714; Fax: +39-081-590-3825
† These authors contributed equally to this work.

Citation: Fusco, R.; Di Bernardo, E.; Piccirillo, A.; Rubulotta, M.R.; Petrosino, T.; Barretta, M.L.; Mattace Raso, M.; Vallone, P.; Raiano, C.; Di Giacomo, R.; et al. Radiomic and Artificial Intelligence Analysis with Textural Metrics Extracted by Contrast-Enhanced Mammography and Dynamic Contrast Magnetic Resonance Imaging to Detect Breast Malignant Lesions. *Curr. Oncol.* 2022, 29, 1947–1966. https://doi.org/10.3390/curroncol29030159

Received: 24 January 2022
Accepted: 10 March 2022
Published: 13 March 2022

Publisher's Note: MDPI stays neutral with regard to jurisdictional claims in published maps and institutional affiliations.

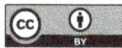

Copyright: © 2022 by the authors. Licensee MDPI, Basel, Switzerland. This article is an open access article distributed under the terms and conditions of the Creative Commons Attribution (CC BY) license (https://creativecommons.org/licenses/by/4.0/).

Abstract: Purpose: The purpose of this study was to discriminate between benign and malignant breast lesions through several classifiers using, as predictors, radiomic metrics extracted from CEM and DCE-MRI images. In order to optimize the analysis, balancing and feature selection procedures were performed. **Methods**: Fifty-four patients with 79 histo-pathologically proven breast lesions (48 malignant lesions and 31 benign lesions) underwent both CEM and DCE-MRI. The lesions were retrospectively analyzed with radiomic and artificial intelligence approaches. Forty-eight textural metrics were extracted, and univariate and multivariate analyses were performed: non-parametric statistical test, receiver operating characteristic (ROC) and machine learning classifiers. **Results:** Considering the single metrics extracted from CEM, the best predictors were KURTOSIS (area under ROC curve (AUC) = 0.71) and SKEWNESS (AUC = 0.71) calculated on late MLO view. Considering the features calculated from DCE-MRI, the best predictors were RANGE (AUC = 0.72), ENERGY (AUC = 0.72), ENTROPY (AUC = 0.70) and GLN (gray-level nonuniformity) of the gray-level run-length matrix (AUC = 0.72). Considering the analysis with classifiers and an unbalanced dataset, no significant results were obtained. After the balancing and feature selection procedures, higher values of accuracy, specificity and AUC were reached. The best performance was obtained considering 18 robust features among all metrics derived from CEM and DCE-MRI, using a linear discriminant analysis (accuracy of 0.84 and AUC = 0.88). **Conclusions:** Classifiers, adjusted with adaptive synthetic sampling and feature selection, allowed for increased diagnostic performance of CEM and DCE-MRI in the differentiation between benign and malignant lesions.

Keywords: contrast-enhanced mammography; magnetic resonance imaging; image enhancement; contrast media; radiomics; artificial intelligence

1. Introduction

In the screening, detection and follow-up of breast cancer, the mammography (MX) was considered the first imaging examination [1,2]. In particular, thanks to the technological improvements achieved by combining digital mammography with techniques that allow low and high energy images to be obtained, and with the administration of iodate contrast agent, it is possible to acquire images that emphasize the vascularity linked to malignant lesions by the contrast agent enhancement. This imaging technique is recognized as contrast-enhanced mammography and exploits the same physiological mechanisms as dynamic contrast-enhanced magnetic resonance imaging (DCE-MRI).

DCE-MRI is an important complementary diagnostic imaging technique that was validated in the screening of high-risk women and dense breasts and in the monitoring of oncological therapies, thanks to its capability of combining morphological and functional information [2,3].

Previous studies have evaluated the sensitivity of CEM compared to conventional digital MX, ultrasound (US) and MRI [4–8]. CEM sensitivity has been reported in the range of 90–100% [5–7], which is significantly higher than the sensitivity of MX or US alone [4–7]. Moreover, CEM allows for the identification of additional occult cancers via mammography to more accurately assess the disease extent, and to guide surgical and treatment planning [8–12].

Radiomics and artificial intelligence approaches have been extensively applied to process both CEM and DCE-MRI in order to increase diagnostic performance in the detection of malignant breast lesions [13,14]. By means of the radiomics approach, it is possible to obtain, from medical images, a large amount of quantitative data that, combined with pattern recognition procedures, allow for the resolution of many clinical issues with high accuracy. Examples of features used in the oncology field are tumor size and shape, as well as intensity, statistical and textural metrics [15–42].

In this study, we designed several classifiers with the aim of discriminating between benign and malignant breast lesions using, as predictors, radiomic metrics extracted from CEM and DCE-MRI images. In order to optimize the analysis, balancing and feature selection procedures were performed.

2. Methods

2.1. Patient Selection

Patients were enrolled in this study, which was approved by the local ethical committee of National Cancer Institute of Naples Pascale Foundation. Fifty four patients (mean age 54.3, range 31–78 years) with 79 histo-pathologically proven breast lesions (48 malignant lesions and 31 benign lesions) (Table 1) underwent both CEM and DCE-MRI. The lesions were retrospectively analyzed with radiomic and artificial intelligence approaches. Breast lesions were categorized based on the American Joint Committee on Cancer staging.

Table 1. Number and corresponding percentage of the total benign or malignant breast lesions.

Benign (31 Lesions)	Number	Percentage Value (%)
Fibrosis	6	19.35
Ductal hyperplasia	8	25.81
Fibroadenoma	9	29.03
Dysplasia	4	12.90
Adenosis	4	12.90
Malignant (48 Lesions)	**Number**	**Percentage Value (%)**
Infiltrating lobular carcinoma	7	14.58
Infiltrating ductal carcinoma	30	62.50
Ductal carcinoma in situ	9	18.75
Tubular Carcinoma	2	4.17

All women gave their written informed consent according to local ethical committee regulations.

Inclusion criteria: patient with known, histologically proven breast lesions who underwent both dual-energy CEM in craniocaudal (CC) and mediolateral oblique (MLO) views and DCE-MRI.

Exclusion criteria were previously reported in [43,44].

2.2. Imaging Protocol

CEM was acquired with the dual-energy mammography system (Hologic's Selenia® Dimensions® Unit, Bedford, MA, USA) as reported in our previous studies [43]. Two minutes after the administration of 1.5 mL/kg body weight of iodinated contrast medium (Visipaque 320; GE Healthcare, Inc., Princeton, NJ, USA) at a rate of 2–3 mL/s, each woman was placed in a CC view. Four and eight minutes after administration of the contrast agent, each breast was compressed in the MLO view: early MLO and late MLO views, respectively.

DCE-MRI was acquired with a 1.5T MR scanner (Magnetom Symphony; Siemens Medical System, Erlangen, Germany) equipped with a dedicated breast coil with 16 channels. Scan settings are reported in our previous study [44]: one series before and nine series after the automatic intravenous injection of 0.1 mmol/kg body weight of a positive paramagnetic contrast material (Gd-DOTA; Dotarem, Guerbet, Roissy CdG CEDEX, France) were acquired.

2.3. Image Processing

Regions of interest were manually segmented, slice by slice, by two expert radiologists, with 25 and 20 years of experience in breast imaging, respectively.

Breast lesions were segmented on dual-energy subtracted images, where contrast uptake was emphasized, both in CC and in MLO, and on the third T1-weighted subtracted series where contrast uptake was emphasized.

Radiomics features were extracted using the Texture Toolbox of MATLAB®, realized by Vallières et al. [45], which includes 48 parameters calculated according to the Image Biomarker Standardization Initiative [46], as previously described in [43,44]. The textural features include both first-order and second-order features; an extra detailed description of each feature has been provided in Appendix A.

2.4. Statistical Analysis

The statistical analysis was performed with RStudio software [47].

To assess variability among radiomic feature values, the intra-class correlation coefficient (ICC) was calculated. A non-parametric Wilcoxon–Mann–Whitney test and receiver operating characteristic (ROC) analysis were performed and the Youden index was calculated to obtain the optimal cut off value for each feature; then, in order to assess analysis results, the area under the ROC curve (AUC), sensitivity (SENS), specificity (SPEC), positive predictive value (PPV), negative predictive value (NPV) and accuracy (ACC) were computed.

Linear classifier (linear discriminant analysis—LDA), decision tree (TREE), k-nearest neighbors (KNN), artificial neural network (NNET) and support vector machine (SVM) using all extracted metrics of textural parameters were used [14]. Configuration settings for each classifier are provided in our previous study [41,43]. The 10-fold cross validation (10-fold CV) and the leave-one-out cross validation (LOOCV) approaches and median values of AUC, accuracy, sensitivity, specificity, PPV and NPV were obtained.

Feature selection with the least absolute shrinkage and selection operator (LASSO) method [48] was performed considering both the λ value with the minimum mean squared error (minMSE) and the largest λ value within one standard error of it (1SE) [49].

In addition, the self-adaptive synthetic over-sampling (SASYNO) approach and the adaptive synthetic sampling (ADASYN) approach, to help balance the classes (malignant and benign), were used [50–55].

The best model was chosen considering the highest area under the ROC curve and highest accuracy.

A p-value < 0.05 was considered as significant.

3. Results

The time interval between CEM and DCE-MRI was 2.5 days as a median value (range 1–16 days).

Table 2 reports the diagnostic performance of significant textural parameters for DCE-MRI and for dual-energy CEM in all views (i.e., CC, early and late MLO view), expressed in terms of AUC and p-value. The best result, considering the single feature in a univariate approach, was reached by the energy, range and GLN_GLRLM extracted on DCE-MRI volume with an AUC of 0.72.

Table 2. Accuracy of significant textural parameters for DCE-MRI and for dual-energy CEM CC, early and late MLO view.

Mammography Projection	Textural Parameters	AUC Values	p-Value
CC-view	IQR	0.67	0.01
	Variance	0.68	0.01
	Correlation	0.69	0.000
MLO view	Kurtosis	0.71	0.000
	Skewness	0.71	0.000
	Textural Parameters	AUC Values	p-Value
	Range	0.72	0.001
	Energy	0.72	0.001
Magnetic Resonance Images	Entropy	0.70	0.003
	GLN_GLRLM	0.72	0.001
	GLN_GLSZM	0.70	0.002

Figure 1 shows ROC curve trends of significant textural features: variance, correlation and IQR for mammography CC projection, kurtosis and skewness for mammography early-MLO projection and range, energy, entropy, GLN_GLRLM and GLN_GLSZM for DCE-MRI images.

Figure 2 shows the boxplots related to the above-mentioned parameters, to separate benign from malignant lesions.

Table 3 reports the performance achieved by the best classifiers designed to discriminate between benign and malignant lesions using CEM and DCE-MRI images.

The best performance, considering the CC view (ACC = 0.71; SENS = 0.71; SPEC = 0.71; PPV = 0.71; NPV = 0.71; AUC = 0.77), was reached with an SVM trained with 10-fold CV and balanced data (with SASYNO function) and a subset of four features (by LASSO and λminMSE). The subset of four robust textural features includes IQR, VARIANCE, CORRELATION and RLV.

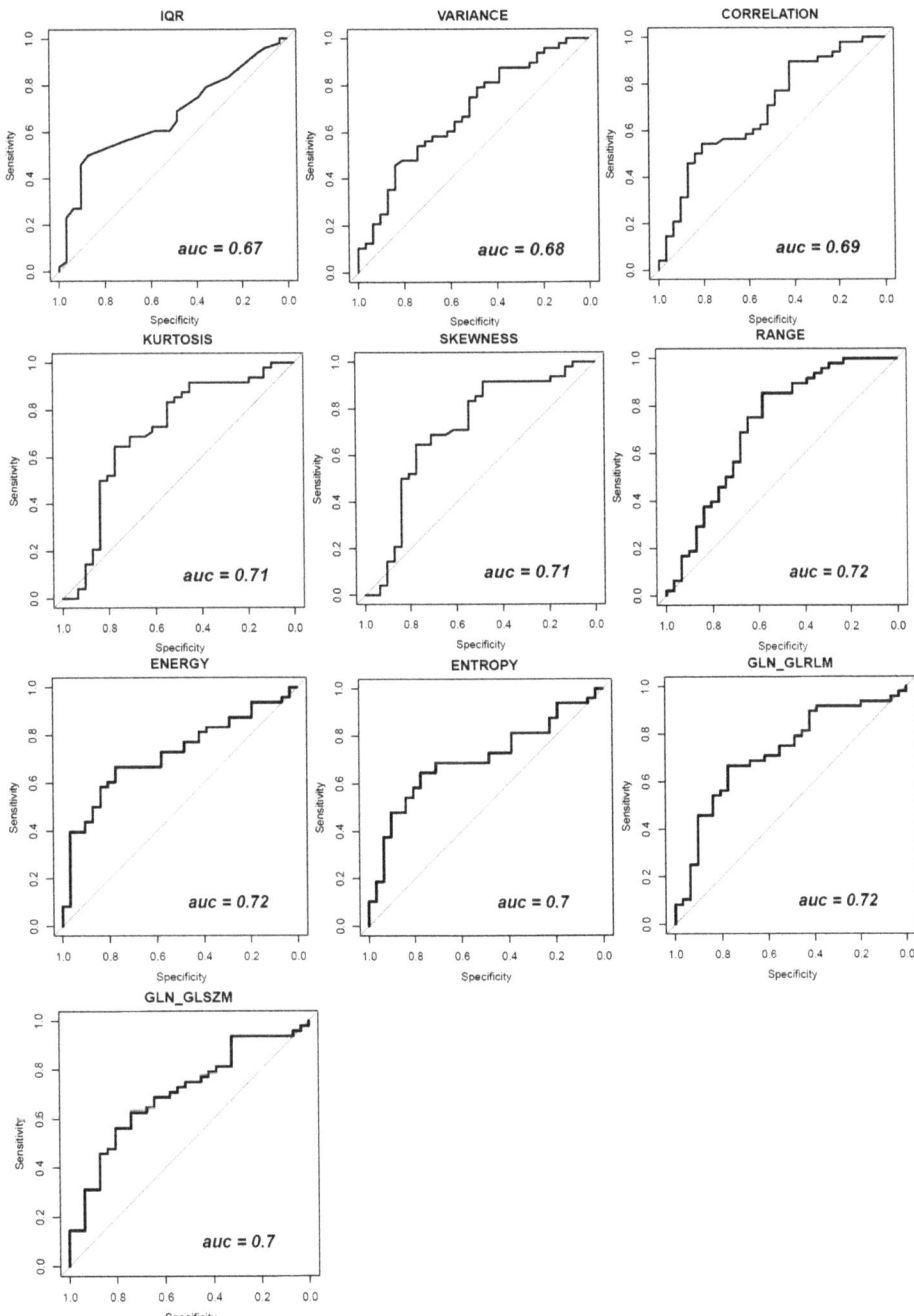

Figure 1. ROC curve trends of significant textural features for DCE-MRI and for dual-energy CEM CC, early and late MLO view.

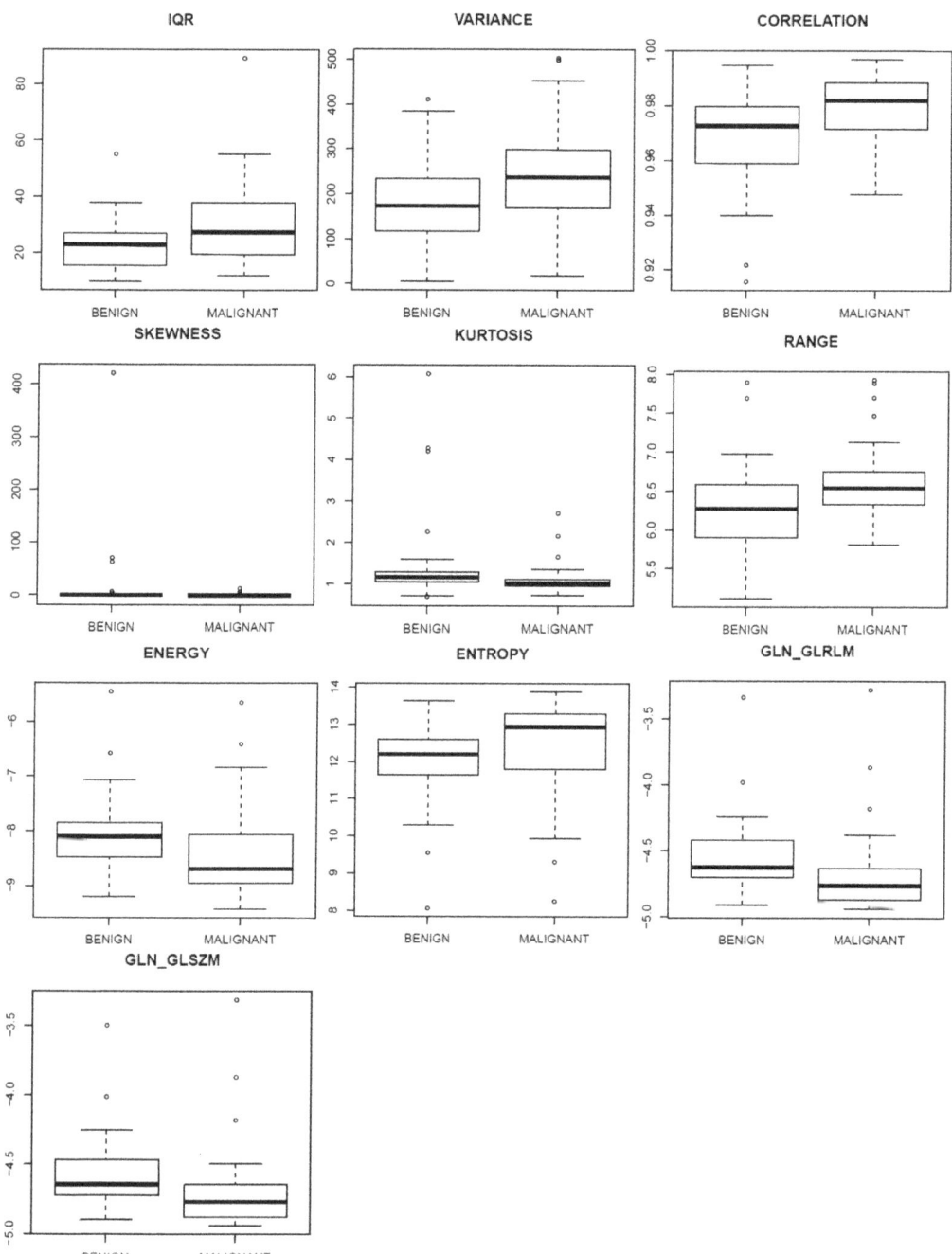

Figure 2. Boxplots of significant textural features for DCE-MRI and for dual-energy CEM CC, early and late MLO view.

Table 3. Performance of the best classifiers designed to discriminate between benign and malignant lesions.

Classifier	Cross-Validation	ACC	SENS	SPEC	PPV	NPV	AUC
\multicolumn{8}{c}{CEM–CC view}							
\multicolumn{8}{c}{Performance of classifiers trained with balanced data (with ADASYN function) and a subset of 34 textural features (AUC ≥ 0.60).}							
TREE	10-fold CV	0.74	0.74	0.78	0.76	0.74	0.73
\multicolumn{8}{c}{Performance of classifiers trained with balanced data (with SASYNO function) and a subset of 4 robust textural features (by LASSO and λ_{minMSE}).}							
LDA	10-fold CV	0.71	0.71	0.71	0.71	0.71	0.76
LDA	LOOCV	0.71	0.71	0.71	0.71	0.71	0.75
SVM	10-fold CV	0.71	0.71	0.71	0.71	0.71	0.77
\multicolumn{8}{c}{Performance of classifiers trained with balanced data (with SASYNO function) and a subset of 3 robust textural features (by LASSO and λ_{1SE}).}							
LDA	10-fold CV	0.71	0.71	0.71	0.71	0.71	0.76
LDA	LOOCV	0.71	0.71	0.71	0.71	0.71	0.75
NNET	10-fold CV	0.70	0.71	0.69	0.69	0.70	0.74
NNET	LOOCV	0.70	0.73	0.67	0.69	0.71	0.74
SVM	10-fold CV	0.71	0.71	0.71	0.71	0.71	0.75
SVM	LOOCV	0.72	0.73	0.71	0.71	0.72	0.76
\multicolumn{8}{c}{CEM–early MLO view}							
\multicolumn{8}{c}{Performance of classifiers trained with balanced data (with ADASYN function) and all 48 textural features}							
LDA	10-fold CV	0.76	0.65	0.87	0.82	0.74	0.73
LDA	LOOCV	0.75	0.60	0.87	0.81	0.72	0.71
\multicolumn{8}{c}{Performance of classifiers trained with balanced data (with ADASYN function) and a subset of 7 robust textural features (by LASSO and λ_{minMSE}).}							
LDA	10-fold CV	0.66	0.54	0.75	0.65	0.65	0.72
LDA	LOOCV	0.66	0.56	0.75	0.66	0.66	0.7
\multicolumn{8}{c}{Performance of classifiers trained with balanced data (with ADASYN function) and a subset of 14 robust textural features (by LASSO and λ_{1SE}).}							
LDA	10 fold CV	0.62	0.52	0.69	0.60	0.62	0.71
LDA	LOOCV	0.66	0.56	0.75	0.66	0.66	0.7
\multicolumn{8}{c}{CEM–late MLO view}							
\multicolumn{8}{c}{Performance of classifiers trained with balanced data (with ADASYN function) and all 48 textural features}							
LDA	10-fold CV	0.78	0.71	0.84	0.79	0.77	0.78
LDA	LOOCV	0.78	0.69	0.86	0.80	0.76	0.77

Table 3. *Cont.*

Classifier	Cross-Validation	ACC	SENS	SPEC	PPV	NPV	AUC
CEM–late MLO view							
Performance of classifiers trained with balanced data (with ADASYN function) and a subset of 17 robust textural features (by LASSO and λ_{minMSE}).							
LDA	10-fold CV	0.75	0.71	0.77	0.72	0.75	0.8
LDA	LOOCV	0.73	0.71	0.75	0.71	0.75	0.8
NNET	10-fold CV	0.72	0.65	0.77	0.70	0.72	0.78
NNET	LOOCV	0.72	0.69	0.75	0.70	0.74	0.72
Performance of classifiers trained with balanced data (with ADASYN function) and a subset of 14 robust textural features (by LASSO and λ_{1SE}).							
LDA	10-fold CV	0.71	0.69	0.71	0.67	0.73	0.78
LDA	LOOCV	0.70	0.69	0.71	0.67	0.73	0.78
NNET	10-fold CV	0.71	0.67	0.75	0.70	0.72	0.74
NNET	LOOCV	0.74	0.69	0.79	0.73	0.75	0.74
CEM–CC + early MLO + late view							
Performance of classifiers trained with balanced data (with ADASYN function) and a subset of 15 robust textural features (by LASSO and λ_{minMSE}).							
LDA	10-fold CV	0.75	0.69	0.81	0.77	0.75	0.82
LDA	LOOCV	0.76	0.71	0.81	0.77	0.76	0.81
NNET	10-fold CV	0.77	0.75	0.80	0.77	0.78	0.79
NNET	LOOCV	0.79	0.75	0.81	0.78	0.79	0.81
SVM	10-fold CV	0.72	0.73	0.70	0.69	0.75	0.79
SVM	LOOCV	0.76	0.73	0.80	0.76	0.77	0.81
Performance of classifiers trained with balanced data (with ADASYN function) and a subset of 8 robust textural features (by LASSO and λ_{1SE}).							
NNET	10-fold CV	0.72	0.73	0.72	0.70	0.75	0.78
DCE-MRI							
Performance of classifiers trained with balanced data (with ADASYN function) and all 48 textural features							
LDA	10-fold CV	0.73	0.69	0.77	0.73	0.73	0.71
LDA	LOOCV	0.70	0.65	0.75	0.70	0.70	0.7
Performance of classifiers trained with balanced data (with SASYNO function) and a subset of 15 robust textural features (by LASSO and λ_{minMSE}).							
SVM	10-fold CV	0.74	0.73	0.75	0.74	0.73	0.72
SVM	LOOCV	0.70	0.69	0.71	0.70	0.69	0.71

The best performance, considering the early-MLO view (ACC = 0.76; SENS = 0.65; SPEC = 0.87; PPV = 0.82; NPV = 0.74; AUC = 0.73), was reached with an LDA trained with 10-fold CV and trained with balanced data (with ADASYN function) and all 48 textural features.

The best performance, considering the late-MLO view (ACC = 0.75; SENS = 0.71; SPEC = 0.77; PPV = 0.72; NPV = 0.75; AUC = 0.80), was reached with an LDA trained with 10-fold CV and balanced data (with ADASYN function) and a subset of 17 features (by LASSO). The subset of 17 robust textural features includes MEAN, MODE, MAD, RANGE,

VARIANCE, CONTRAST, CORRELATION, SRLGE, LRLGE, RLV, SZE, SZLGE, SZHGE, GLV_GLSZM, BUSYNESS, COMPLEXITY and STRENGTH.

The best performance, considering all three mammographic projections (ACC = 0.79; SENS = 0.75; SPEC = 0.81; PPV = 0.78; NPV = 0.79; AUC = 0.81), was reached with an NNET trained with LOOCV and balanced data (with ADASYN function) and a subset of 15 features (by LASSO). The subset of 15 robust textural features includes IQR, VARIANCE, CORRELATION, LRHGE, GLV_GLRLM and SZLGE among textural features extracted from CC view; MODE, CONTRAST and GLV_GLRLM among textural features extracted from early-MLO view; MODE, STD, RANGE, IQR, CORRELATIOND and COMPLEXITY among textural features extracted from late-MLO view.

With regard to DCE-MRI images, the best performance (ACC = 0.74; SENS = 0.73; SPEC = 0.75; PPV = 0.74; NPV = 0.73; AUC = 0.72) was reached with an SVM trained with 10-fold CV and balanced data (with SASYNO function) and a subset of 15 features (by LASSO and λminMSE). The subset of 15 robust textural features includes MODE, MEDIAN, STD, MAD, ENTROPY, SUM AVERAGE, SRE, GLN_GLRLM, SRHGE, LZE, ZSN, ZP, LZHGE, GLV_GLSZM and ZSV.

Table 4 reports the performance achieved by the best classifiers to discriminate benign from malignant lesions when features extracted from CEM and DCE-MRI were combined. The best results overall (ACC = 0.84; SENS = 0.73; SPEC = 0.92; PPV = 0.90; NPV = 0.79; AUC = 0.88) were obtained considering a subset of 18 textural features extracted from all three mammographic views (CC, early MLO and late MLO) and DCE-MRI with an LDA trained with 10-fold CV and with balanced data (with ADASYN function). The subset of 18 robust textural features (by LASSO and λminMSE) includes IQR, VARIANCE, CORRELATION, LRHGE, GLV_GLRLM and RLV among textural features extracted from CC mammographic view; MODE and CONTRAST among textural features extracted from early-MLO mammographic view; STD, RANGE, CORRELATION and COMPLEXITY among textural features extracted from late-MLO mammographic view; RANGE, KURTOSIS, AUTOCORRELATION, LRHGE, LZE and GLV_GLSZM among textural features extracted from DCE-MRI images.

Table 4. Performance achieved by the best classifiers to discriminate between benign and malignant lesions for combined CEM and DCE-MRI.

Classifier	Cross-Validation	ACC	SENS	SPEC	PPV	NPV	AUC
Performance for classifiers trained with balanced data (with ADASYN function) and a subset of 18 robust textural features (by LASSO and λ_{minMSE}).							
LDA	10-fold CV	0.84	0.73	0.92	0.90	0.79	0.88
	LOOCV	0.80	0.71	0.88	0.85	0.77	0.87
SVM	10-fold CV	0.84	0.81	0.87	0.85	0.83	0.86
	LOOCV	0.83	0.79	0.87	0.84	0.82	0.86
Performance for classifiers trained with balanced data (with SASYNO function) and a subset of 3 robust textural features (by LASSO and λ_{minMSE}).							
LDA	10-fold CV	0.79	0.79	0.79	0.79	0.79	0.88
	LOOCV	0.79	0.79	0.79	0.79	0.79	0.89
SVM	10-fold CV	0.80	0.79	0.79	0.79	0.79	0.86
	LOOCV	0.79	0.77	0.81	0.80	0.78	0.87

Figure 3 shows the ROC curves of the best classifier obtained combining features from CEM and DCE-MRI.

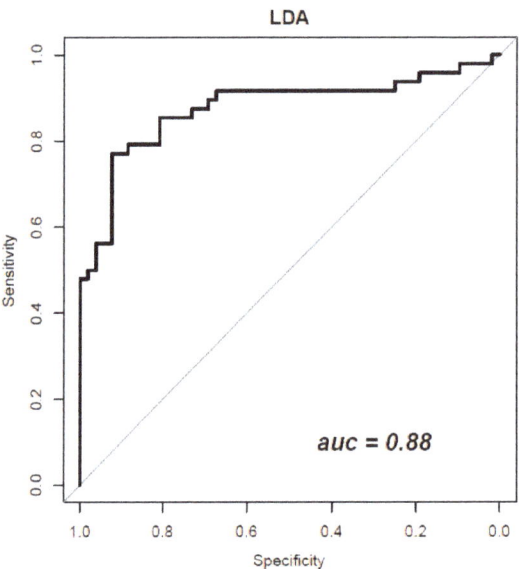

Figure 3. LDA classifier ROC curve trained with 18 robust radiomic features from CEM and DCE-MRI.

4. Discussion

Using texture features from dual-energy CEM and DCE-MRI, considered both individually and in combination, we aimed to evaluate radiomic analysis in discriminating between malignant and benign breast lesions.

In recent years, many studies have addressed the problem of breast lesion classification by using several feature categories such as textural and morphological features, in combination with different machine learning approaches, based on CEM and on DCE-MRI images analysis considered separately [30–41,56–60].

Marino et al. [61] investigated the potential of radiomic analysis of both CEM and DCE-MRI of the breast for the non-invasive assessment of tumor invasiveness, hormone receptor status and tumor grade in patients with primary breast cancer. This retrospective study included 48 female patients with 49 biopsy-proven breast cancers who underwent pretreatment breast CEM and MRI. Radiomic analysis was performed by using MaZda software. Radiomic parameters were correlated with tumor histology (invasive vs. non-invasive), hormonal status (HR+ vs. HR−) and grading (low grade G1 + G2 vs. high grade G3). CEM radiomics analysis yielded classification accuracies of up to 92% for invasive vs. non-invasive breast cancers, 95.6% for HR+ vs. HR− breast cancers and 77.8% for G1 + G2 vs. G3 invasive cancers. MRI radiomics analysis yielded classification accuracies of up to 90% for invasive vs. non-invasive breast cancers, 82.6% for HR+ vs. HR− breast cancers and 77.8% for G1 + G2 vs. G3 cancers. Their study, however, did not reported the combination of radiomic features extracted from CEM and DCE-MRI.

Jiang et al. [62] noninvasively evaluated the use of intratumoral and peritumoral regions from full-field digital mammography (DM), digital breast tomosynthesis (DBT) and dynamic contrast-enhanced and diffusion-weighted (DW) magnetic resonance imaging images separately and combined to predict the Ki-67 level based on radiomics. Their results demonstrated that the combined intra- and peritumoral radiomic signatures improved the AUC compared with the intra- or peritumoral radiomic signature in each modality. The nomogram incorporating the multi-model radiomics signature, age and lymph node metastasis status achieved the best prediction performance in the training (AUC = 0.922) and validation (AUC = 0.866) cohorts.

Zhao et al. [63] constructed radiomic models from DCE-MRI and mammography for the values in the diagnosis of breast cancer, reporting an accuracy of the individual model of 83.2% for DCE-MRI, 75.7% for mammography lesion, 64.4% for mammography margin and 77.2% for lesion + margin. When all features were combined, the accuracy increased to 89.6%.

Niu et al. [64] evaluated digital mammography, DBT, DCE- and DW-MRI, individually and combined, for the values in the diagnosis of breast cancer. They reported that the radiomic signature derived from DBT plus DM generated a lower AUC and sensitivity, but a higher specificity compared with that from DCE plus DWI. The nomogram integrating the combined radiomic signature, age and menstruation status achieved the best diagnostic performance in the training (AUC = 0.975) and validation (AUC = 0.983) cohorts.

Our results demonstrated that, considering the single metrics extracted from CEM, the best predictors were KURTOSIS (area under ROC curve (AUC) = 0.71) and SKEWNESS (AUC = 0.71) calculated on late MLO view. Considering the features calculated from DCE-MRI, the best predictors were RANGE (AUC = 0.72), ENERGY (AUC = 0.72), ENTROPY (AUC = 0.70) and GLN (Gray-Level Nonuniformity) of the gray-level run-length matrix (AUC = 0.72).

Considering the analysis with classifiers and the unbalanced dataset, no significant results were obtained. After the balancing and feature selection procedures, higher values of accuracy, specificity and AUC were reached. The best performance was obtained considering 18 robust features among all metrics derived from CEM and DCE-MRI, using a linear discriminant analysis (accuracy of 0.84 and AUC = 0.88).

This study had some limitations. The small cohort of studied patients represents a preliminary result to validate increasing the cohort of patients. Manual segmentation was time-consuming and could be operator-dependent and lose reproducibility; however, an automatic segmentation considering possible multicentric lesions or background parenchymal enhancement could be difficult to perform. In this study, the histological differences of tumors were not considered. This could improve the performance in the classification problem and allow for the classification of breast lesions according to grading and histotype.

Both DCE-MRI and CEM provide functional information on neoplastic neo-angiogenesis. CEM is an attractive alternative when MRI is not available, contraindicated or poorly tolerated. However, at our institution, a study protocol to compare DCE-MRI and CEM in staging and follow-up in breast cancer is still ongoing. Therefore, a future endpoint could be to design separate classifiers for CEM and DCE-MRI images and then merge the results in specific clinical settings, such as during patient follow-up in cases of suspicious local recurrence.

5. Conclusions

In conclusion, classifiers adjusted with adaptive synthetic sampling and feature selection allowed for increased diagnostic performance of CEM and DCE-MRI in the differentiation between benign and malignant lesions.

Author Contributions: Formal analysis, R.F., E.D.B. and A.P. (Adele Piccirillo); Investigation, V.G., M.R.R., T.P., M.L.B., M.M.R., P.V., C.R., C.S., F.A., G.S., M.D.B. and A.P. (Antonella Petrillo); Methodology, R.F., E.D.B., A.P. (Adele Piccirillo), V.G., M.R.R., T.P., M.L.B., R.D.G. and A.P. (Antonella Petrillo); Writing–original draft, R.F.; Writing—review and editing, R.F. All authors have read and agreed to the published version of the manuscript.

Funding: This research received no external funding.

Institutional Review Board Statement: The study was approved by the Ethics Committee of the National Cancer Institute of Naples Pascale Foundation (Deliberation N. 617 of 9 August 2016).

Informed Consent Statement: Each patient signed the informed consent.

Data Availability Statement: Data are available at link https://zenodo.org/record/6344730#.YixvazXSK3A (accessed on 20 January 2022).

Acknowledgments: The authors are grateful to Alessandra Trocino, librarian at the National Cancer Institute of Naples, Italy. Moreover, for the collaboration, the authors are grateful for the research support of Paolo Pariate, Martina Totaro and Andrea Esposito of the Radiology Division at Istituto Nazionale Tumori IRCCS Fondazione Pascale–IRCCS di Napoli, I-80131 Naples, Italy.

Conflicts of Interest: The authors declare no conflicts of interest.

Appendix A. Definition of Textural Features

Appendix A.1. First-Order Gray-Level Statistics

First-order gray-level statistics describe the distribution of gray values within the volume. Let X denote the 3-D image matrix with N voxels, P the first order histogram, $P(i)$ the fraction of voxels with intensity level i and Nl the number of discrete intensity levels.

- Mean, the mean gray level of X.

$$mean = \frac{1}{N} \sum_{i=1}^{N} X(i)$$

- Mode, the most frequent element(s) of array X.
- Median, the sample median of X or the 50th percentile of X.
- Standard deviation (STD)

$$STD = \left(\frac{1}{N-1} \sum_{i=1}^{N} (X(i) - \overline{X})^2 \right)^{1/2}$$

- Mean Absolute Deviation (MAD), the mean of the absolute deviation of all voxel intensities around the mean intensity value.

$$MAD = \frac{1}{N} \sum_{i=1}^{N} |X(i) - \overline{X}|$$

- Range, the range of intensity values of X.

$$range = \max(X) - \min(X)$$

where $\max(X)$ is the maximum intensity value of X and $\min(X)$ is the minimum intensity value of X.

- Interquartile range (IQR), the interquartile range is defined as the 75th minus the 25th percentile of X.
- Kurtosis:

$$kurtosis = \frac{\frac{1}{N} \sum_{i=1}^{N} (X(i) - \overline{X})^4}{\left(\sqrt{\frac{1}{N} \sum_{i=1}^{N} (X(i) - \overline{X})^2} \right)^2}$$

where $\overline{X}$ is the mean of X.

- Variance, Variance is the square of the standard deviation:

$$variance = \frac{1}{N-1} \sum_{i=1}^{N} (X(i) - \overline{X})^2$$

where $\overline{X}$ is the mean of X.

- Skewness:

$$skewness = \frac{\frac{1}{N}\sum_{i=1}^{N}(X(i)-\overline{X})^3}{\left(\sqrt{\frac{1}{N}\sum_{i=1}^{N}(X(i)-\overline{X})^2}\right)^3}$$

where $\overline{X}$ is the mean of X.

Appendix A.2. Gray Level Co-Occurrence Matrix (GLCM)

A normalized GLCM is defined as $P(i,j;\delta,\alpha)$, a metric with size $N_g \times N_g$ describing the second-order joint probability function of an image, where the (i,j)th element represents the number of times the combination of intensity levels i and j occur in two pixels in the image, that are separated by a distance of δ pixels in direction α and N_g is the maximum discrete intensity level in the image. Let:

- $P(i,j)$ be the normalized (i.e., $\sum P(i,j) = 1$) co-occurrence matrix, generalized for any δ and α,
- $p_x(i) = \sum_{j=1}^{N_g} P(i,j)$,
- $p_y(j) = \sum_{i=1}^{N_g} P(i,j)$,
- μ_x be the mean of p_x, where $\mu_x = \sum_{i=1}^{N_g}\sum_{j=1}^{N_g} iP(i,j)$,
- μ_y be the mean of p_y, where $\mu_y = \sum_{i=1}^{N_g}\sum_{j=1}^{N_g} jP(i,j)$,
- σ_x be the standard deviation of p_x, where $\sigma_x = \sum_{i=1}^{N_g}\sum_{j=1}^{N_g} P(i,j)(i-\mu_x)^2$,
- σ_y be the standard deviation of p_y, where $\sigma_y = \sum_{i=1}^{N_g}\sum_{j=1}^{N_g} P(i,j)(j-\mu_y)^2$.

- Energy

$$energy = \sum_{i=1}^{N_g}\sum_{j=1}^{N_g}[P(i,j)]^2$$

- Contrast

$$contrast = \sum_{i=1}^{N_g}\sum_{j=1}^{N_g}|i-j|^2 P(i,j)$$

- Entropy

$$entropy = -\sum_{i=1}^{N_g}\sum_{j=1}^{N_g} P(i,j)log_2[P(i,j)]$$

- Homogeneity

$$homogeneity = \sum_{i=1}^{N_g}\sum_{j=1}^{N_g}\frac{P(i,j)}{1+|i-j|}$$

- Correlation

$$correlation = \frac{\sum_{i=1}^{N_g}\sum_{j=1}^{N_g} ijP(i,j) - \mu_x\mu_y}{\sigma_x\sigma_y}$$

- Sum Average

$$sum\ average = \frac{1}{N_g \times N_g}\sum_{i=1}^{N_g}\sum_{j=1}^{N_g}[iP(i,j) + jP(i,j)]$$

- Dissimilarity

$$dissimilarity = \sum_{i=1}^{N_g}\sum_{j=1}^{N_g}|i-j|P(i,j)$$

- Autocorrelation

$$autocorrelation = \sum_{i=1}^{N_g} \sum_{j=1}^{N_g} ijP(i,j)$$

Appendix A.3. Gray Level Run-Length Matrix (GLRLM)

Run-length metrics quantify gray level runs in an image. A gray level run is defined as the length in number of pixels, of consecutive pixels that have the same gray level value. In a gray level run length matrix $p(i,j|\theta)$, the (i,j)th element describes the number of times j a gray level i appears consecutively in the direction specified by θ. Let:

- $p(i,j)$ be the (i,j)th entry in the given run-length matrix p, generalized for any direction θ,
- N_g be the number of discrete intensity values in the image,
- N_r be the maximum run length,
- N_s be the total numbers of runs, where $N_s = \sum_{i=1}^{N_g} \sum_{j=1}^{N_r} p(i,j)$,
- p_r be the sum distribution of the number of runs with run length j, where $p_r(j) = \sum_{i=1}^{N_g} p(i,j)$,
- p_g be the sum distribution of the number of runs with run length i, where $p_g(i) = \sum_{j=1}^{N_r} p(i,j)$,
- N_p be the number of voxels in the image, where $N_p = \sum_{j=1}^{N_r} jp_r$,
- μ_r be the mean run length, where $\mu_r = \sum_{i=1}^{N_g} \sum_{j=1}^{N_r} jp_n(i,j)$,
- μ_g be the mean gray level, where $\mu_g = \sum_{i=1}^{N_g} \sum_{j=1}^{N_r} ip_n(i,j)$.

- Short-Run Emphasis (SRE)

$$SRE = \sum_{j=1}^{N_r} \frac{p_r}{j^2}$$

- Long-Run Emphasis (LRE)

$$LRE = \sum_{j=1}^{N_r} j^2 p_r$$

- Gray Level Nonuniformity (GLN)

$$GLN = \sum_{i=1}^{N_g} p_g{}^2$$

- Run-Length Nonuniformity (RLN)

$$RLN = \sum_{j=1}^{N_r} p_r{}^2$$

- Run Percentage (RP)

$$RP = \frac{N_s}{N_p}$$

- Low Gray Level Run Emphasis (LGRE)

$$LGRE = \sum_{i=1}^{N_g} \frac{p_g}{i^2}$$

- High Gray Level Run Emphasis (HGRE)

$$HGRE = \sum_{i=1}^{N_g} i^2 p_g$$

- Short-Run Low Gray Level Emphasis (SRLGE)

$$SRLGE = \sum_{i=1}^{N_g} \sum_{j=1}^{N_r} \frac{p(i,j)}{i^2 j^2}$$

- Short-Run High Gray Level Emphasis (SRHGE)

$$SRHGE = \sum_{i=1}^{N_g} \sum_{j=1}^{N_r} \frac{p(i,j)i^2}{j^2}$$

- Long-Run Low Gray Level Emphasis (LRLGE)

$$LRLGE = \sum_{i=1}^{N_g} \sum_{j=1}^{N_r} \frac{p(i,j)j^2}{i^2}$$

- Long-Run High Gray Level Emphasis (LRHGE)

$$LRHGE = \sum_{i=1}^{N_g} \sum_{j=1}^{N_r} p(i,j)i^2 j^2$$

- Gray Level Variance (GLV)

$$GLV = \frac{1}{N_g \times N_r} \sum_{i=1}^{N_g} \sum_{j=1}^{N_r} (ip(i,j) - \mu_g)^2$$

- Run-Length Variance (RLV)

$$RLV = \frac{1}{N_g \times N_r} \sum_{i=1}^{N_g} \sum_{j=1}^{N_r} (jp(i,j) - \mu_r)^2$$

Appendix A.4. Gray Level Size Zone Matrix (GLSZM)

A gray level size zone matrix describes the amount of homogeneous connected areas within the volume, of a certain size and intensity. The (i,j) entry of the GLSZM $p(i,j)$ is the number of connected areas of gray level (i.e., intensity value) i and size j. GLSZM features therefore describe homogeneous areas within the tumor volume, describing tumor heterogeneity at a regional scale [5]. Let:

- $p(i,j)$ be the (i,j)th entry in the given GLSZM p,
- N_g be the number of discrete intensity values in the image,
- N_z be the size of the largest, homogeneous region in the volume of interest,
- N_s be the total number of homogeneous regions (zones), where $N_s = \sum_{i=1}^{N_g} \sum_{j=1}^{N_z} p(i,j)$,
- p_z be the sum distribution of the number of zones with size j, where $p_z(j) = \sum_{i=1}^{N_g} p(i,j)$,
- p_g be the sum distribution of the number of zones with gray level i, where $p_g(i) = \sum_{j=1}^{N_z} p(i,j)$,
- N_p be the number of voxels in the image, where $N_p = \sum_{j=1}^{N_z} j p_r$,

- μ_r be the mean zone size, where $\mu_r = \sum_{i=1}^{N_g} \sum_{j=1}^{N_z} jp(i,j|\theta)$,
- μ_g be the mean gray level, where $\mu_g = \sum_{i=1}^{N_g} \sum_{j=1}^{N_z} ip(i,j|\theta)$.

- Small Zone Emphasis (SZE)

$$SZE = \sum_{j=1}^{N_z} \frac{p_z}{j^2}$$

- Large Zone Emphasis (LZE)

$$LZE = \sum_{j=1}^{N_z} j^2 p_z$$

- Gray Level Nonuniformity (GLN)

$$GLN = \sum_{i=1}^{N_g} p_g{}^2$$

- Zone Size Nonuniformity (ZSN)

$$ZSN = \sum_{i=1}^{N_g} p_z{}^2$$

- Zone Percentage (ZP)

$$ZP = \frac{N_s}{N_p}$$

- Low Gray Level Zone Emphasis (LGZE)

$$LGZE = \sum_{i=1}^{N_g} \frac{p_g}{i^2}$$

- High Gray Level Zone Emphasis (HGZE)

$$HGZE = \sum_{i=1}^{N_g} i^2 p_g$$

- Small Zone Low Gray Level Emphasis (SZLGE)

$$SZLGE = \sum_{i=1}^{N_g} \sum_{j=1}^{N_z} \frac{p(i,j)}{i^2 j^2}$$

- Small Zone High Gray Level Emphasis (SZHGE)

$$SZHGE = \sum_{i=1}^{N_g} \sum_{j=1}^{N_z} \frac{p(i,j)i^2}{j^2}$$

- Large Zone Low Gray Level Emphasis (LZLGE)

$$LZLGE = \sum_{i=1}^{N_g} \sum_{j=1}^{N_z} \frac{p(i,j)j^2}{i^2}$$

- Large Zone High Gray Level Emphasis (LZHGE)

$$LZHGE = \sum_{i=1}^{N_g} \sum_{j=1}^{N_z} p(i,j) j^2 i^2$$

- Gray Level Variance (GLV)

$$GLV = \frac{1}{N_g \times N_z} \sum_{i=1}^{N_g} \sum_{j=1}^{N_z} (ip(i,j) - \mu_g)^2$$

- Zone Size Variance (ZSV)

$$ZSV = \frac{1}{N_g \times N_z} \sum_{i=1}^{N_g} \sum_{j=1}^{N_z} (jp(i,j) - \mu_z)^2$$

Appendix A.5. Neighborhood Gray Tone Difference Matrix (NGTDM)

The ith entry of the NGTDM $s(i|d)$ is the sum of gray level differences of voxels with intensity i and the average intensity A_i of their neighboring voxels within a distance d. Let:

- n_i be the number of voxels with gray level i,
- $N = \sum n_i$ be the total number of voxels,
- $s(i) = \begin{cases} \sum_{n_i} |i - A_i| \text{ for } n_i > 0 \\ 0 \text{ otherwise} \end{cases}$ be generalized for any distance d,
- N_g be the maximum discrete intensity level in the image,
- $p(i) = \frac{n_i}{N}$ be the probability of gray level i,
- N_p be the total number of gray levels present in the image.

- Coarseness:

$$coarseness = \left[\varepsilon + \sum_{n=1}^{N_g} p(i)s(i)\right]^{-1}$$

where ε is a small number to prevent coarseness from becoming infinite.

- Contrast

$$contrast = \left(\frac{1}{N_p(1-N_p)} \sum_{i=1}^{N_g} \sum_{j=1}^{N_g} p(i)p(j)(i-j)^2\right) \left(\frac{1}{N} \sum_{i=1}^{N_g} s(i)\right)$$

- Busyness

$$busyness = \frac{\sum_{i=1}^{N_g} p(i)s(i)}{\sum_{i=1}^{N_g} \sum_{j=1}^{N_g} |ip(i) - jp(j)|}, \qquad p(i) \neq 0, \, p(j) \neq 0$$

- Complexity

$$complexity = \sum_{i=1}^{N_g} \sum_{j=1}^{N_g} |i-j| \frac{p(i)s(i) + p(j)s(j)}{N(p(i)+p(j))}, \qquad p(i) \neq 0, \, p(j) \neq 0$$

- Strength

$$strength = \frac{\sum_{i=1}^{N_g} \sum_{j=1}^{N_g} [p(i)+p(j)](i-j)^2}{\varepsilon + \sum_{n=1}^{N_g} s(i)}, \qquad p(i) \neq 0, \, p(j) \neq 0$$

where ε is a small number to prevent strength from becoming infinite.

References

1. Patel, B.K.; Lobbes, M.; Lewin, J. Contrast Enhanced Spectral Mammography: A Review. *Semin. Ultrasound CT MRI* **2018**, *39*, 70–79. [CrossRef]
2. Heywang-Köbrunner, S.; Viehweg, P.; Heinig, A.; Küchler, C. Contrast-enhanced MRI of the breast: Accuracy, value, controversies, solutions. *Eur. J. Radiol.* **1997**, *24*, 94–108. [CrossRef]
3. Viehweg, P.; Paprosch, I.; Strassinopoulou, M.; Heywang-Köbrunner, S.H. Contrast-enhanced magnetic resonance imaging of the breast: Interpretation guidelines. *Top. Magn. Reson. Imaging* **1998**, *9*, 17–43. [CrossRef] [PubMed]
4. Dromain, C.; Balleyguier, C.; Muller, S.; Mathieu, M.-C.; Rochard, F.; Opolon, P.; Sigal, R. Evaluation of Tumor Angiogenesis of Breast Carcinoma Using Contrast-Enhanced Digital Mammography. *Am. J. Roentgenol.* **2006**, *187*, 528–537. [CrossRef] [PubMed]
5. Baltzer, P.A.; Bickel, H.; Spick, C.; Wengert, G.; Woitek, R.; Kapetas, P.; Clauser, P.; Helbich, T.H.; Pinker, K. Potential of Noncontrast Magnetic Resonance Imaging with Diffusion-Weighted Imaging in Characterization of Breast Lesions. *Investig. Radiol.* **2018**, *53*, 229–235. [CrossRef] [PubMed]
6. Pinker, K.; Moy, L.; Sutton, E.J.; Mann, R.; Weber, M.; Thakur, S.; Jochelson, M.S.; Bago-Horvath, Z.; Morris, E.A.; Baltzer, P.A.; et al. Diffusion-Weighted Imaging with Apparent Diffusion Coefficient Mapping for Breast Cancer Detection as a Stand-Alone Parameter: Comparison with Dynamic Contrast-Enhanced and Multiparametric Magnetic Resonance Imaging. *Investig. Radiol.* **2018**, *53*, 587–595. [CrossRef]
7. Liu, Z.; Feng, B.; Li, C.; Chen, Y.; Chen, Q.; Li, X.; Guan, J.; Chen, X.; Cui, E.; Li, R.; et al. Preoperative prediction of lymphovascular invasion in invasive breast cancer with dynamic contrast-enhanced-MRI-based radiomics. *J. Magn. Reson. Imaging* **2019**, *50*, 847–857. [CrossRef]
8. Li, L.; Roth, R.; Germaine, P.; Ren, S.; Lee, M.; Hunter, K.; Tinney, E.; Liao, L. Contrast-enhanced spectral mammography (CESM) versus breast magnetic resonance imaging (MRI): A retrospective comparison in 66 breast lesions. *Diagn. Interv. Imaging* **2017**, *98*, 113–123. [CrossRef]
9. Fallenberg, E.M.; Dromain, C.; Diekmann, F.; Engelken, F.; Krohn, M.; Singh, J.M.; Ingold-Heppner, B.; Winzer, K.J.; Bick, U.; Renz, D.M. Contrast-enhanced spectral mammography versus MRI: Initial results in the detection of breast cancer and assessment of tumour size. *Eur. Radiol.* **2014**, *24*, 256–264. [CrossRef]
10. Lewin, J.M.; Isaacs, P.K.; Vance, V.; Larke, F.J. Dual-Energy Contrast-enhanced Digital Subtraction Mammography: Feasibility. *Radiology* **2003**, *229*, 261–268. [CrossRef]
11. Jochelson, M.S.; Dershaw, D.D.; Sung, J.; Heerdt, A.; Thornton, C.; Moskowitz, C.S.; Ferrara, J.; Morris, E. Bilateral Contrast-enhanced Dual-Energy Digital Mammography: Feasibility and Comparison with Conventional Digital Mammography and MR Imaging in Women with Known Breast Carcinoma. *Radiology* **2013**, *266*, 743–751. [CrossRef] [PubMed]
12. Tagliafico, A.S.; Bignotti, B.; Rossi, F.; Signori, A.; Sormani, M.P.; Valdora, F.; Calabrese, M.; Houssami, N. Diagnostic performance of contrast-enhanced spectral mammography: Systematic review and meta-analysis. *Breast* **2016**, *28*, 13–19. [CrossRef] [PubMed]
13. Liney, G.P.; Sreenivas, M.; Gibbs, P.; Bsc, R.G.-A.; Turnbull, L.W. Breast lesion analysis of shape technique: Semiautomated vs. manual morphological description. *J. Magn. Reson. Imaging* **2006**, *23*, 493–498. [CrossRef] [PubMed]
14. Fusco, R.; Sansone, M.; Filice, S.; Carone, G.; Amato, D.M.; Sansone, C.; Petrillo, A. Pattern Recognition Approaches for Breast Cancer DCE-MRI Classification: A Systematic Review. *J. Med. Biol. Eng.* **2016**, *36*, 449–459. [CrossRef]
15. Nie, K.; Chen, J.-H.; Yu, H.J.; Chu, Y.; Nalcioglu, O.; Su, M.-Y. Quantitative Analysis of Lesion Morphology and Texture Features for Diagnostic Prediction in Breast MRI. *Acad. Radiol.* **2008**, *15*, 1513–1525. [CrossRef] [PubMed]
16. Hu, H.-T.; Shan, Q.-Y.; Chen, S.-L.; Li, B.; Feng, S.-T.; Xu, E.-J.; Li, X.; Long, J.-Y.; Xie, X.-Y.; Lu, M.-D.; et al. CT-based radiomics for preoperative prediction of early recurrent hepatocellular carcinoma: Technical reproducibility of acquisition and scanners. *Radiol. Med.* **2020**, *125*, 697–705. [CrossRef] [PubMed]
17. Rossi, F.; Bignotti, B.; Bianchi, L.; Picasso, R.; Martinoli, C.; Tagliafico, A.S. Radiomics of peripheral nerves MRI in mild carpal and cubital tunnel syndrome. *Radiol. Med.* **2019**, *125*, 197–203. [CrossRef]
18. Santone, A.; Brunese, M.C.; Donnarumma, F.; Guerriero, P.; Mercaldo, F.; Reginelli, A.; Miele, V.; Giovagnoni, A.; Brunese, L. Radiomic features for prostate cancer grade detection through formal verification. *Radiol. Med.* **2021**, *126*, 688–697. [CrossRef]
19. Fusco, R.; Sansone, M.; Filice, S.; Granata, V.; Catalano, O.; Amato, D.M.; Di Bonito, M.; D'Aiuto, M.; Capasso, I.; Rinaldo, M.; et al. Integration of DCE-MRI and DW-MRI Quantitative Parameters for Breast Lesion Classification. *BioMed Res. Int.* **2015**, *2015*, 237863. [CrossRef]
20. Zhang, Y.; Zhu, Y.; Zhang, K.; Liu, Y.; Cui, J.; Tao, J.; Wang, Y.; Wang, S. Invasive ductal breast cancer: Preoperative predict Ki-67 index based on radiomics of ADC maps. *Radiol. Med.* **2020**, *125*, 109–116. [CrossRef]
21. Chianca, V.; Albano, D.; Messina, C.; Vincenzo, G.; Rizzo, S.; Del Grande, F.; Sconfienza, L.M. An update in musculoskeletal tumors: From quantitative imaging to radiomics. *Radiol. Med.* **2021**, *126*, 1095–1105. [CrossRef] [PubMed]
22. Kirienko, M.; Ninatti, G.; Cozzi, L.; Voulaz, E.; Gennaro, N.; Barajon, I.; Ricci, F.; Carlo-Stella, C.; Zucali, P.; Sollini, M.; et al. Computed tomography (CT)-derived radiomic features differentiate prevascular mediastinum masses as thymic neoplasms versus lymphomas. *Radiol. Med.* **2020**, *125*, 951–960. [CrossRef]
23. Karmazanovsky, G.; Gruzdev, I.; Tikhonova, V.; Kondratyev, E.; Revishvili, A. Computed tomography-based radiomics approach in pancreatic tumors characterization. *Radiol. Med.* **2021**, *126*, 1388–1395. [CrossRef] [PubMed]

24. Cellina, M.; Pirovano, M.; Ciocca, M.; Gibelli, D.; Floridi, C.; Oliva, G. Radiomic analysis of the optic nerve at the first episode of acute optic neuritis: An indicator of optic nerve pathology and a predictor of visual recovery? *Radiol. Med.* **2021**, *126*, 698–706. [CrossRef]
25. Benedetti, G.; Mori, M.; Panzeri, M.M.; Barbera, M.; Palumbo, D.; Sini, C.; Muffatti, F.; Andreasi, V.; Steidler, S.; Doglioni, C.; et al. CT-derived radiomic features to discriminate histologic characteristics of pancreatic neuroendocrine tumors. *Radiol. Med.* **2021**, *126*, 745–760. [CrossRef] [PubMed]
26. Nazari, M.; Shiri, I.; Hajianfar, G.; Oveisi, N.; Abdollahi, H.; Deevband, M.R.; Oveisi, M.; Zaidi, H. Noninvasive Fuhrman grading of clear cell renal cell carcinoma using computed tomography radiomic features and machine learning. *Radiol. Med.* **2020**, *125*, 754–762. [CrossRef] [PubMed]
27. Crivelli, P.; Ledda, R.E.; Parascandolo, N.; Fara, A.; Soro, D.; Conti, M. A New Challenge for Radiologists: Radiomics in Breast Cancer. *BioMed Res. Int.* **2018**, *2018*, 6120703. [CrossRef] [PubMed]
28. Maglogiannis, I.; Zafiropoulos, E.; Anagnostopoulos, I. An intelligent system for automated breast cancer diagnosis and prognosis using SVM based classifiers. *Appl. Intell.* **2007**, *30*, 24–36. [CrossRef]
29. Zheng, Y.; Englander, S.; Baloch, S.; Zacharaki, E.I.; Fan, Y.; Schnall, M.D.; Shen, D. STEP: Spatiotemporal enhancement pattern for MR-based breast tumor diagnosis. *Med. Phys.* **2009**, *36*, 3192–3204. [CrossRef]
30. Lambin, P.; Rios-Velazquez, E.; Leijenaar, R.; Carvalho, S.; van Stiphout, R.G.P.M.; Granton, P.; Zegers, C.M.L.; Gillies, R.; Boellard, R.; Dekker, A.; et al. Radiomics: Extracting more information from medical images using advanced feature analysis. *Eur. J. Cancer* **2012**, *48*, 441–446. [CrossRef]
31. Sinha, S.; Ms, F.A.L.-Q.; Debruhl, N.D.; Sayre, J.; Farria, D.; Gorczyca, D.P.; Bassett, L.W. Multifeature analysis of Gd-enhanced MR images of breast lesions. *J. Magn. Reson. Imaging* **1997**, *7*, 1016–1026. [CrossRef]
32. Vomweg, T.W.; Buscema, P.M.; Kauczor, H.U.; Teifke, A.; Intraligi, M.; Terzi, S.; Heussel, C.P.; Achenbach, T.; Rieker, O.; Mayer, D.; et al. Improved artificial neural networks in prediction of malignancy of lesions in contrast-enhanced MR-mammography. *Med. Phys.* **2003**, *30*, 2350–2359. [CrossRef] [PubMed]
33. Sathya, D.J.; Geetha, K. Mass classification in breast DCE-MR images using an artificial neural network trained via a bee colony optimization algorithm. *ScienceAsia* **2013**, *39*, 294. [CrossRef]
34. Sathya, J.; Geetha, K. Experimental Investigation of Classification Algorithms for Predicting Lesion Type on Breast DCE-MR Images. *Int. J. Comput. Appl.* **2013**, *82*, 1–8. [CrossRef]
35. Fusco, R.; Sansone, M.; Petrillo, A.; Sansone, C. A Multiple Classifier System for Classification of Breast Lesions Using Dynamic and Morphological Features in DCE-MRI. In *Joint IAPR International Workshops on Statistical Techniques in Pattern Recognition (SPR) and Structural and Syntactic Pattern Recognition (SSPR)*; Springer: Berlin/Heidelberg, Germany, 2012; pp. 684–692. [CrossRef]
36. Degenhard, A.; Tanner, C.; Hayes, C.; Hawkes, D.J.; O Leach, M. The UK MRI Breast Screening Study Comparison between radiological and artificial neural network diagnosis in clinical screening. *Physiol. Meas.* **2002**, *23*, 727–739. [CrossRef]
37. Haralick, R.M.; Shanmugam, K.; Dinstein, I.H. Textural Features for Image Classification. *IEEE Trans. Syst. Man Cybern.* **1973**, *SMC-3*, 610–621. [CrossRef]
38. Fusco, R.; Sansone, M.; Sansone, C.; Petrillo, A. Segmentation and classification of breast lesions using dynamic and textural features in Dynamic Contrast Enhanced-Magnetic Resonance Imaging. In Proceedings of the 25th IEEE International Symposium on Computer-Based Medical Systems (CBMS), Rome, Italy, 20–22 June 2012; pp. 1–4.
39. Abdolmaleki, P.; Buadu, L.D.; Naderimansh, H. Feature extraction and classification of breast cancer on dynamic magnetic resonance imaging using artificial neural network. *Cancer Lett.* **2001**, *171*, 183–191. [CrossRef]
40. Agner, S.C.; Soman, S.; Libfeld, E.; McDonald, M.; Thomas, K.; Englander, S.; Rosen, M.A.; Chin, D.; Nosher, J.; Madabhushi, A. Textural Kinetics: A Novel Dynamic Contrast-Enhanced (DCE)-MRI Feature for Breast Lesion Classification. *J. Digit. Imaging* **2010**, *24*, 446–463. [CrossRef]
41. Levman, J.; Leung, T.; Causer, P.; Plewes, D.; Martel, A.L. Classification of dynamic contrast-enhanced magnetic resonance breast lesions by support vector machines. *IEEE Trans. Med. Imaging* **2008**, *27*, 688–696. [CrossRef]
42. Levman, J.; Martel, A.L. Computer-aided diagnosis of breast cancer from magnetic resonance imaging examinations by custom radial basis function vector machine. In Proceedings of the 2010 Annual International Conference of the IEEE Engineering in Medicine and Biology, Buenos Aires, Argentina, 30 August–4 September 2010; Volume 2010, pp. 5577–5580.
43. Fusco, R.; Piccirillo, A.; Sansone, M.; Granata, V.; Rubulotta, M.; Petrosino, T.; Barretta, M.; Vallone, P.; Di Giacomo, R.; Esposito, E.; et al. Radiomics and Artificial Intelligence Analysis with Textural Metrics Extracted by Contrast-Enhanced Mammography in the Breast Lesions Classification. *Diagnostics* **2021**, *11*, 815. [CrossRef]
44. Fusco, R.; Piccirillo, A.; Sansone, M.; Granata, V.; Vallone, P.; Barretta, M.L.; Petrosino, T.; Siani, C.; Di Giacomo, R.; Di Bonito, M.; et al. Radiomic and Artificial Intelligence Analysis with Textural Metrics, Morphological and Dynamic Perfusion Features Extracted by Dynamic Contrast-Enhanced Magnetic Resonance Imaging in the Classification of Breast Lesions. *Appl. Sci.* **2021**, *11*, 1880. [CrossRef]
45. Vallières, M.; Freeman, C.R.; Skamene, S.R.; El Naqa, I. A radiomics model from joint FDG-PET and MRI texture features for the prediction of lung metastases in soft-tissue sarcomas of the extremities. *Phys. Med. Biol.* **2015**, *60*, 5471–5496. [CrossRef]
46. Zwanenburg, A.; Vallières, M.; Abdalah, M.A.; Aerts, H.J.W.L.; Andrearczyk, V.; Apte, A.; Ashrafinia, S.; Bakas, S.; Beukinga, R.J.; Boellaard, R.; et al. The Image Biomarker Standardization Initiative: Standardized Quantitative Radiomics for High-Throughput Image-based Phenotyping. *Radiology* **2020**, *295*, 328–338. [CrossRef]

47. R-Tools Technology Inc. Available online: https://www.r-tt.com/ (accessed on 15 October 2020).
48. Tibshirani, R. The lasso Method for Variable Selection in the Cox Model. *Statist. Med.* **1997**, *16*, 385–395. [CrossRef]
49. Tibshirani, R. Regression Shrinkage and Selection Via the Lasso. *J. R. Stat. Soc. Ser. B Statist. Methodol.* **1996**, *58*, 267–288. [CrossRef]
50. Bruce, P.; Bruce, A. *Practical Statistics for Data Scientists*; O'Reilly Media, Inc.: Newton, MA, USA, 2017.
51. James, G.; Witten, D.; Hastie, T.; Tibshirani, R. *An Introduction to Statistical Learning*; Springer: New York, NY, USA, 2013; Volume 112, p. 18.
52. Wang, Q.; Luo, Z.; Huang, J.; Feng, Y.; Liu, Z. A Novel Ensemble Method for Imbalanced Data Learning: Bagging of Extrapolation-SMOTE SVM. *Comput. Intell. Neurosci.* **2017**, *2017*, 1827016. [CrossRef] [PubMed]
53. Gu, X.; Angelov, P.P.; Soares, E.A. A self-adaptive synthetic over-sampling technique for imbalanced classification. *Int. J. Intell. Syst.* **2020**, *35*, 923–943. [CrossRef]
54. Chen, Z.; Lin, T.; Xia, X.; Xu, H.; Ding, S. A synthetic neighborhood generation-based ensemble learning for the imbalanced data classification. *Appl. Intell.* **2017**, *48*, 2441–2457. [CrossRef]
55. He, H.; Bai, Y.; Garcia, E.A.; Li, S. ADASYN: Adaptive synthetic sampling approach for imbalanced learning. In Proceedings of the 2008 IEEE International Joint Conference on Neural Networks (IEEE World Congress on Computational Intelligence), Hong Kong, China, 1–6 June 2008; pp. 1322–1328.
56. Bernardi, D.; Belli, P.; Benelli, E.; Brancato, B.; Bucchi, L.; Calabrese, M.; Carbonaro, L.A.; Caumo, F.; Cavallo-Marincola, B.; Clauser, P.; et al. Digital breast tomosynthesis (DBT): Recommendations from the Italian College of Breast Radiologists (ICBR) by the Italian Society of Medical Radiology (SIRM) and the Italian Group for Mammography Screening (GISMa). *Radiol. Med.* **2017**, *122*, 723–730. [CrossRef] [PubMed]
57. Bucchi, L.; Belli, P.; Benelli, E.; Bernardi, D.; Brancato, B.; Calabrese, M.; Carbonaro, L.A.; Caumo, F.; Cavallo-Marincola, B.; Clauser, P.; et al. Recommendations for breast imaging follow-up of women with a previous history of breast cancer: Position paper from the Italian Group for Mammography Screening (GISMa) and the Italian College of Breast Radiologists (ICBR) by SIRM. *Radiol. Med.* **2016**, *121*, 891–896. [CrossRef] [PubMed]
58. Losurdo, L.; Fanizzi, A.; Basile, T.M.A.; Bellotti, R.; Bottigli, U.; Dentamaro, R.; Didonna, V.; Lorusso, V.; Massafra, R.; Tamborra, P.; et al. Radiomics Analysis on Contrast-Enhanced Spectral Mammography Images for Breast Cancer Diagnosis: A Pilot Study. *Entropy* **2019**, *21*, 1110. [CrossRef]
59. Fanizzi, A.; Losurdo, L.; Basile, T.M.A.; Bellotti, R.; Bottigli, U.; Delogu, P.; Diacono, D.; Didonna, V.; Fausto, A.; Lombardi, A.; et al. Fully Automated Support System for Diagnosis of Breast Cancer in Contrast-Enhanced Spectral Mammography Images. *J. Clin. Med.* **2019**, *8*, 891. [CrossRef] [PubMed]
60. La Forgia, D.; Fanizzi, A.; Campobasso, F.; Bellotti, R.; Didonna, V.; Lorusso, V.; Moschetta, M.; Massafra, R.; Tamborra, P.; Tangaro, S.; et al. Radiomic Analysis in Contrast-Enhanced Spectral Mammography for Predicting Breast Cancer Histological Outcome. *Diagnostics* **2020**, *10*, 708. [CrossRef] [PubMed]
61. Marino, M.A.; Leithner, D.; Sung, J.; Avendano, D.; Morris, E.A.; Pinker, K.; Jochelson, M.S. Radiomics for Tumor Characterization in Breast Cancer Patients: A Feasibility Study Comparing Contrast-Enhanced Mammography and Magnetic Resonance Imaging. *Diagnostics* **2020**, *10*, 492. [CrossRef]
62. Jiang, T.; Song, J.; Wang, X.; Niu, S.; Zhao, N.; Dong, Y.; Wang, X.; Luo, Y.; Jiang, X. Intratumoral and Peritumoral Analysis of Mammography, Tomosynthesis, and Multiparametric MRI for Predicting Ki-67 Level in Breast Cancer: A Radiomics-Based Study. *Mol. Imaging Biol.* **2021**, 1–10. [CrossRef]
63. Zhao, Y.-F.; Chen, Z.; Zhang, Y.; Zhou, J.; Chen, J.-H.; Lee, K.E.; Combs, F.J.; Parajuli, R.; Mehta, R.S.; Wang, M.; et al. Diagnosis of Breast Cancer Using Radiomics Models Built Based on Dynamic Contrast Enhanced MRI Combined with Mammography. *Front. Oncol.* **2021**, *11*, 774248. [CrossRef]
64. Niu, S.; Wang, X.; Zhao, N.; Liu, G.; Kan, Y.; Dong, Y.; Cui, E.-N.; Luo, Y.; Yu, T.; Jiang, X. Radiomic Evaluations of the Diagnostic Performance of DM, DBT, DCE MRI, DWI, and Their Combination for the Diagnosisof Breast Cancer. *Front. Oncol.* **2021**, *11*, 725922. [CrossRef]

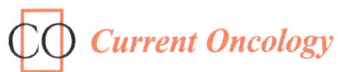

Article

Contrast-Enhanced Spectral Mammography Assessment of Patients Treated with Neoadjuvant Chemotherapy for Breast Cancer

Katarzyna Steinhof-Radwańska [1,*], Anna Grażyńska [2], Andrzej Lorek [3], Iwona Gisterek [4], Anna Barczyk-Gutowska [1], Agnieszka Bobola [4], Karolina Okas [2], Zuzanna Lelek [2], Irmina Morawska [2], Jakub Potoczny [2], Paweł Niemiec [5] and Karol Szyluk [6]

[1] Department of Radiology and Nuclear Medicine, Prof. Kornel Gibiński Independent Public Central Clinical Hospital, Medical University of Silesia, Medyków 18, 40-514 Katowice, Poland; abarczykgutkowska@gmail.com

[2] Students' Scientific Society, Department of Radiology and Nuclear Medicine, Medical University of Silesia, Medyków 18, 40-514 Katowice, Poland; grazynska.anna@gmail.com (A.G.); karolina.okas@o2.pl (K.O.); zuzkalelek@gmail.com (Z.L.); irmina.morawska@gmail.com (I.M.); potocznyjakub123@gmail.com (J.P.)

[3] Department of Oncological Surgery, Prof. Kornel Gibiński Independent Public Central Clinical Hospital, Medical University of Silesia, Medyków 18, 40-514 Katowice, Poland; ajlorek@O2.pl

[4] Department of Oncology and Radiotherapy, Prof. Kornel Gibiński Independent Public Central Clinical Hospital, Medical University of Silesia, Medyków 18, 40-514 Katowice, Poland; igisterek@sum.edu.pl (I.G.); bobola.agnieszka@gmail.com (A.B.)

[5] Department of Biochemistry and Medical Genetics, School of Health Sciences in Katowice, Medical University of Silesia, Medyków 18, 40-752 Katowice, Poland; pniemiec@sum.edu.pl

[6] 1st Department of Orthopaedic and Trauma Surgery, District Hospital of Orthopaedics and Trauma Surgery, Bytomska 62, 41-940 Piekary Śląskie, Poland; szyluk@urazowka.piekary.pl

* Correspondence: kasia.steinhof@gmail.com; Tel.: +48-32-358-1350

Abstract: Background: Evaluating the tumor response to neoadjuvant chemotherapy is key to planning further therapy of breast cancer. Our study aimed to evaluate the effectiveness of low-energy and subtraction contrast-enhanced spectral mammography (CESM) images in the detection of complete response (CR) for neoadjuvant chemotherapy (NAC) in breast cancer. Methods: A total of 63 female patients were qualified for our retrospective analysis. Low-energy and subtraction CESM images just before the beginning of NAC and as a follow-up examination 2 weeks before the end of chemotherapy were compared with one another and assessed for compliance with the postoperative histopathological examination (HP). The response to preoperative chemotherapy was evaluated based on the RECIST 1.1 criteria (Response Evaluation Criteria in Solid Tumors). Results: Low-energy images tend to overestimate residual lesions (6.28 mm) and subtraction images tend to underestimate them (2.75 mm). The sensitivity of low-energy images in forecasting CR amounted to 33.33%, while the specificity was 92.86%. In the case of subtraction CESM, the sensitivity amounted to 85.71% and the specificity to 71.42%. Conclusions: CESM is characterized by high sensitivity in the assessment of CR after NAC. The use of only morphological assessment is insufficient. CESM correlates well with the size of residual lesions on histopathological examination but tends to underestimate the dimensions.

Keywords: contrast-enhanced spectral mammography; breast cancer; neoadjuvant chemotherapy; complete response; response evaluation criteria in solid tumors

1. Introduction

Neoadjuvant chemotherapy (NAC) is currently one of the basic methods of treatment of locally advanced breast cancer [1,2]. The main advantage of NAC use is the possibility of reducing the mass of previously inoperable tumors to allow surgical intervention. In the case of massive yet operable tumors, NAC provides a decrease of their mass to a size that makes conservative surgical treatment possible. Thus, a better cosmetic effect will be achieved and fewer post-operative complications will be present [3–5]. Besides reducing the tumor mass and enabling thereby offering better conditions for local treatment (breast-conserving therapy (BCT)), NAC provides unique opportunities for in vivo chemotherapeutic evaluation of cancer cells' sensitivity, as well as for the search for new biomarkers of therapeutic response. In addition to locally advanced breast cancers, NAC has applications in some molecular subtypes of breast cancer. It is recommended for the following kinds of cancer patients: hormone receptor positive/human epidermal growth factor receptor 2 negative (HR+/HER2-) low and high risk, human epidermal growth factor receptor 2 positive (HER2+) and triple negative breast cancer (TNBC) of any size and stage. NAC is also a method of choice in cases of inflammatory breast cancer (IBC) [6–8].

Consequently, in the event of poor response and progression of the disease, NAC offers a chance to alter the treatment scheme or refer a specific patient for surgical treatment. Apart from the predictive and prognostic factors known to date, including staging, grading, HER2 status, hormone receptors status, and Ki-67% index, the therapeutic response of the tumor to NAC provides information about the patient's prognosis [9–11]. Achieving complete response (CR) upon completion of neoadjuvant therapy and surgical resection is associated with improved survival rates. CR was approved by the US Food and Drug Administration (FDA) in 2020 as the final point of clinical studies in the neoadjuvant therapy of early breast cancer with high recurrence risk [12]. However, it has to be mentioned that NAC response parameters can differ among patients due to the internal heterogeneity of tumors caused by molecular features, their clinical status, and morphological appearance. It is estimated that approximately 10–35% of female patients diagnosed with breast cancer remain chemotherapy-resistant, while in 5% NAC is completely non-reactive and leads to the disease progression [13]. In cases of such patients, NAC is a method of much lower efficacy: it deteriorates prognosis, delays surgical intervention, and increases the overall cost of therapy. Most recent research indicates its unsatisfactory results in decreasing or removing metastatic sites [11,14,15]. Despite the limitations described above, NAC is widely used in breast cancer therapy. It is estimated that approximately 7–27% of female patients suffering from breast cancer in Europe, the USA, and Australia undergo NAC treatment [2].

Evaluating the tumor response to NAC is key to planning further therapy. Underestimation of residual lesions after NAC can lead to incomplete tumor resection during surgery. This can lead to relapse or a need for reoperation. On the other hand, overestimation may result in overly radical surgical intervention, which can lead to much more serious complications. The gold standard of NAC response analysis is still histopathological examination. However, such examinations are conducted postoperatively. Due to this, it is crucial to determine and find reliable, non-invasive, and effective imaging diagnostic methods to assess NAC response in tumors.

The diagnostic imaging techniques currently used to assess response to NAC are conventional mammography (MG), ultrasound (US), photon emission tomography, and magnetic resonance imaging (MRI) with contrast enhancement (CE-MRI). CE-MRI is considered to be the most effective of these methods [16,17]. Multiple studies have shown that dynamic contrast-enhanced MRI is the optimal imaging tool to determine disease response, with a sensitivity reaching 90%, specificity of 60% to 100%, and accuracy of approximately 91%. However, CE-MRI remains an expensive method with limited access in local diagnostic centers. Patients with contraindications and who are unable to tolerate examination conditions (i.e., claustrophobia, psychic comfort, old-type pacemakers) cannot undergo such examinations [18–22]. Furthermore, some research shows that MRI may under- as well as overestimate the size of residual lesions in 18% of cases [23]. Considering all these aspects, the search for new, more efficient, and potent diagnostic methods is still important.

Contrast-enhanced spectral mammography (CESM) is a novel technique intensively developed in the last few years. This diagnostic method was accepted by the FDA for clinical use in the United States in 2011. During CESM examination, approximately 2 min after contrast administration (chelated iodine-based X-ray contrast agent), dual-energy mammography is performed. During one examination, two images are acquired: one resembling conventional mammography (low-energy images of equal or noninferior quality to those of standard digital mammography) and another—the subtraction image—demonstrating areas of increased contrast enhancement (like in the case of the CE-MRI that uses Gadolinium-based contrast dose) [24,25]. Another advantage of CESM is that it provides both the anatomical and morphological characteristics of the lesions in the breast and regions of increased neoangiogenesis. CESM is characterized by comparable or even better sensitivity and a higher negative predictive value (NPV) and positive predictive value (PPV). Moreover, in contrast to MRI, CESM allows the visualization of microcalcifications [26,27]. Due to the much shorter examination time, lower costs, higher comfort, and low anxiety involved, patients tend to cooperate more fully and prefer CESM to MRI [28].

Consequently, the use of CESM in the evaluation of response to NAC is justified, bearing in mind the efficiency of this method, which is comparable to CE-MRI. According to the European Society of Breast Cancer (EUSOBI) recommendation in 2017, CESM can be considered as an alternative to contrast-enhanced MRI in the case of contraindications to MRI. CESM is a younger and less-studied technique than MRI. In CESM, there is an extra radiation dose of approximately 20%, but both images—low- and high-energy—still imply an X-ray dose below the recommended dose for mammography. In patients treated with neoadjuvant chemotherapy for breast cancer when a CESM examination is planned, additional MG can be avoided, with the possibility of saving the radiation dose [29].

Therefore, our study aimed to evaluate the effectiveness of low-energy and subtraction CESM images in the detection of CR for neoadjuvant chemotherapy in breast cancer. In addition, we decided to correlate the residual changes assessed with CESM low-energy and subtraction images.

2. Materials and Methods

A total of 63 female patients (mean age of 53.32 ± 9.47 years; ages ranged from 33 to 75 years) were qualified for our retrospective analysis. Between 2016 and 2019 they were put forward for NAC due to breast cancer in the University Clinical Center of the Medical University of Silesia in Katowice, Poland. Inclusion criteria encompassed: a diagnosis of breast cancer (based on core needle biopsy), minimal stage of T1N+, age of more than 18 years, completion of NAC treatment, surgery after NAC, and a complete set of imaging examinations—CESM; ultrasonography (US) of the breast, lymph nodes, and abdomen; and chest X-ray. Exclusion criteria were as follows: known BRCA1 or BRCA2 mutation (to provide the highest radioprotection), pregnancy, anaphylaxis or anaphylactoid reaction to a contrast agent in medical history, e-GFR of less than 60 mL/min, chronic kidney disease in stage 3 or higher, and incomplete NAC. Patients with significant post-biopsy changes (e.g., hemorrhage) affecting image quality were also excluded. A full description of the study group is in Table 1.

Table 1. Patients and tumors characteristics.

Characteristics	Number	Percentage
Number of Patients	63	100%
Age, years (median ± SD)	53.32 ± 9.47	-
Menopause		
Before	27	42.86
After	36	57.14
Molecular characteristics		
LumA	5	8.06
LumB	34	54.84
TNBC1-Jan	24	38.71
Type of tumor		

Table 1. *Cont.*

Characteristics	Number	Percentage
Mixed IDC/ILC	6	9.50
ILC	6	9.50
IDC	51	80.95
TNM stage upon diagnosis		
T1N+	2	3.17
T2N0	13	20.63
T2N+	13	20.63
T3N0	11	17.46
T3N+	16	25.40
T4N0	3	4.76
T4N+	5	7.94

Abbreviations: IDC—invasive ductal carcinoma; ILC—invasive lobular carcinoma; LumA—luminal A breast cancer; LumB—luminal B breast cancer; TNBC—triple-negative breast cancer; TNM—T, N, and M status.

Due to the retrospective nature of this study, the local ethics committee of the Medical University of Silesia repealed the requirement for informed consent (decision number PCN/0022/KB/157/20). All the test procedures were carried out in compliance with the ethical principles of the 1964 Helsinki Declaration and its subsequent amendments.

2.1. Neoadjuvant Systemic Therapy

After the end of breast cancer diagnosis, each patient's final decision concerning the proper treatment was made by the multidisciplinary breast cancer team (BCU) unit, taking into account patients' preferences. Following the decision by the BCU team, 98% of patients received chemotherapy based on anthracyclines and taxanes (for a period of 12 weeks), including 30% in the "dose-dense" regimen. Only one patient did not receive anthracyclines due to a limited dose of anthracyclines in earlier treatment of Hodgkin's disease. Due to the lack of public funding for trastuzumab in this center in the years 2016–2019 (no drug prescription government program), all the cancer patients with positive HER2 were treated outside our center and were not included in this analysis.

2.2. CESM Examination

All CESM examinations were performed in our hospital. They were carried out with the use of a digital mammography device dedicated to performing dual-energy CESM acquisitions (SenoBright, GE Healthcare, 3000 N. Grandview Blvd., Waukesha, WI, USA). An intravenous injection of 1.5 mL/kg of body mass of non-ionic contrast agent was performed using a power injector at a rate of 3 mL/s with a bolus chaser of 30 mL of saline. In CESM mode, the device automatically performed a pair of exposures (low- and high-energy) in each view. Specific image processing of low-energy and high-energy images was done. This processing aimed to obtain subtraction images to highlight contrast enhancement and suppress structured noise due to fibroglandular breast tissue. The morphological information obtained from low-energy images of CESM is similar to the morphological information given by standard mammography and the functional information obtained from subtraction images of CESM visualizes the vascularization of breast lesions [24,25,30]. For each view, the CESM technique made it possible to obtain two images: a low-energy acquisition at 26–30 kVp and a high-energy acquisition at 45–49 kVp, with these values depending on breast density and thickness. Motion blur could be sometimes observed on subtraction images due to movements between the acquisition of low- and high-energy images. All of the images obtained were in the DICOM format [31]. The total examination time was usually 10 min. After examination, the patients were observed for approximately 30 min for any adverse reactions that may have occurred after administration of the contrast agent.

2.3. Imaging Interpretation

All CESM examinations were carried out two times: just before the beginning of NAC and as a follow-up examination 2 weeks before the end of chemotherapy to evaluate its effect (and to inform decisions about possible changes in therapeutic strategies). For our retrospective analysis, we performed renewed CESM image evaluations with every patient. Such evaluations were made separately by two different radiologists with 20 years of experience and a minimum of 5 years' experience in CESM image interpretation. Radiologists were blinded from each other and from the results of histopathological examination. CESM images were assessed according to the Breast Imaging-Reporting and Data System (BI-RADS) scale. Three measurements were taken in the CC and MLO projections, while the statistical analysis encompassed one—i.e., the largest dimension of the tumor. The tumor dimensions were compared while analyzing:

- Low-energy images from two consecutive contrast-enhanced spectral mammograms (taken before the start and at completion of neoadjuvant chemotherapy);
- Subtraction images from two consecutive contrast-enhanced spectral mammograms (taken before the start and at completion of neoadjuvant chemotherapy).

The response to preoperative chemotherapy was evaluated based on the Response Evaluation Criteria in Solid Tumors (RECIST) 1.1 criteria. The response was classified as follows: complete response (CR, disappearance of all lesions); partial response (PR, $\geq$30% dimensional reduction), stable disease (SD, <30% dimensional reduction/<20% dimensional increase), and progressive disease (PD, $\geq$20% dimensional increase) [17,32]. For this article, PR, SD, and PD have been classified as "non-CR".

After surgery, a comparison of the NAC response, evaluated with the use of CESM (both low-energy and spectral images), to the histopathological study results was undertaken. Our analysis of histopathology (HP) was used as a "golden standard" against which the effectiveness of both CESM image types in NAC response detection could be analyzed.

2.4. Histopathological Examination

The histopathological examination was conducted in the Histopathology Laboratory of our center by two pathologists with broad experience in breast cancer diagnostics. The greatest dimension of the tumor, necessary for determining the T descriptor in the pTNM classification apart from the macroscopic measurement, was verified histopathologically. This verification was undertaken using a microscope and the Olympus Cell Sens Dimension® software (Japan, 2013). Tumors up to 2 cm were excised whole, serially, on a cross-sectional basis with a margin of 0.2 to 0.4 cm and embedded in a paraffin block after each cross-section. Tumors measuring over 2 cm that could not fit within a single paraffin block were divided into two or more parts by making parallel cuts of the lesion. Next, they were marked in pairs with ink of the same color and the individual layers were given numbers to allow for the restoration of the largest section of the tumor. The T value of the tumor was the total of the parallel measurements of the particular parts of the lesion.

2.5. Statistical Analysis

Tumors that underwent histopathology examination were used as the "gold standard" and compared to the tumor sizes derived from CESM images. The normality of the distribution was assessed using the Shapiro–Wilk test and the continuous variables were summarized using the arithmetic mean with standard deviation for data following a normal distribution or a median with quartiles 1 and 3 for data demonstrating anon-normal distribution. Comparison of four respective aspects referring to the maximal tumor dimension (defined as the maximum of three dimensions measured in the CESM and histopathology) included the Pearson's correlation coefficient (R-value) in order to measure the strength of the relationship between low-energy and subtraction images of CESM measurements. Paired *t*-tests were used to assess mean differences between each analyzed study participant. The correlations of data are illustrated by plotting the actual measurements while all paired measurements for each patient are summarized using paired

3. Results

Before neoadjuvant chemotherapy, the average size of the tumors varied from 34.4 mm for low-energy CESM to 34.3 mm for CESM subtraction images. After neoadjuvant chemotherapy, their average sizes were 17.6 mm for low-energy images and 8.5 mm for CESM subtraction images. The average size of the lesions in the histopathological examination was 11.1 mm (Table 2). The average reduction of the tumors reached 52.22% of the initial tumor mass based on low-energy images, and this even reached 78.76% in the case of CESM subtraction images.

Table 2. Dimensions of the lesions before and after neoadjuvant chemotherapy for low-energy and subtraction CESM images and histopathological examination.

	Minimal Dimension	Maximal Dimension	Mean ± SD
PL-E CESM (mm)	15.0	77.0	34.4 ± 12.6
NL-E CESM (mm)	0.0	80.0	17.6 ± 15.4
PS CESM (mm)	8.0	100.0	34.3 ± 17.4
NS CESM (mm)	0.0	66.0	8.5 ± 12.0
NHP (mm)	0.0	65.0	11.1 ± 12.8

Abbreviations: PL-E CESM—low-energy CESM images prior to NAC; NL-E CESM—low-energy CESM images after NAC; PS CESM—subtraction CESM images prior to NAC; NS CESM—subtraction CESM images after NAC; NHP—histopathological examination after NAC.

When comparing the maximum tumor dimensions before neoadjuvant chemotherapy for low-energy and subtraction CESM images, a high degree of correlation in the Spearman's analysis ($R = 0.89$, $p < 0.01$) was noticed. When the comparison between the maximum tumor dimensions after neoadjuvant therapy for low-energy and subtraction CESM images is considered, the correlation between the results can be described as moderate ($R = 0.57$, $p < 0.01$) (Figure 1).

A certain correlation, defined as moderate ($R = 0.44$, $p < 0.01$), can also be observed upon the comparison of the maximum tumor reductions for low-energy and subtraction CESM images. In terms of comparing the measurements of the maximum size for low-energy and subtraction CESM images following NAC and the maximum size in the histopathological examination, there was a low level of correlation for low-energy CESM images ($R = 0.26$, $p < 0.04$) and a high level of correlation for subtraction CESM images ($R = 0.67$, $p < 0.01$) (Figure 2).

Both pairs of images tended to imprecisely estimate the sizes of residual lesions. In the case of low-energy images, the size of these lesions was overestimated (the average overestimation value was 6.28 mm), whereas in the case of subtraction CESM images, residual lesions were underestimated (the average underestimation value was 2.75 mm).

According to the RECIST 1.1 guidelines, the low-energy images with morphological assessment only revealed 15.87% CR ($n = 10$) and 84.13% non-CR ($n = 53$). In the case of subtraction CESM images, these parameters were 47.62% ($n = 30$) and 52.38% ($n = 33$), respectively. Histopathological examination demonstrated CR in 33.33% ($n = 21$) of cases and non-CRs in 66.67% ($n = 42$). A detailed description of the particular responses to NAC can be found in Table 3.

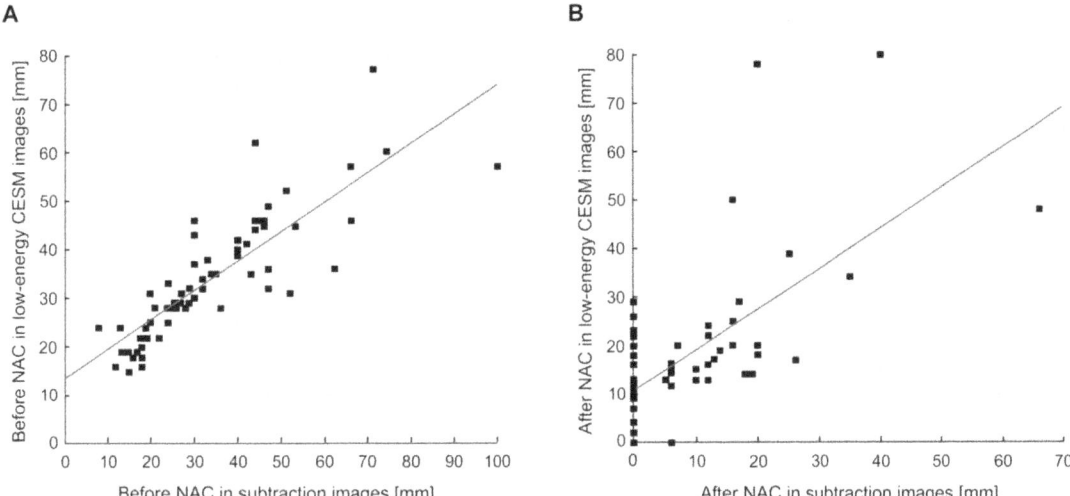

Figure 1. Correlations between: (**A**) the maximum tumor size before NAC in low-energy and subtraction CESM images: R = 0.89, $p < 0.01$; (**B**) the maximum tumor size after NAC in low-energy and subtraction CESM images: R = 0.57, $p < 0.01$.

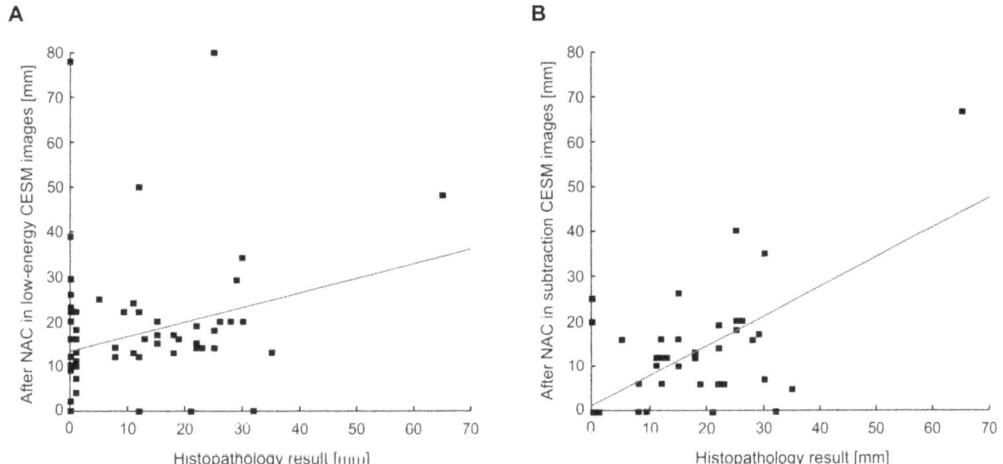

Figure 2. Correlations between: (**A**) the maximum tumor sizes after NAC in low-energy CESM images and in histopathology results: R = 0.26, $p < 0.04$; (**B**) the maximum tumor sizes after NAC in low-energy CESM images and in histopathology results: R = 0.67, $p < 0.01$.

Table 3. Individual therapeutic responses to NAC using low-energy and subtraction CESM images.

	Low-Energy Images		Subtraction Images	
	n	%	n	%
CR	10	15.87	30	47.62
PR	43	68.25	31	49.20
SD	9	14.29	2	3.17
PD	1	1.59	0	0

Abbreviations: CR—complete response; PR—partial response; SD—stable disease; PD—progressive disease.

In the histopathological examination for invasive ductal carcinoma (IDC), a CR of 39.22% (20 out of 51 of tumors) could be achieved, whereas for invasive lobular carcinoma (ILC) it was 16.67% (1 out of 6 tumors). In the case of mixed IDC/ILC, CR was not achieved in any of the tumors. In Table 4, differences in the NAC response depending on the type of breast cancer analyzed by CESM and histopathological examination are shown.

Table 4. Differences in NAC response depending on the type of breast cancer.

Pathological Response to NAC	IDC (n = 51)			Mixed IDC/ILC (n = 6)			ILC (n = 6)		
	Low-Energy CESM Images	Subtraction CESM Images	HP	Low-Energy CESM Images	Subtraction CESM Images	HP	Low-Energy CESM Images	Subtraction CESM Images	HP
CR	8	25	20	0	2	0	2	3	1
Non-CR	43	26	31	6	4	6	4	3	5

Abbreviations: CR—complete response; IDC—invasive ductal carcinoma; ILC—invasive lobular carcinoma; HP—histopathology examination.

Comparing the two types of CESM images to the histopathological examination, Table 5 presents the sensitivity, specificity, negative predictive value (NPV), and positive predictive value (PPV) of both images in the prediction of the CR. The sensitivity of low-energy images in forecasting CR amounted to 33.33%, while its specificity was 92.86%. In the case of the subtraction CESM images, the sensitivity amounted to 85.71% and the specificity to 71.42%.

Table 5. Diagnostic performance indexes for the assessment of complete (CR) and non-complete response (PR, SD, PD) according to RECIST 1.1 criteria using low-energy and subtraction CESM images compared to histopathology results.

Assessment	RECIST 1.1	Histopathology CR	Histopathology Non-CR (PR, SD, PD)	
Low-energy CESM images	CR	7	3	PPV: 70.0% 95% CI: 0.35–0.93
	Non-CR (PR, SD, PD)	14	39	NPV: 73.58% 95% CI: 0.60–0.85
		Sensitivity: 33.33% 95% CI: 0.15–0.57	Specificity: 92.86% 95% CI: 0.81–0.99	
Subtraction CESM images	CR	18	12	PPV: 60.00% 95% CI: 0.41–0.77
	Non-CR (PR, SD, PD)	3	30	NPV: 90.90% 95% CI: 0.76–0.98
		Sensitivity: 85.71% 95% CI: 0.64–0.97	Specificity: 71.42% 95% CI: 0.55–0.84	

Abbreviations: CR—complete response; PR—partial response; SD—stable disease; PD—progressive disease; PPV—positive predictive value; NPV—negative predictive value.

Figure 3 presents the differences in ROC curves for low-energy and subtraction CESM images in detecting CR.

Figures 4 and 5 present an assessment of the therapeutic responses in two pairs of CESM images.

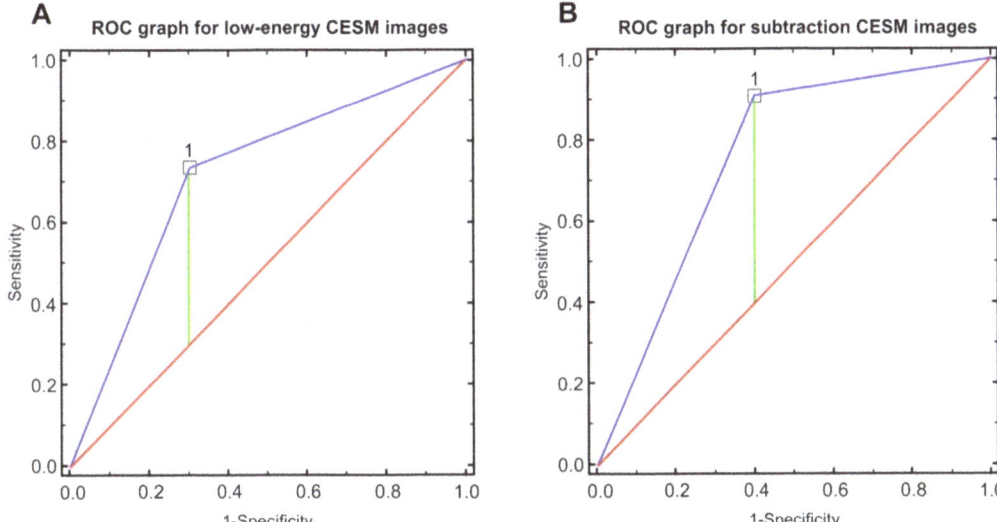

Figure 3. ROC curves based on the tested diagnostic methods (Youden Index:0.44, proposed cut-off point: 1.00): (**A**) for low-energy CESM images, the value of the AUC field was 0.718 at a standard error of 0.091 and $p < 0.0172$; (**B**) for subtraction CESM images, the value of the AUC field was 0.755 at a standard error of 0.064 and $p < 0.0001$.

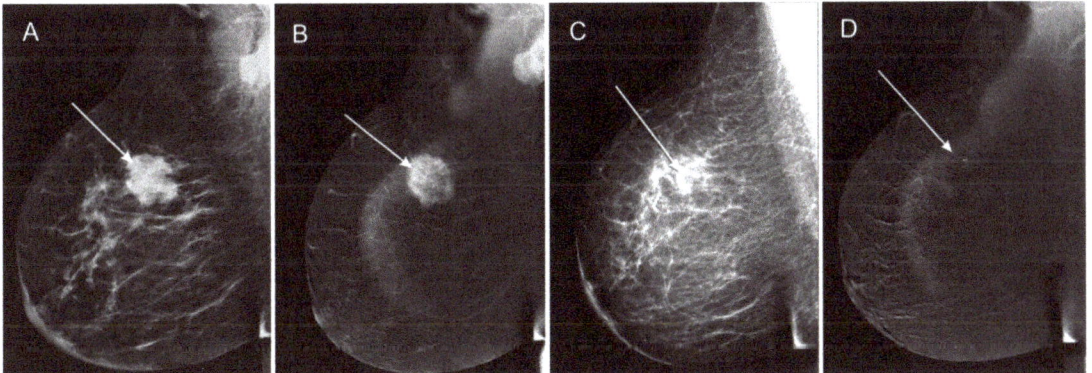

Figure 4. Assessment of therapeutic response in low-energy MLO (**A**,**C**) and subtraction MLO (**B**,**D**). Before NAC, a tumor can be seen in the upper outer quadrant of the right breast with high density and polycyclic outlines, accompanied by enlarged lymph nodes in the axillary fossa (**A**), revealing pathological contrast enhancement in subtraction CESM images (**B**). Following NAC, in the tumor field, there is a visible focal asymmetry, with a density lower than the residual glandular tissue (**C**), without pathological contrast enhancement (**D**). Based on the low-energy images, the therapeutic response was classified as partial response (PR). Based on the subtraction images, the therapeutic response was classified as complete response (CR), which was acknowledged in the HP examination.

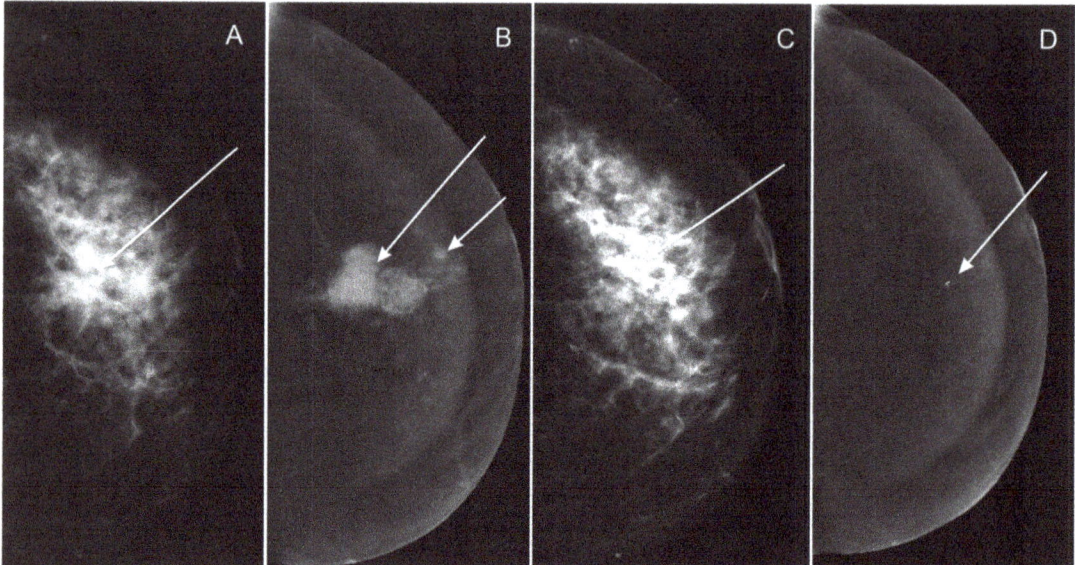

Figure 5. Assessment of therapeutic response in low-energy CESM CC images (**A,C**) and subtraction CESM CC images (**B,D**) before NAC (IDC LumB, G2 T3N1) showing irregular infiltration on the border of the outer quadrants of the left breast with high density (**A**), revealing pathological contrast enhancement on subtraction CESM images (**B**). Additionally, satellite foci are visible in subtraction CESM images, which were confirmed in core-needle biopsy (smaller arrow) (**B**). Following NAC, there was a visible focal asymmetry, with a density slightly lower than the infiltration before NAC (**C**), shown again without pathological contrast enhancement (**D**). Based on the low-energy CESM images, the therapeutic response was classified as stable disease (SD). Based on the subtraction CESM images, the therapeutic response was classified as complete response (CR), which was acknowledged in the HP examination.

4. Discussion

Early assessment of NAC response to breast cancer and correct differentiation between patients with the complete pathological response (pCR) and without NAC response is the key point in NAC therapy. Proper evaluation is crucial to the future clinical perspectives and therapy for each patient. Obtaining complete pathological response results in better event-free survival (EFS) and overall survival (OS) rates [33,34].

In our study, the sensitivity of low-energy images in forecasting CR reached 33.33%, the specificity was 92.86%, the PPV was 70%, and the NPV was 73.58%. After the conversion of subtraction images, the sensitivity of CESM in CR detection in a group of patients after NAC was 85.71%, its specificity was 71.42%, the PPV was 60%, and the NPV was 90.90%. Similar results for subtraction CESM images have been acquired by other authors such as Patel et al. [35] (64 patients, sensitivity: 95%, specificity: 66.7%, PPV: 55.9%, NPV: 96.7%), Iotti et al. [36] (46 patients, sensitivity: 100%, specificity: 84%, PPV: 57%, NPV: 100%), and Barra et al. [37] (33 patients, sensitivity: 76%, specificity: 62.5%, PPV: 86%, NPV: 45.4%). All mentioned studies, including ours, showed that, in the assessment of the CR following NAC, subtraction CESM images reached significantly higher sensitivity. Unfortunately, their specificity was lower. These results demonstrate that imaging techniques, even after intravenous administration of a contrast agent, may not differentiate between residual infiltration lesions and co-existing inflammatory/reactive lesions. A similar problem occurs with MRI, which tends to underestimate residual changes [23].

In their meta-analysis, Tang et al. [38] demonstrated that the pooled sensitivity, specificity, positive likelihood ratio (PLR), negative likelihood ratio (NLR), and diagnostic odds ratio (DOR) of the pathological response of breast cancer to NAC assessed by CESM were:

0.83 (95% CI, 0.66–0.93), 0.82 (95% CI, 0.68–0.91), 4.66 (95% CI, 2.59–8.41), 0.20 (95% CI, 0.10–0.43), and 22.91 (95% CI, 8.66–60.62), respectively. The same parameters for MRI, which is considered to be the best method for assessing response to NAC, were as follows: sensitivity: 0.77 (95% CI, 0.67–0.84), specificity: 0.82 (95% CI, 0.73–0.89), PLR: 4.35 (95% CI, 3.00–6.33), NLR: 0.28 (95%CI, 0.20–0.39), and DOR: 15.48 (95% CI, 9.97–24.03). Based on these findings, it can be concluded that CESM has the same specificity and higher sensitivity than MRI and is more accurate in the pathological evaluation of NAC response in breast cancer treatment.

The largest pretreatment tumor dimensions in our analysis of low-energy and subtraction CESM images were similar and there was a statistical difference between these modalities ($R = 0.89$, $p = 0.01$). However, these differences became significant following neoadjuvant chemotherapy ($R = 0.55$, $p = 0.01$). This was because post-NAC tumors reduce their density and then become difficult to distinguish from glandular tissue based on morphological images alone. On the other hand, the functional information provided by CESM in subtraction images showed that the residual infiltration was visible, and the type of breast tissue did not affect its visualization. Moreover, in our study, the comparison of the measurement of the maximal sizes of residual changes after NAC, evaluated using CESM subtraction images and histopathology, showed a high correlation ($R = 0.67$, $p = 0.01$). Iotti et al. [36], while comparing the sizes of tumors after NAC with a histopathological examination, proved that CESM showed greater coherence with histopathology than MRI (Lin's coefficient were 0.81 and 0.59, respectively). In contrast, Patel et al. [35] achieved the opposite results, where MRI showed higher compatibility with histopathology than CESM (Lin's concordance coefficient was 0.75 for CESM and 0.76 for MRI; Pearson's correlation was 0.77 for CESM and 0.80 for MRI). The lack of consistency between researchers indicates the need for further research—multicenter, on a larger group of patients, using equipment available on the market from various companies.

In our study, Low-energy images tended to overestimate the dimensions of residual lesions following NAC, while subtraction CESM images tended to underestimate them. Similar results were acquired by Patel et al. [35] and Iotti et al. [36], where CESM and histopathology results underestimated the size of post-NAC tumors by 5mm and 4.1mm, respectively. It should also be emphasized that the underestimation of the dimensions of residual lesions in our study had no impact on the scope of surgical treatment. Since CESM is a method involving vascularization of the tumor foci, the effect of excessive reduction in vascularization around the tumor during NAC may account for the weaker enhancement of the residual tumor mass on follow-up CESM, underestimating the actual dimension of residual lesions. A similar problem arises with MRI, which tends to underestimate residual lesions in follow-up examinations [35,36]. Over-or underestimation of residual disease can also be a result of the fact that, due to neoadjuvant chemotherapy, induction of cellular changes leading to the elimination of cancerous cells occurs before the decrease in tumor size [39,40]. Moreover, after the eradication of cancerous cells in the region of the tumor, the residual mass visible on radiological images may still be present. It consists of fibrotic tissue left after the therapy. To overcome this problem, Xing et al. [41] and Moustafa et al. [42] suggested relying not only on RECIST 1.1 criteria in the evaluation of NAC response but also creating a special mathematical model. It consists of a combination of the measurement of the largest diameter of the target lesion together with subjective identification of the difference in the intensity of the contrast uptake before and after NAC. After that, a combination of the summation of the number of pixels and their intensity within the area of interest before and after NAC is included in this model. It should be noted that, after using this method, CESM remained a method of high sensitivity and specificity in the evaluation of NAC response. Such results prove that CESM is one of the best methods for diagnostic imaging available for the analysis of the response to neoadjuvant chemotherapy.

The histological and molecular heterogeneity of tumors cannot be evaluated with a simple examination with a contrast medium, and biopsies are limited, especially in large tumors. The need to better define the heterogeneity of tumors will involve the aid of new methodologies currently under study, such as radiomics. Radiomics in MRI can be more effective in the diagnosis of breast cancer and in the histological and morphological assessment of tumors. For CESM, a radiomics model achieved a significantly better discriminative ability compared to the standard clinical model (AUC, 0.81 vs. 0.55, $p < 0.01$) [43–45]. In recent years, it has also been suggested to use background parenchymal enhancement (BPE) in the assessment of responses to NAC, which describes the enhancement of the normal breast tissue related to physiological vascularization. La Forgia et al., indicated that BPE is an important aspect that conditions the diagnosis and that it is a potential predictive factor in the response to neoadjuvant cancer therapies in graphic contrast examinations, as already confirmed in MRI and CESM examinations [46–48].

CESM, while being a relatively novel diagnostic imaging technique, has become a useful tool in diagnosing and evaluating breast cancer stages. Subtraction images improve the diagnostic specificity of low-energy images, providing more precise measurement of tumor size as well as the possibility of identifying multifocal diseases, especially in women with dense breast tissue. Thus, the effectiveness of CESM in breast cancer diagnosis is comparable to MRI and is a promising tool to serve as a basic imaging technique in patients with symptomatic breast cancer or for the detection of multifocal and multicentric breast cancers [49–51]. As we have shown in our study, CESM is also a useful and effective method in assessing the pathological response to NAC. Post-NAC treatment monitoring is extremely important for planning surgical treatment, reducing the number of mutilating mastectomies, and replacing them with breast-conserving surgeries. However, the most accurate measurements possible should be made to avoid underestimating the size of the tumor and increasing the extent of the operation. The advantage of CESM over other methods so far available is its precise definition of the tumor before NAC thanks to the directly integrated visualization of suspicious calcifications in the low-energy images and enhancement in the recombined images, which is not possible with MRI [52].

Our study had several limitations. Firstly, this single-institution research was carried out on a relatively small number of female patients due to the limited number of qualifications for NAC. Moreover, all CESM examinations were conducted on a single vendor system. Finally, we did not include patients with HER2-positive cancer in our study due to the lack of public funding for trastuzumab in this center in the years from2016–2019 (no drug prescription government program). There is a need for multi-institutional studies with larger groups of patients free of the limitations described above in the future.

5. Conclusions

Due to the possibility of assessing vascularity, CESM is characterized by high sensitivity in the assessment of CR after NAC. The use of morphological assessment alone is insufficient. CESM correlates well with the sizes of residual lesions from histopathological examination but tends to underestimate the dimensions.

Author Contributions: Conceptualization, A.G. and K.S.-R.; methodology, A.G., K.S.-R., and A.B.-G.; software, K.S.-R. and A.L.; validation, A.L., K.S., and K.S.-R.; formal analysis, A.L., A.B., P.N., and K.S.-R.; investigation, A.L., A.B., K.S.-R., and A.B.-G.; writing—original draft preparation, A.L., K.S.-R., A.G., K.O., Z.L., and I.M.; writing—review and editing, K.S., P.N., A.L., K.S.-R., and A.G.; design of the manuscript, A.G., P.N., K.S.-R., and A.L.; translation, J.P.; supervision, I.G. and K.S. All authors have read and agreed to the published version of the manuscript.

Funding: This research received no external funding.

Institutional Review Board Statement: Due to the retrospective nature of this study, the local ethics committee of the Medical University of Silesia repealed the requirement for informed consent (decision number PCN/0022/KB/157/20). All the test procedures were carried out in compliance with the ethical principles of the 1964 Helsinki Declaration and its subsequent amendments.

Informed Consent Statement: Not applicable.

Data Availability Statement: Data are available upon special request.

Conflicts of Interest: The authors declare no conflict of interest.

References

1. Gradishar, W.J.; Anderson, B.O.; Balassanian, R.; Blair, S.L.; Burstein, H.J.; Cyr, A.; Elias, A.D.; Farrar, W.B.; Forero, A.; Giordano, S.H.; et al. Breast Cancer, Version 4.2017, NCCN Clinical Practice Guidelines in Oncology. *J. Natl. Compr. Cancer Netw.* **2018**, *16*, 310–320. [CrossRef] [PubMed]
2. Cancer Research UK. Cancer Statistics. Breast Cancer. 2017. Available online: http://www.cancerresearchuk.org/health-professional/cancer-statistics/statistics-by-cancer-type/breast-cancer (accessed on 6 July 2021).
3. Gao, W.; Guo, N.; Dong, T. Diffusion-Weighted Imaging in Monitoring the Pathological Response to Neoadjuvant Chemotherapy in Patients with Breast Cancer: A Meta-Analysis. *World J. Surg. Oncol.* **2018**, *16*, 145. [CrossRef]
4. Masuda, N.; Lee, S.-J.; Ohtani, S.; Im, Y.-H.; Lee, E.-S.; Yokota, I.; Kuroi, K.; Im, S.-A.; Park, B.-W.; Kim, S.-B.; et al. Adjuvant Capecitabine for Breast Cancer after Preoperative Chemotherapy. *N. Engl. J. Med.* **2017**, *376*, 2147–2159. [CrossRef] [PubMed]
5. Curigliano, G.; Burstein, H.J.; Winer, E.P.; Gnant, M.; Dubsky, P.; Loibl, S.; Colleoni, M.; Regan, M.M.; Piccart-Gebhart, M.; Senn, H.-J.; et al. De-Escalating and Escalating Treatments for Early-Stage Breast Cancer: The St. Gallen International Expert Consensus Conference on the Primary Therapy of Early Breast Cancer 2017. *Ann. Oncol.* **2017**, *28*, 1700–1712. [CrossRef] [PubMed]
6. Cardoso, F.; Kyriakides, S.; Ohno, S.; Penault-Llorca, F.; Poortmans, P.; Rubio, I.T.; Zackrisson, S.; Senkus, E. Early Breast Cancer: ESMO Clinical Practice Guidelines for Diagnosis, Treatment and Follow-Up. *Ann. Oncol.* **2019**, *30*, 1194–1220. [CrossRef] [PubMed]
7. Ditsch, N.; Untch, M.; Thill, M.; Müller, V.; Janni, W.; Albert, U.-S.; Bauerfeind, I.; Blohmer, J.; Budach, W.; Dall, P.; et al. AGO Recommendations for the Diagnosis and Treatment of Patients with Early Breast Cancer: Update 2019. *Breast Care* **2019**, *14*, 224–245. [CrossRef]
8. Korde, L.A.; Somerfield, M.R.; Carey, L.A.; Crews, J.R.; Denduluri, N.; Hwang, E.S.; Khan, S.A.; Loibl, S.; Morris, E.A.; Perez, A.; et al. Neoadjuvant Chemotherapy, Endocrine Therapy, and Targeted Therapy for Breast Cancer: ASCO Guideline. *J. Clin. Oncol. Off. J. Am. Soc. Clin. Oncol.* **2021**, *39*, 1485–1505. [CrossRef]
9. Morigi, C. Highlights of the 16th St Gallen International Breast Cancer Conference, Vienna, Austria, 20–23 March 2019: Personalised Treatments for Patients with Early Breast Cancer. *Ecancermedicalscience* **2019**, *13*, 924. [CrossRef]
10. Bevers, T.B.; Helvie, M.; Bonaccio, E.; Calhoun, K.E.; Daly, M.B.; Farrar, W.B.; Garber, J.E.; Gray, R.; Greenberg, C.C.; Greenup, R.; et al. Breast Cancer Screening and Diagnosis, Version 3.2018, NCCN Clinical Practice Guidelines in Oncology. *J. Natl. Compr. Cancer Netw.* **2018**, *16*, 1362–1389. [CrossRef]
11. Werutsky, G.; Untch, M.; Hanusch, C.; Fasching, P.A.; Blohmer, J.-U.; Seiler, S.; Denkert, C.; Tesch, H.; Jackisch, C.; Gerber, B.; et al. Locoregional Recurrence Risk after Neoadjuvant Chemotherapy: A Pooled Analysis of Nine Prospective Neoadjuvant Breast Cancer Trials. *Eur. J. Cancer* **2020**, *130*, 92–101. [CrossRef]
12. United States Food and Drug Administration. Pathological Complete Response in Neoadjuvant Treatment of High-Risk Early-Stage Breast Cancer: Use as an Endpoint to Support Accelerated Approval Guidance for Industry. Available online: https://www.fda.gov/regulatory-information/search-fda-guidance-documents/pathological-complete-response-neoadjuvant-treatment-high-risk-early-stage-breast-cancer-use (accessed on 10 July 2021).
13. Colleoni, M.; Goldhirsch, A. Neoadjuvant Chemotherapy for Breast Cancer: Any Progress? *Lancet Oncol.* **2014**, *15*, 131–132. [CrossRef]
14. Vaidya, J.S.; Massarut, S.; Vaidya, H.J.; Alexander, E.C.; Richards, T.; Caris, J.A.; Sirohi, B.; Tobias, J.S. Rethinking Neoadjuvant Chemotherapy for Breast Cancer. *BMJ* **2018**, *360*, j5913. [CrossRef] [PubMed]
15. Coleman, W.B.; Anders, C.K. Discerning Clinical Responses in Breast Cancer Based on Molecular Signatures. *Am. J. Pathol.* **2017**, *187*, 2199–2207. [CrossRef] [PubMed]
16. Moo, T.-A.; Sanford, R.; Dang, C.; Morrow, M. Overview of Breast Cancer Therapy. *PET Clin.* **2018**, *13*, 339–354. [CrossRef] [PubMed]
17. Wang, H.; Mao, X. Evaluation of the Efficacy of Neoadjuvant Chemotherapy for Breast Cancer. *Drug Des. Dev. Ther.* **2020**, *14*, 2423–2433. [CrossRef] [PubMed]
18. Choi, W.J.; Kim, H.H.; Cha, J.H.; Shin, H.J.; Chae, E.Y. Comparison of Pathologic Response Evaluation Systems After Neoadjuvant Chemotherapy in Breast Cancers: Correlation with Computer-Aided Diagnosis of MRI Features. *Am. J. Roentgenol.* **2019**, *213*, 944–952. [CrossRef]
19. Taydas, O.; Durhan, G.; Akpinar, M.G.; Basaran Demirkazik, F. Comparison of MRI and US in Tumor Size Evaluation of Breast Cancer Patients Receiving Neoadjuvant Chemotherapy. *Eur. J. Breast Health* **2019**, *15*, 119–124. [CrossRef]
20. Negrão, E.M.S.; Souza, J.A.; Marques, E.F.; Bitencourt, A.G.V. Breast Cancer Phenotype Influences MRI Response Evaluation after Neoadjuvant Chemotherapy. *Eur. J. Radiol.* **2019**, *120*, 108701. [CrossRef]
21. Goorts, B.; Dreuning, K.M.A.; Houwers, J.B.; Kooreman, L.F.S.; Boerma, E.-J.G.; Mann, R.M.; Lobbes, M.B.I.; Smidt, M.L. MRI-Based Response Patterns during Neoadjuvant Chemotherapy Can Predict Pathological (Complete) Response in Patients with Breast Cancer. *Breast Cancer Res.* **2018**, *20*, 34. [CrossRef]

22. Yoshikawa, K.; Ishida, M.; Kan, N.; Yanai, H.; Tsuta, K.; Sekimoto, M.; Sugie, T. Direct Comparison of Magnetic Resonance Imaging and Pathological Shrinkage Patterns of Triple-Negative Breast Cancer after Neoadjuvant Chemotherapy. *World J. Surg. Onc.* **2020**, *18*, 177. [CrossRef]
23. Vriens, B.E.P.J.; de Vries, B.; Lobbes, M.B.I.; van Gastel, S.M.; van den Berkmortel, F.W.P.J.; Smilde, T.J.; van Warmerdam, L.J.C.; de Boer, M.; van Spronsen, D.J.; Smidt, M.L.; et al. Ultrasound Is at Least as Good as Magnetic Resonance Imaging in Predicting Tumour Size Post-Neoadjuvant Chemotherapy in Breast Cancer. *Eur. J. Cancer* **2016**, *52*, 67–76. [CrossRef]
24. Lalji, U.C.; Jeukens, C.R.L.P.N.; Houben, I.; Nelemans, P.J.; van Engen, R.E.; van Wylick, E.; Beets-Tan, R.G.H.; Wildberger, J.E.; Paulis, L.E.; Lobbes, M.B.I. Evaluation of Low-Energy Contrast-Enhanced Spectral Mammography Images by Comparing Them to Full-Field Digital Mammography Using EUREF Image Quality Criteria. *Eur. Radiol.* **2015**, *25*, 2813–2820. [CrossRef]
25. Jochelson, M.S.; Lobbes, M.B.I. Contrast-Enhanced Mammography: State of the Art. *Radiology* **2021**, *299*, 36–48. [CrossRef]
26. Xing, D.; Lv, Y.; Sun, B.; Xie, H.; Dong, J.; Hao, C.; Chen, Q.; Chi, X. Diagnostic Value of Contrast-Enhanced Spectral Mammography in Comparison to Magnetic Resonance Imaging in Breast Lesions. *J. Comput. Assist. Tomogr.* **2019**, *43*, 245–251. [CrossRef] [PubMed]
27. Fallenberg, E.M.; Schmitzberger, F.F.; Amer, H.; Ingold-Heppner, B.; Balleyguier, C.; Diekmann, F.; Engelken, F.; Mann, R.M.; Renz, D.M.; Bick, U.; et al. Contrast-Enhanced Spectral Mammography vs. Mammography and MRI—Clinical Performance in a Multi-Reader Evaluation. *Eur. Radiol.* **2017**, *27*, 2752–2764. [CrossRef] [PubMed]
28. Hobbs, M.M.; Taylor, D.B.; Buzynski, S.; Peake, R.E. Contrast-Enhanced Spectral Mammography (CESM) and Contrast Enhanced MRI (CEMRI): Patient Preferences and Tolerance: CESM and CEMRI Preferences and Tolerance. *J. Med. Imaging Radiat. Oncol.* **2015**, *59*, 300–305. [CrossRef] [PubMed]
29. Sardanelli, F.; Fallenberg, E.M.; Clauser, P.; Trimboli, R.M.; Camps-Herrero, J.; Helbich, T.H.; Forrai, G.; for the European Society of Breast Imaging (EUSOBI), with Language Review by Europa Donna—The European Breast Cancer Coalition. Mammography: An Update of the EUSOBI Recommendations on Information for Women. *Insights Imaging* **2017**, *8*, 11–18. [CrossRef]
30. La Forgia, D.; Catino, A.; Dentamaro, R.; Galetta, D.; Gatta, G.; Losurdo, L.; Massafra, R.; Scattone, A.; Tangaro, S.; Fanizzi, A. Role of the contrast-enhanced spectral mammography for the diagnosis of breast metastases from extramammary neoplasms. *J. BUON* **2019**, *24*, 1360–1366. [PubMed]
31. Fanizzi, A.; Losurdo, L.; Basile, T.M.A.; Bellotti, R.; Bottigli, U.; Delogu, P.; Diacono, D.; Didonna, V.; Fausto, A.; Lombardi, A.; et al. Fully Automated Support System for Diagnosis of Breast Cancer in Contrast-Enhanced Spectral Mammography Images. *J. Clin. Med.* **2019**, *8*, 891. [CrossRef] [PubMed]
32. Litière, S.; Collette, S.; de Vries, E.G.E.; Seymour, L.; Bogaerts, J. RECIST—Learning from the Past to Build the Future. *Nat. Rev. Clin. Oncol.* **2017**, *14*, 187–192. [CrossRef]
33. Cortazar, P.; Zhang, L.; Untch, M.; Mehta, K.; Costantino, J.P.; Wolmark, N.; Bonnefoi, H.; Cameron, D.; Gianni, L.; Valagussa, P.; et al. Pathological Complete Response and Long-Term Clinical Benefit in Breast Cancer: The CTNeoBC Pooled Analysis. *Lancet* **2014**, *384*, 164–172. [CrossRef]
34. Ahmed, S.H. Safety of neoadjuvant chemotherapy for the treatment of breast cancer. *Expert Opin. Drug Saf.* **2019**, *18*, 817–827. [CrossRef]
35. Patel, B.K.; Hilal, T.; Covington, M.; Zhang, N.; Kosiorek, H.E.; Lobbes, M.; Northfelt, D.W.; Pockaj, B.A. Contrast-enhanced spectral mammography is comparable to mri in the assessment of residual breast cancer following neoadjuvant systemic therapy. *Ann. Surg. Oncol.* **2018**, *25*, 1350–1356. [CrossRef]
36. Iotti, V.; Ravaioli, S.; Vacondio, R.; Coriani, C.; Caffarri, S.; Sghedoni, R.; Nitrosi, A.; Ragazzi, M.; Gasparini, E.; Masini, C.; et al. Contrast-enhanced spectral mammography in neoadjuvant chemotherapy monitoring: A comparison with breast magnetic resonance imaging. *Breast Cancer Res.* **2017**, *19*, 106. [CrossRef] [PubMed]
37. Barra, F.R.; Sobrinho, A.B.; Barra, R.R.; Magalhães, M.T.; Aguiar, L.R.; de Albuquerque, G.F.L.; Costa, R.P.; Farage, L.; Pratesi, R. Contrast-enhanced mammography (CEM) for detecting residual disease after neoadjuvant chemotherapy: A comparison with breast magnetic resonance imaging (MRI). *BioMed Res. Int.* **2018**, *2018*, 8531916. [CrossRef] [PubMed]
38. Tang, S.; Xiang, C.; Yang, Q. The Diagnostic Performance of CESM and CE-MRI in Evaluating the Pathological Response to Neoadjuvant Therapy in Breast Cancer: A Systematic Review and Meta-Analysis. *Br. J. Radiol.* **2020**, *93*, 20200301. [CrossRef]
39. Fowler, A.M.; Mankoff, D.A.; Joe, B.N. Imaging Neoadjuvant Therapy Response in Breast Cancer. *Radiology* **2017**, *285*, 358–375. [CrossRef]
40. Fasching, P.A.; Gass, P.; Hein, A. Neoadjuvant Treatment of Breast Cancer—Advances and Limitations. *Breast Care* **2016**, *11*, 313–314. [CrossRef]
41. Xing, D.; Mao, N.; Dong, J.; Ma, H.; Chen, Q.; Lv, Y. Quantitative Analysis of Contrast Enhanced Spectral Mammography Grey Value for Early Prediction of Pathological Response of Breast Cancer to Neoadjuvant Chemotherapy. *Sci. Rep.* **2021**, *11*, 5892. [CrossRef]
42. Moustafa, A.F.I.; Kamal, R.M.; Gomaa, M.M.M.; Mostafa, S.; Mubarak, R.; El-Adawy, M. Quantitative Mathematical Objective Evaluation of Contrast-Enhanced Spectral Mammogram in the Assessment of Response to Neoadjuvant Chemotherapy and Prediction of Residual Disease in Breast Cancer. *Egypt. J. Radiol. Nucl. Med.* **2019**, *50*, 44. [CrossRef]
43. Massafra, R.; Bove, S.; Lorusso, V.; Biafora, A.; Comes, M.C.; Didonna, V.; Diotaiuti, S.; Fanizzi, A.; Nardone, A.; Nolasco, A.; et al. Radiomic Feature Reduction Approach to Predict Breast Cancer by Contrast-Enhanced Spectral Mammography Images. *Diagnostics* **2021**, *11*, 684. [CrossRef]

44. Wang, Z.; Lin, F.; Ma, H.; Shi, Y.; Dong, J.; Yang, P.; Zhang, K.; Guo, N.; Zhang, R.; Cui, J.; et al. Contrast-Enhanced Spectral Mammography-Based Radiomics Nomogram for the Prediction of Neoadjuvant Chemotherapy-Insensitive Breast Cancers. *Front. Oncol.* **2021**, *11*, 605230. [CrossRef]
45. Conti, A.; Duggento, A.; Indovina, I.; Guerrisi, M.; Toschi, N. Radiomics in Breast Cancer Classification and Prediction. *Semin. Cancer Biol.* **2021**, *72*, 238–250. [CrossRef]
46. La Forgia, D.; Vestito, A.; Lasciarrea, M.; Comes, M.C.; Diotaiuti, S.; Giotta, F.; Latorre, A.; Lorusso, V.; Massafra, R.; Palmiotti, G.; et al. Response Predictivity to Neoadjuvant Therapies in Breast Cancer: A Qualitative Analysis of Background Parenchymal Enhancement in DCE-MRI. *J. Pers. Med.* **2021**, *11*, 256. [CrossRef] [PubMed]
47. Teixeira, S.R.C.; de Camargo Júnior, H.S.A.; Cabello, C. Background Parenchymal Enhancement: Behavior during Neoadjuvant Chemotherapy for Breast Cancer and Relationship with a Pathological Complete Response. *Radiol. Bras.* **2020**, *53*, 95–104. [CrossRef] [PubMed]
48. Arasu, V.A.; Miglioretti, D.L.; Sprague, B.L.; Alsheik, N.H.; Buist, D.S.M.; Henderson, L.M.; Herschorn, S.D.; Lee, J.M.; Onega, T.; Rauscher, G.H.; et al. Population-Based Assessment of the Association Between Magnetic Resonance Imaging Background Parenchymal Enhancement and Future Primary Breast Cancer Risk. *J. Clin. Oncol.* **2019**, *37*, 954–963. [CrossRef] [PubMed]
49. Lorek, A.; Steinhof-Radwańska, K.; Barczyk-Gutkowska, A.; Zarębski, W.; Paleń, P.; Szyluk, K.; Lorek, J.; Grażyńska, A.; Niemiec, P.; Gisterek, I. The Usefulness of Spectral Mammography in Surgical Planning of Breast Cancer Treatment—Analysis of 999 Patients with Primary Operable Breast Cancer. *Curr. Oncol.* **2021**, *28*, 232. [CrossRef] [PubMed]
50. Alexander, S.; Dulku, G.; Hashoul, S.; Taylor, D.B. Practical Uses of Contrast-enhanced Spectral Mammography in Daily Work: A Pictorial Review. *J. Med. Imaging Radiat. Oncol.* **2019**, *63*, 473–478. [CrossRef]
51. Richter, V.; Hatterman, V.; Preibsch, H.; Bahrs, S.D.; Hahn, M.; Nikolaou, K.; Wiesinger, B. Contrast-Enhanced Spectral Mammography in Patients with MRI Contraindications. *Acta Radiol.* **2018**, *59*, 798–805. [CrossRef]
52. Iotti, V.; Ragazzi, M.; Besutti, G.; Marchesi, V.; Ravaioli, S.; Falco, G.; Coiro, S.; Bisagni, A.; Gasparini, E.; Giorgi Rossi, P.; et al. Accuracy and Reproducibility of Contrast-Enhanced Mammography in the Assessment of Response to Neoadjuvant Chemotherapy in Breast Cancer Patients with Calcifications in the Tumor Bed. *Diagnostics* **2021**, *11*, 435. [CrossRef]

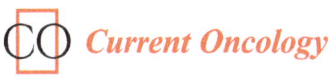

Review

The Impact of Dense Breasts on the Stage of Breast Cancer at Diagnosis: A Review and Options for Supplemental Screening

Paula B. Gordon

Department of Radiology, Faculty of Medicine, University of British Columbia, 505-750 West Broadway, Vancouver, BC V5Z 1H4, Canada; pbgordon@mac.com

Abstract: The purpose of breast cancer screening is to find cancers early to reduce mortality and to allow successful treatment with less aggressive therapy. Mammography is the gold standard for breast cancer screening. Its efficacy in reducing mortality from breast cancer was proven in randomized controlled trials (RCTs) conducted from the early 1960s to the mid 1990s. Panels that recommend breast cancer screening guidelines have traditionally relied on the old RCTs, which did not include considerations of breast density, race/ethnicity, current hormone therapy, and other risk factors. Women do not all benefit equally from mammography. Mortality reduction is significantly lower in women with dense breasts because normal dense tissue can mask cancers on mammograms. Moreover, women with dense breasts are known to be at increased risk. To provide equity, breast cancer screening guidelines should be created with the goal of maximizing mortality reduction and allowing less aggressive therapy, which may include decreasing the interval between screening mammograms and recommending consideration of supplemental screening for women with dense breasts. This review will address the issue of dense breasts and the impact on the stage of breast cancer at the time of diagnosis, and discuss options for supplemental screening.

Keywords: mammography; breast ultrasound; breast density; breast cancer screening; interval cancer; mortality reduction; breast MRI; digital breast tomosynthesis; molecular breast imaging; contrast-enhanced mammography

1. Background: Screening Mammography

The purpose of breast cancer screening is to find cancers early to reduce mortality and to allow successful treatment with less aggressive therapy. Mammography is the gold standard for breast screening. The randomized controlled trials (RCTs), carried out from the early 1960s to the mid 1990s showed a significant decrease in breast cancer deaths in women invited to screening. The magnitude of mortality reduction was shown to be considerably higher among women who actually participated in mammography screening regularly. Coldman et al. showed 40% mortality reduction overall, and 44% reduction in women aged 40–49 [1]. In Sweden, Tabár et al. showed that women aged 40–69 who participated in organized screening were 60% less likely to die of breast cancer in the 10 years following diagnosis, and 47% less likely within 20 years [2]. In a review of European studies, Broeders et al. showed that the relative reduction in breast cancer mortality for women who actually participated in screening was 38% based on incidence-based mortality studies and 48% based on case control studies [3].

2. What Is Breast Density?

Breast density refers to the proportions of fibroglandular tissue and fat in women's breasts, as seen on a mammogram. Unlike imaging of other organs, there is marked variability of the appearance of normal breast tissue, ranging from no dense tissue and almost all fat, to almost no fat, and all dense tissue. Breast density is divided into four categories in the American College of Radiology Breast Imaging and Data System (ACR BI-RADS) 5th edition. A—almost entirely fat, B—scattered fibroglandular densities,

C—heterogeneously dense, D—extremely dense (Figure 1). Categories A and B are considered non-dense, and categories C and D are considered dense. Having dense breasts is normal and common: Among women aged 40 years or older, approximately 43% have dense breasts: 36% have Category C density, and 7% have Category D [4]. Han et al. found that women with a family history of breast cancer were more likely to have dense breasts than women with no family history [5].

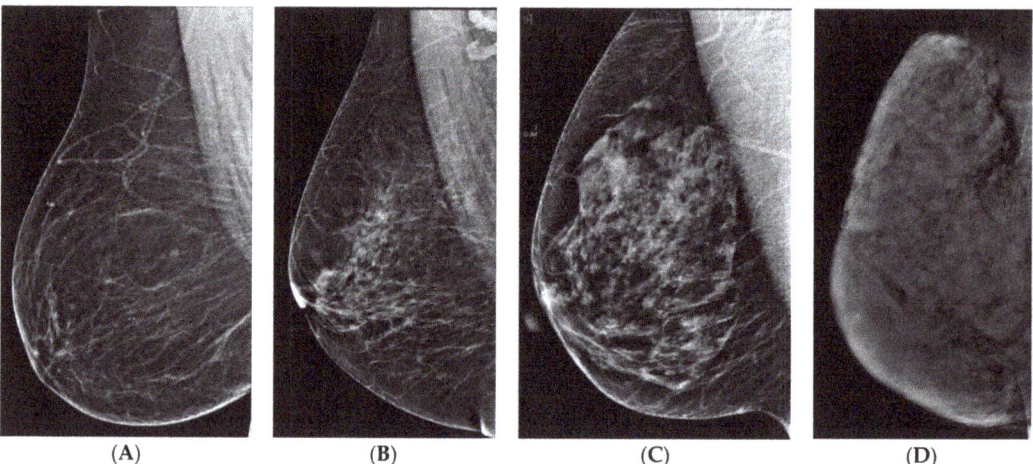

Figure 1. ACR BI-RADS 5th edition density categories: (**A**) Category A—almost entirely fat, (**B**) Category B—scattered fibroglandular densities, (**C**) Category C—heterogeneously dense, (**D**) Category D—extremely dense.

3. What Is the Significance of Dense Breasts?

There are two risks associated with dense breasts. The more important risk [with respect to screening performance] is the masking of cancers on mammograms, because they can be obscured in normal dense tissue [6,7]. Mammographic sensitivity is inversely proportional to the degree of breast density. Sensitivity for digital mammography is 79.9% overall, but almost 100% in Category A, 83.9% for Category B, 72.9% for Category C, and 50% for Category D [8]. Stated another way, as many as 50% of cancers are missed on mammograms in women with Category D. This explains why women do not all benefit equally from mammography (Figure 2).

Mortality reduction is significantly lower in women with dense breasts. Using data from the Nijmegen (Dutch) screening program, Van der Waal et al. showed 41% mortality reduction in women with fatty breasts (that they defined as <25% dense) but only 13% mortality reduction in women with dense breasts (that they defined as >25% dense) [9]. Chiu et al. showed that women with dense breasts had significantly increased breast cancer mortality (RR = 1.91) after adjusting for other risk factors [10].

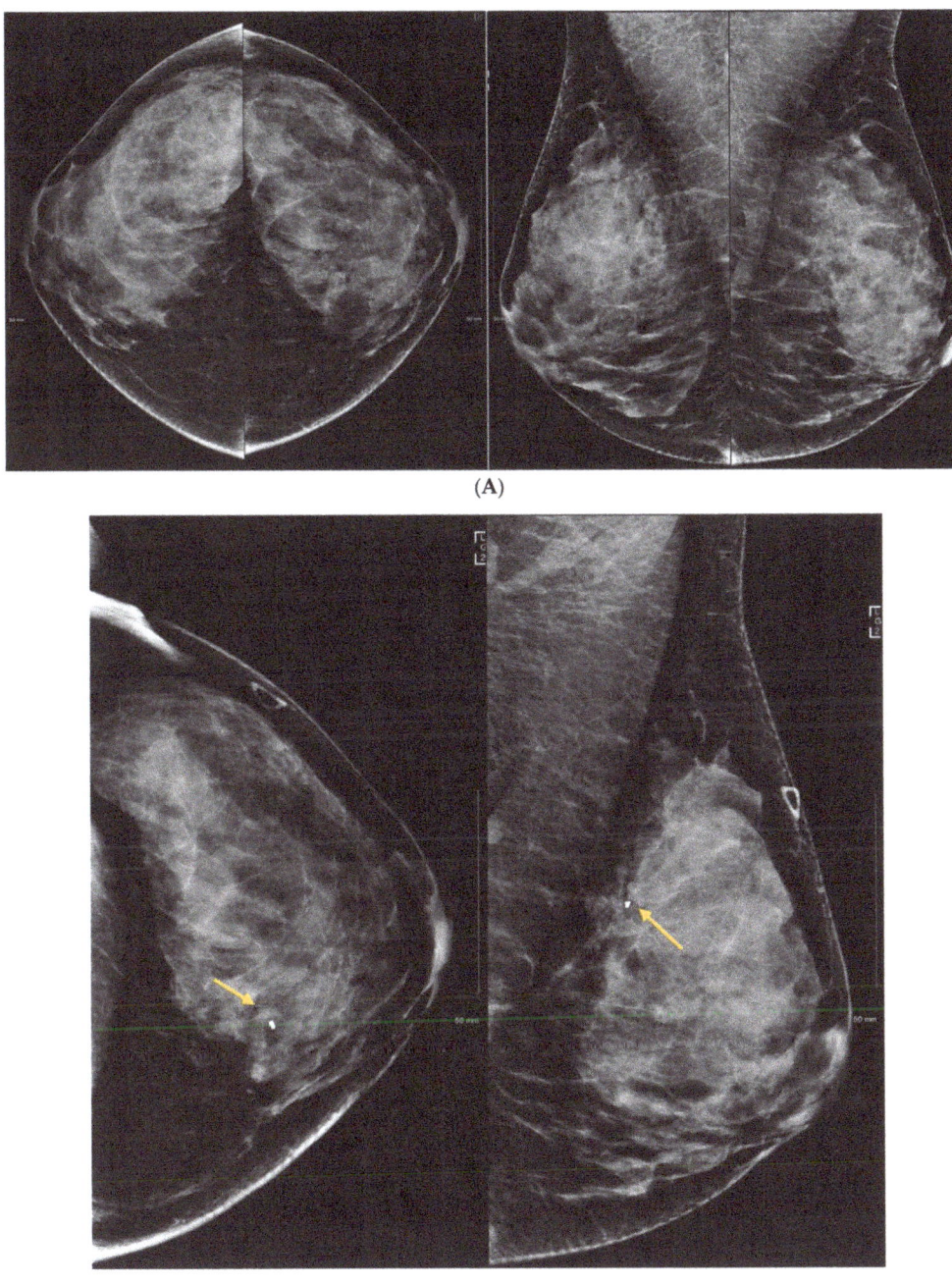

Figure 2. *Cont.*

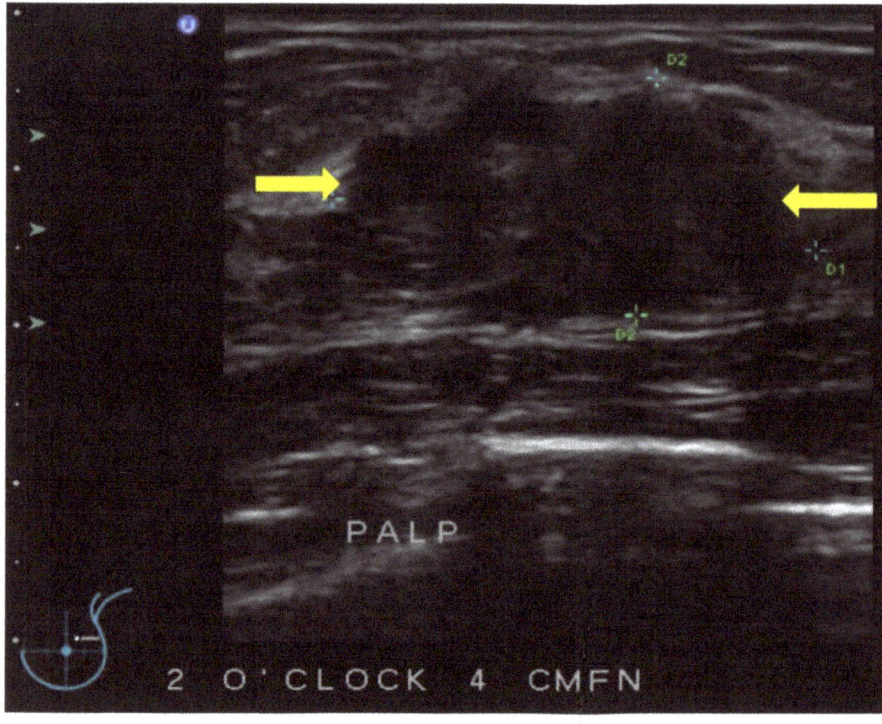

(C)

Figure 2. (**A**) Routine screening mammogram in a 50-year-old woman with screening Density Category D. Calcifications were seen in the left upper inner quadrant (not shown) for which stereotactic core biopsy showed atypical ductal hyperplasia. Surgical excision was planned. Eight months later she returned with a palpable lump in the left upper outer quadrant. (**B**) Left mammography was performed with a triangular skin marker taped at the site of the lump. The post biopsy marker clip was seen (arrow), but no abnormality was seen at the site of the lump on full field digital mammography (FFDM) or on digital breast tomosynthesis (not shown). (**C**) Ultrasound showed a 3.2 cm mass (arrows) and abnormal axillary nodes (not shown). Core biopsy confirmed invasive ductal carcinoma. This is an interval cancer.

The other risk for women with dense breasts is an increased risk of getting breast cancer, but the magnitude of increased risk varies, possibly in part because of the different ways of measuring density. Engmann et al. found that high breast density was the most prevalent risk factor for both premenopausal and postmenopausal women [11]. Boyd et al., using a semi-quantitative method called interactive thresholding to determine breast density found that women with dense breasts were up to six times higher risk than women of the same age with little or no density [12]. Using a five-category scale of percentage breast density, McCormack and dos Santos Silva, in a meta-analysis of 42 studies using three different density-grading methods, found increasing risk of breast cancer, with 4–6 times higher risk for women with >75% density compared to those with <5% [13]. Bertrand et al., pooling data from six studies where density was calculated by the same interactive thresholding method described by Boyd, found that women with high breast density (>51%) are twice as likely to develop breast cancer as women with average density (11–25%) [14]. It should be noted that the use of >51% most closely resembles a combination of BI-RADS Categories C and D. Using data from the Kopparberg randomized controlled trial in Sweden, Chiu et al. demonstrated increased breast cancer incidence for women with high breast density (defined as pattern IV or V by the Tabár classification) after adjusting for other risk factors [10,15].

Breast density is also a biomarker for predicting response to neo-adjuvant chemotherapy. Skarping et al. showed that premenopausal women with high mammographic density respond poorly to neoadjuvant chemotherapy [16].

Woodard et al. found that women with Category D breasts who have been treated for breast cancer had lower Oncotype DX test recurrence scores than women with Category A breasts [17]. This would seem counterintuitive, but they theorized that it might be due to "deregulation of adipose tissue signaling pathways within the breast microenvironment, leading to local aromatization of androgens to estrogens that may promote tumor recurrence."

However, Huang et al., in a case-control study showed a higher risk of locoregional recurrence for women with Categories C and D after modified radical mastectomy [18] and Eriksson et al. found that high mammographic density (defined as >25% density) was associated with increased risk of local and locoregional recurrence compared to women with <25% density, but was not associated with distant metastasis nor survival [19].

Dense tissue also limits detection of recurrent breast cancer in treated women.

4. Density and Interval Cancers

Interval cancers (ICs) are those detected in the interval between planned screening mammograms, i.e., after a negative screening mammogram. Some ICs arise because they are rapidly growing, and were not visible on the prior mammogram but are visible on the mammogram performed at the time of diagnosis ("true IC") [20]. Some may have been present, but not seen because of poor technique or positioning (the cancer was not included on the image), not seen because of masking by dense breast tissue, or visible in retrospect but not detected or misinterpreted by the screener ("false negative").

ICs are more common in younger women, women with a family history of breast cancer and women on menopausal hormone therapy. They tend to be larger and higher grade than screen-detected cancers, more likely estrogen receptor negative (ER-)and progesterone receptor negative (PR-negative), more likely mucinous and lobular histology, more likely with nodal metastases at the time of diagnosis, and with a higher proliferation index [14,19–25].

The interval cancer rate will vary according to the breast cancer incidence in a given population, how ICs are determined, whether initial or subsequent screening round, and the length of time between screens. Longer intervals between screening examinations lead to increased IC rates. Screening programs will have varying targets for ICs depending on their screening interval. Jurisdictions that screen every 2–3 years may accept a higher IC rate than programs that screen annually. Lehman et al. reviewed performance measures in the Breast Cancer Consortium from 2007 to 2013 and found an IC rate of 0.8/1000 within 12 months of a negative mammogram [26]. Houssami and Hunter reviewed 24 screening programs globally, most of which screen biennially, and found that 20–25% of ICs are false negative, but IC rates are lower for annual screening intervals and higher for triennial screening. IC rates ranged from 8.4 to 21.1 per 10,000 screens, with the larger proportion of the estimate occurring in year two of a two-yearly interval [22]. Seely et al. showed that in Canada, jurisdictions that offer only biennial mammograms to women with dense breasts have 63% higher interval cancer rates than those that offer annual mammography [27].

High breast density is associated with an increased risk of interval cancers [7,28–30]. Interval cancers are 13–31 times more likely in Category D breasts than in category A [6,30,31]. Van der Waal et al. showed that the proportion of women with dense breasts among interval cases ranged from 38.7% to 54.5%, but ranged from 20.7% to 30.5% in screen-detected cases in the Dutch screening program [9]. ICs in women with dense breasts are 2–3.5 more lethal than in women with non-dense breasts [9,32].

An important goal of breast cancer screening is to minimize ICs in women of all breast densities. Research, including artificial intelligence, is underway to determine which women are at risk of interval cancers. Several imaging modalities, including ultrasound (US), digital breast tomosynthesis (DBT), magnetic resonance imaging (MRI), contrast-enhanced mammography (CEM) and molecular breast imaging (MBI) are capable of detecting cancers missed on mammograms.

The efficacy of any imaging modality should ideally be shown by decreased mortality in RCTs. Unlike in therapeutic trials, these take decades to mature, since for lower mortality to be evident requires that there be deaths in the control group. Because of improvements in therapy, women in the control group might not die for many years, or even decades, meaning that by the time RCT results are available, the technology used in the trials may be obsolete. Kuhl and Baltzer argue that efficacy should be determined by surrogate measures such as decreased rates of ICs and advanced cancers [33]. This should be reasonable, especially given that using surrogate endpoints has been shown to underestimate benefit [34], and it would allow the introduction of life-saving technology sooner. Moreover, what really is of importance to an individual woman in the shared decision-making process regarding participation in supplemental screening is not the outcome of a trial where there was noncompliance among women in the study group, and contamination by women in the control group, but rather the outcome for women who did participate.

5. Ultrasound (US)

Ultrasound (US) uses sound waves to image tissue. It uses no ionizing radiation, and intravenous contrast is not required. It was used for abdominal and pelvic imaging in the 1970s and early 1980s. Breast ultrasound was attempted then with the available lower frequency transducers, and the possibility of screening with US was explored, but was unsuccessful [35,36]. With the development of high-frequency transducers in the mid 1980s, it was possible to use US in the breast: initially for cyst/solid differentiation [37], and then benign/malignant differentiation [38,39]. Since the first demonstration of US-detection of cancers missed on mammograms in 1995 [40], numerous single center studies confirmed the potential of US as a supplemental screen for women with dense breasts [41–45]. Summarizing these, 94% of the cancers were invasive, and 70% of them were 1 cm or smaller in size. Ninety percent were stage 0 or stage I and 90.5% of the women with sonographically-detected cancers had either heterogeneously dense or extremely dense parenchyma [46]. These studies showed a biopsy rate of 3%, and 11% of the biopsies showed malignancy. Seven percent of women had short-interval follow-up. Overall, the incremental cancer detection rate (ICDR) was 3.5 cancers/1000 screens. This increased cancer detection was of invasive cancers, so concern regarding "overdiagnosis" of DCIS did not apply.

The Avon-ACRIN (American College of Radiology) 6666 multicenter study recruited 2809 women at 21 sites, who were at increased risk and who had dense breast tissue in at least one quadrant, to have three consecutive screening examinations with mammography and breast US. The goal was to determine the ICDR of annual breast ultrasound screening, and all participants were offered breast MRI at the conclusion of the study. They found that US and MRI both detected cancers missed on mammography, at the cost of low specificity. ICDR and positive predictive value (PPV) for US was 5.3/1000 and 11% in the first year, and 3.7/1000 and 16% in the second and third years, averaging 4.3/1000 and 14% overall. Of the cancers seen only on US, 94% were invasive with a median size of 10 mm, and 96% of those staged were node negative. MRI detected an additional 14.7/1000 after negative US and mammography [47].

False alarms, i.e., women recalled for additional tests at screening but found to be benign after diagnostic workup, cause anxiety for women. Those that are determined to be "probably benign," for which surveillance can be recommended instead of biopsy, incur costs and use appointment slots that could be used for more urgent cases. Barr et al. investigated the outcomes of 745 BI-RADS 3 masses in the Avon ACRIN 6666 trial, and found 6 cancers (0.8%). Only one of the cancers had suspicious changes at 6-month follow-up, so it is reasonable to drop the necessity of a 6-month US and recommend a 1-year diagnostic follow-up for BI-RADS category 3 lesions detected at screening US [48].

In 2009, Connecticut was the first state to enact breast density notification legislation, and to perform high volume supplemental US screening. Hooley reported the initial experience with technologist-performed US, which showed ICDR of 3.2 cancers/1000 prevalence screens. PPV was 6.5% [49]. At RSNA 2016, Philpotts et al. reported on the outcomes during their 5th-year and showed ICDR of 2.6 cancers/1000 screens, with a much-improved PPV of 25% [50]. Elsewhere in Connecticut, Weigert and Steenbergen reported on their first year of screening US: ICDR was 3.25 cancers/1000 screens with a PPV of 6.7% [51]. Their 4th year showed stable ICDR of 3.3 cancers/1000 and much-improved PPV 20.1% [52]. Currently, there is insurance coverage for supplemental ultrasound screening in 12 states and the District of Columbia, but the laws vary by state, and out-of-pocket costs may apply [53].

Breast density notification is also underway in in Canada. In response to patient advocacy, the first of several provinces started notifying all women of their breast density on their screening mammography reports in 2018 [54]. Coverage by public health insurance followed in early 2019 [55]. Women in British Columbia with category C and D densities and no other risk factors may attend supplemental US screening, with a referral from their physician or nurse practitioner. Wu and Warren reported on the first year of screening US after insurance coverage started, and showed ICDR of 7/1000, with average tumor size of 9 mm (all node negative), biopsy rate of 1.3% and PPV of 42% (Figure 3). Importantly, 40% of the cancers were found in women with no risk factors other than dense breasts [56]. Sixty percent of the cancers were found in women with category C density [57]. This is relevant, as some have suggested that supplemental screening should be rationed to only the smaller percentage of women with extremely dense breasts.

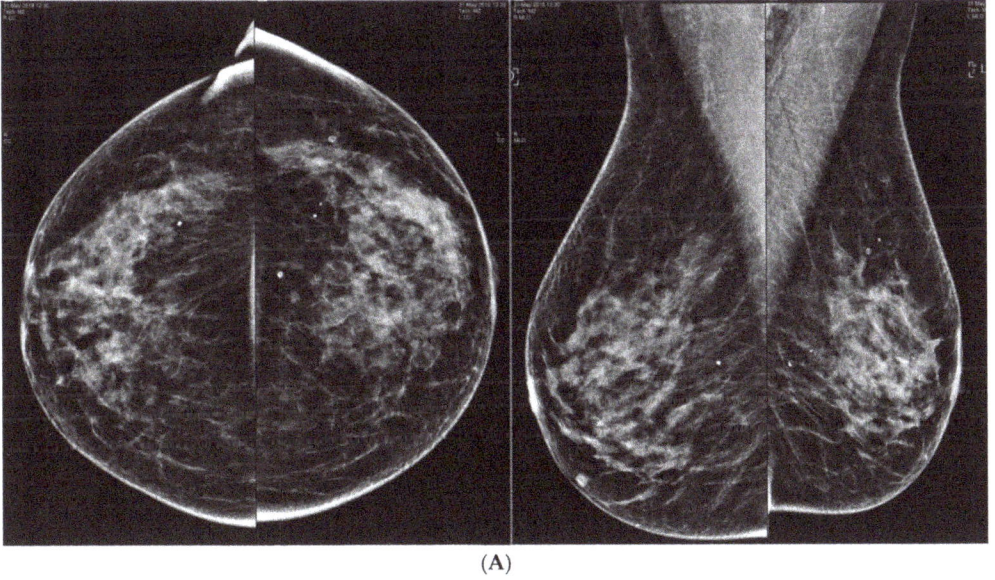

(A)

Figure 3. *Cont.*

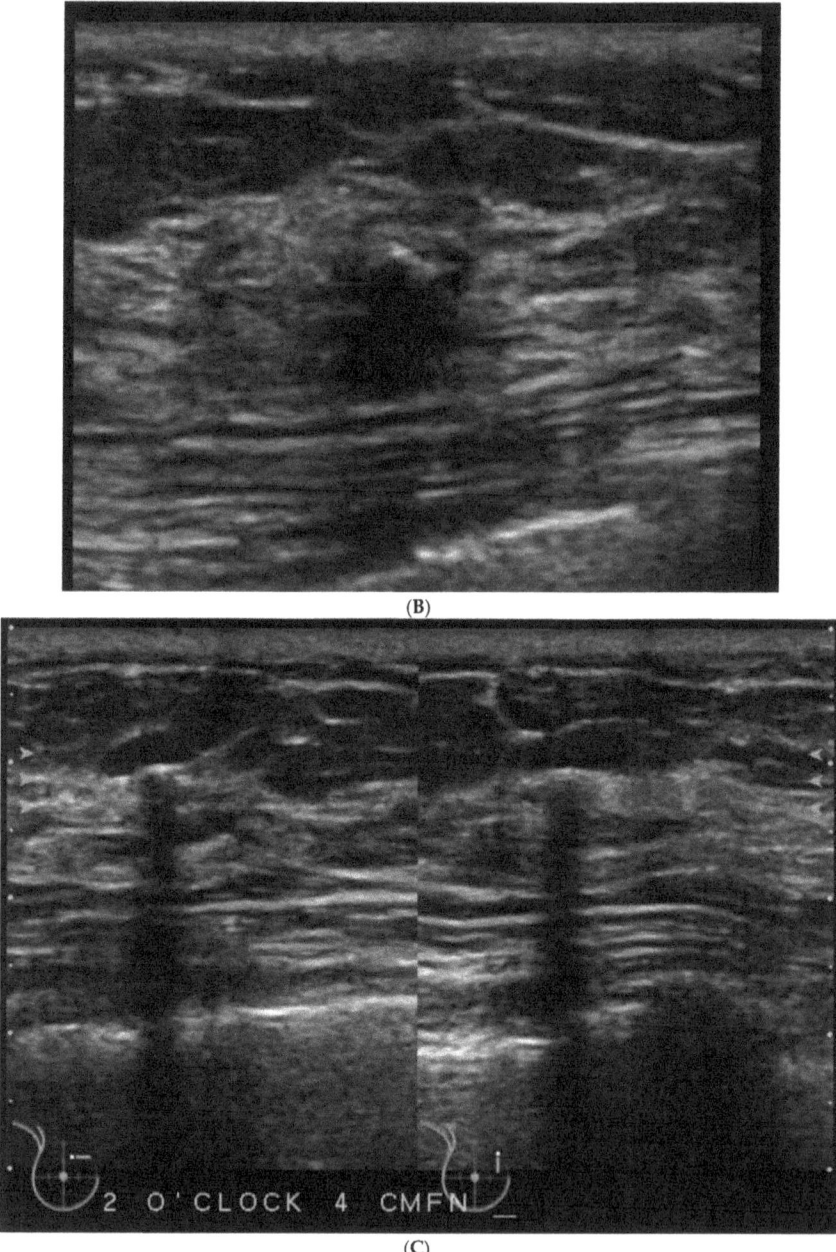

Figure 3. (**A**) Negative screening mammogram in a 73-year-old woman with category C density. Screening ultrasound showed masses in (**B**) left and (**C**) right breasts. Tomosynthesis is not part of the screening mammography program, but was performed after masses were found on US, but was also negative (not shown). Mass on left showed invasive lobular carcinoma on core biopsy. Mass on right showed atypical lobular hyperplasia.

Acknowledging the importance of increasing ICDRs and reducing ICs, Corsetti et al. reported on a retrospective cohort of 8865 women studied from 2001–2006. Women with non-dense breasts had mammography alone, and women with dense breasts had mammography and US. After one year, CDR was 6.3/1000 screens in the mammogram group, and 8.3/1000 screens in the mammogram plus US group. Overall, there was no significant difference in the IC rate: 1.0/1000 in women with non-dense breasts, and 1.1/1000 in women with dense breasts. The ICs were early stage (in situ or small invasive) cancers, and almost all were node-negative. They admitted that cancers not seen on mammography may or may not progress to become ICs, and that reducing ICs might not reduce mortality, and stated the importance of an RCT [58].

An RCT of screening US, the Japan Strategic Anti-cancer Randomized Trial (J-START), is underway in Japan. From July 2007 to March 2011, 72,998 women aged 40–49 of all breast densities were enrolled at 42 study sites and divided into 2 equal groups, one having mammography alone (control group), and the other having mammography plus US (intervention group) annually for 2 years. In a preliminary publication, sensitivity was significantly higher in the intervention group than in the control group (91·1% vs. 77·0%; $p = 0.0004$). Specificity was significantly lower (87·7% vs. 91·4%; $p < 0.0001$). More cancers were detected in the intervention group (184 vs. 117; $p = 0.0003$) and were more frequently stage 0 and I (144 vs. 79; $p = 0.0194$). Fewer ICs were detected in the intervention group 18 vs. 35; ($p = 0.034$) [59]. Further follow-up is anticipated in the near future.

Harada-Shoji et al. did a secondary analysis of the J-START trial to determine the effect of breast density on outcome of adding ultrasound to mammography. The unexpected finding that women with non-dense breasts benefitted equally to women with dense breasts, indicates that there is room for improvement in screening women of all densities in this younger age group [60]. As Kuhl points out, it is noteworthy that there was a greater proportion of women with dense breasts in the study compared with Western women: 68% vs. 43% [4], and the peak incidence of breast cancer in Japan is much younger than in women in the USA or Europe: aged 40–49 vs. 60–69 [61,62]. So not surprisingly, Kuhl sees this study as a reminder that there is a need for research on improved screening strategies for women of all breast densities [62]. Her work in 2017 showed that supplemental MRI screening in average-risk women of all breast densities detected 22.6 cancers/1000 prevalent screens and 6.9/1000 incident screens with no interval cancers, and the MRI-detected cancers were high-grade in 41.7% of cases at prevalence screening and 46.0% of cases at incidence screening [63].

Ohnuki et al. addressed the lower specificity in the intervention group that arose in the J-START trial, as a result of further examination being required in all positive cases classified by either mammography or ultrasound. They developed an overall assessment system of combined mammography and adjunctive ultrasound for breast cancer screening which lowered recall rates by 16–53% [64]. For example: if mammography showed a mass requiring recall, but concurrent US showed a benign lesion, then recall could be avoided.

Initially performed as a hand-held examination, automated US equipment using large footprint transducers was developed, and tested in the Somo-Insight multicenter trial, where 15,318 average-risk women with Category C and D density were recruited. The ICDR was 1.9 cancers/1000 women, but with an increased recall rate over mammography of 285/1000 [65].

Kelly et al. used a device with a small-footprint hand-held type transducer attached to an automated articulated arm. The images were acquired with the transducer moved in overlapping vertical rows and were viewed in cine loops. The ICDR was 3.6 cancers/1000; recall rate was 7.2%; PPV 38% [66].

Berg and Vourtsis reviewed ICDR in hand-held and automated breast ultrasound, and reported similar ICDRs averaging 2.1–2.7/1000 for physician- and technologist-performed examinations, but the ranges are wide. This may be due to the differences in the time periods encompassed. The averages using hand-held included studies date from 1995, so the earlier studies were performed with more primitive technology. The automated studies were from 2010–2018, so used more advanced technology [67].

Observational data showing surrogate markers of tumor size and lymph node status indicates that supplemental US finds the same kinds of cancers that led to decreased mortality in the RCTs of mammography. It has been shown that using surrogate markers underestimates benefits [34]. Nevertheless, task forces in Canada and the USA do not recommend supplemental screening for women with dense breasts, because they decline to consider data other than RCTs. This underscores the value of the J-START trial.

Supplemental US screening is available in some locations in Canada [68], the USA [69], and Europe [70]. Currently, there is insurance coverage in 12 American states and the District of Columbia, but the details vary by state [53]. Shared, informed decision-making is recommended to ensure that women are aware of and prepared for possible recall. The data used for shared decision-making should include all available information, including observational studies. In France and Austria supplemental US screening is part of organized screening programs [70].

Whether to perform supplemental ultrasound concurrently with screening mammography, or alternating with it should take patient convenience into account, and Ohnuki's demonstration of improved specificity is also a consideration [65]. However, where screening mammography is performed only biennially, alternating the ultrasound with mammography (each modality every 2 years) allows more frequent screening, and the opportunity for earlier detection.

6. Digital Breast Tomosynthesis (DBT)

DBT is a quasi-three-dimensional technique, where multiple low-dose images are obtained over a range of angles, and reconstructed in slices [71]. It received United States Food and Drug Administration (FDA) approval in 2011. Initially, DBT was performed in addition to digital mammography. Increasingly, if is performed with "synthetic two-dimensional (2D)," which reduces dose by half [72].

DBT increases cancer detection by reducing superimposition, thereby unmasking abnormalities that are obscured by overlapping tissue [73–75], and these are maintained beyond the prevalence round [76]. Invasive lobular cancers in particular, are more conspicuous because of increased visibility of spiculation and architectural distortion [73,77]. The additional cancers detected are invasive, not DCIS, which minimizes "overdiagnosis". DBT reduces recalls by confirming that many apparent abnormalities are artifactual, caused by summation of normal structures [78]. Figure 4 shows an example of a women screened with only 2D digital mammography, where an asymmetry was seen on one view only. Her diagnostic examination was performed with DBT, which confirmed the screening finding to be summation artifact, but also unmasked a cancer that was missed on the 2D screening study.

DBT is widely used in opportunistic screening in the USA. As of 1March 2022, 82% of facilities had DBT units and 45% of all accredited units were DBT in the United States [79]. There is legislation in 17 states and the District of Columbia requiring insurance coverage for DBT screening, but the details of coverage vary by state [53]. However, beyond state law mandates for tomosynthesis coverage, nearly every major insurer in the United States now covers DBT, although out of pocket costs may apply.

DBT is not used in any of the organized screening programs in Canada, but is available for women participating in the TMIST trial in six Canadian cities [80]. It is used in some European countries either in organized screening or opportunistically [70]. The ongoing TMIST trial aims to determine whether DBT reduces advanced cancers, defined as: those with distant metastases, positive lymph nodes, or invasive cancer of greater than 20 mm. Invasive cancer greater than 10 mm but less than 20 mm in size are considered advanced cancer if they are either triple negative or human epidermal growth factor receptor 2 positive (HER2+) [81]. So far, ICs have not shown to be reduced [82,83].

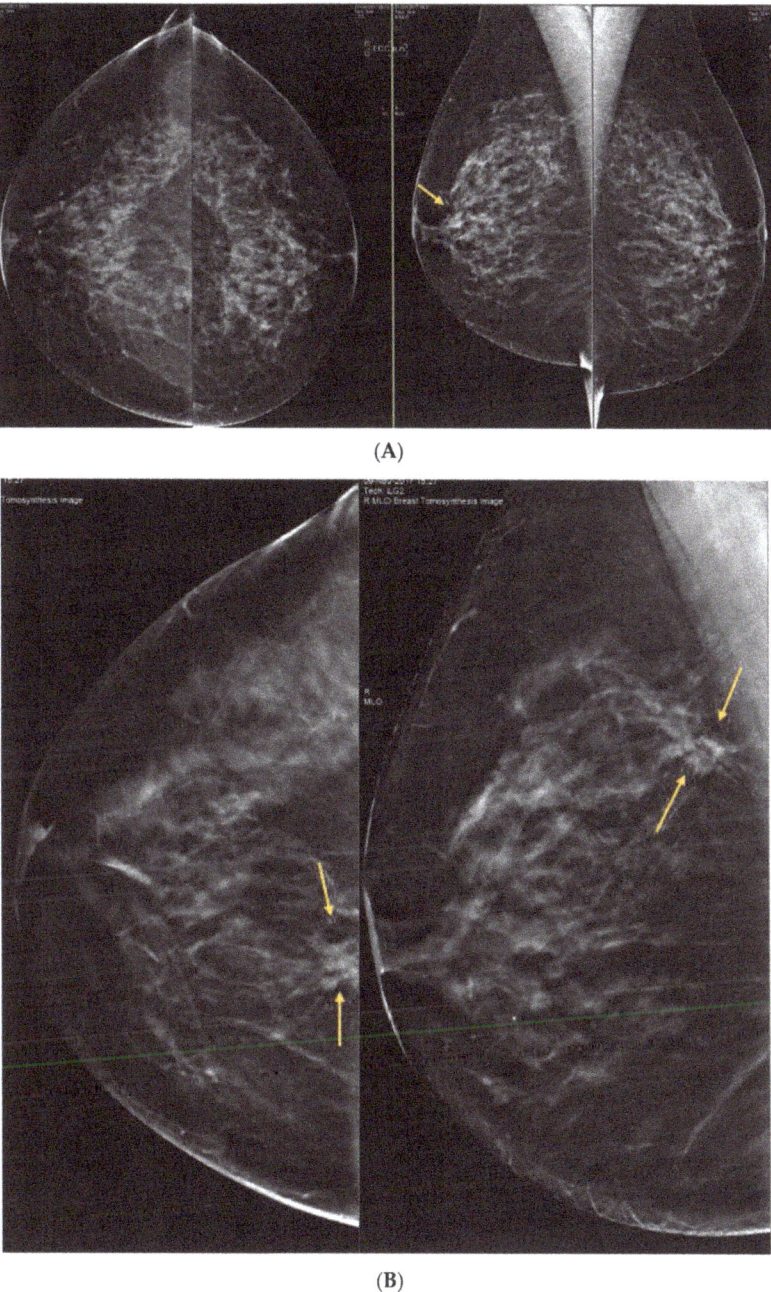

Figure 4. Cont.

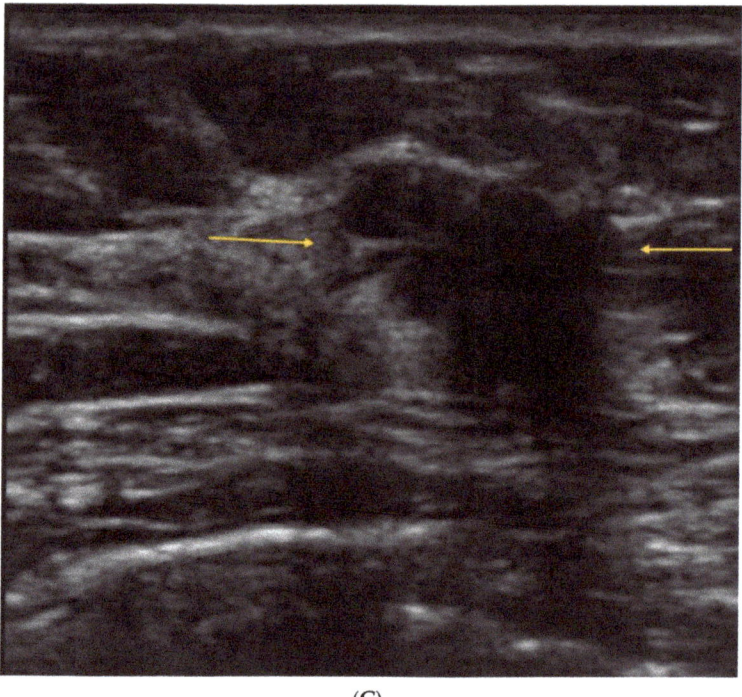

(**C**)

Figure 4. Illustration of DBT resolving an asymmetry seen at 2D screening mammography in the right retroareolar region, and unmasking a cancer in the right upper inner quadrant, not seen on the 2D mammogram. (**A**) This 58-year-old woman had a questionable asymmetry seen on her 2D screening mammogram on the right mediolateral oblique (MLO) view in the retroareolar region (arrow). (**B**) DBT was performed and the asymmetry was shown to be normal tissue, but a spiculated mass was seen in the right upper inner quadrant posteriorly (arrows). (**C**) A correlate was seen on US (arrows), for which histology showed invasive ductal carcinoma.

Rafferty et al. studied the effectiveness of DBT according to breast density, and documented that it is most beneficial in heterogeneously dense breasts, but adds no significant cancer detection in extremely dense breasts [84]. So DBT does not obviate the need for supplemental screening for women with dense breasts (see Figure 2). The ASTOUND trial prospectively compared DBT and US in mammographically-negative dense breasts. US detected almost twice as many additional cancers as DBT at a similar recall rate [85,86]. Figure 5 shows a cancer seen only on DBT, even in a relatively fatty area in a category B breast. US was performed to determine whether a correlate would allow an US-guided core biopsy. The DBT-detected cancer was not seen on the US, and was biopsied with DBT-guidance, but the US revealed a second cancer that was not seen on the DBT, and it was biopsied with US-guidance. Figure 6 shows 3 cancers missed on DBT, but seen with US.

There is significant disparity in breast cancer screening. Although black women have a lower incidence of breast cancer compared with white women, they have higher breast cancer mortality [87,88]. This may be due, in part, because on average, black women have higher breast density than white women [89] and are diagnosed with advanced disease more often [87,88,90]. TMIST will compare how breast density affects the detection of advanced cancer between digital mammography and DBT [81].

DBT has been called "a better mammogram", and this claim is borne out in its improved sensitivity and specificity compared to digital mammography. It does not, however bring equity in breast cancer screening in women with dense breasts.

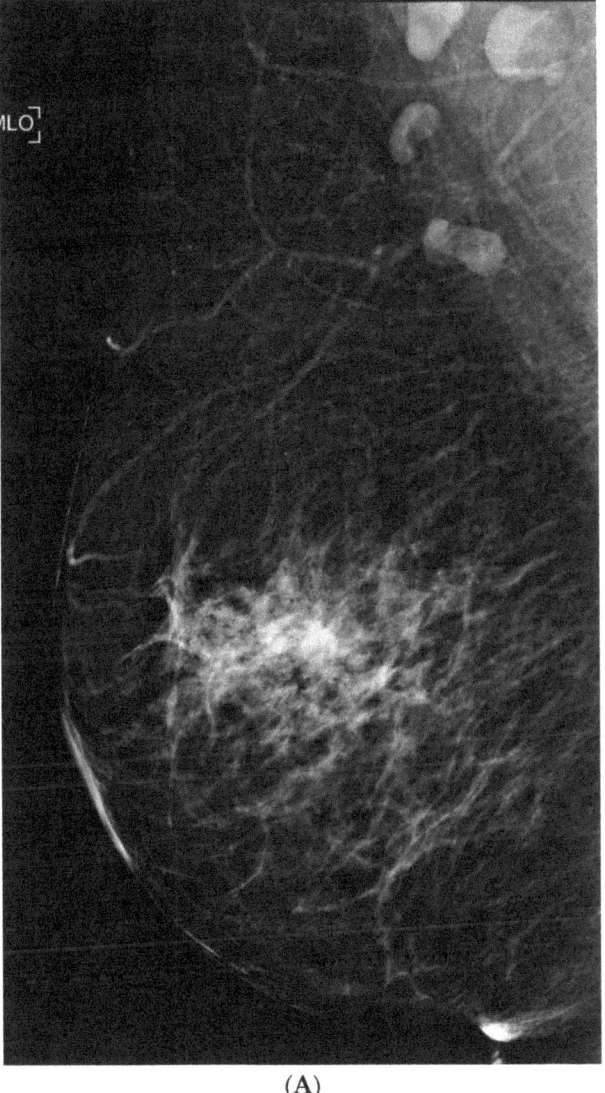

(A)

Figure 5. *Cont.*

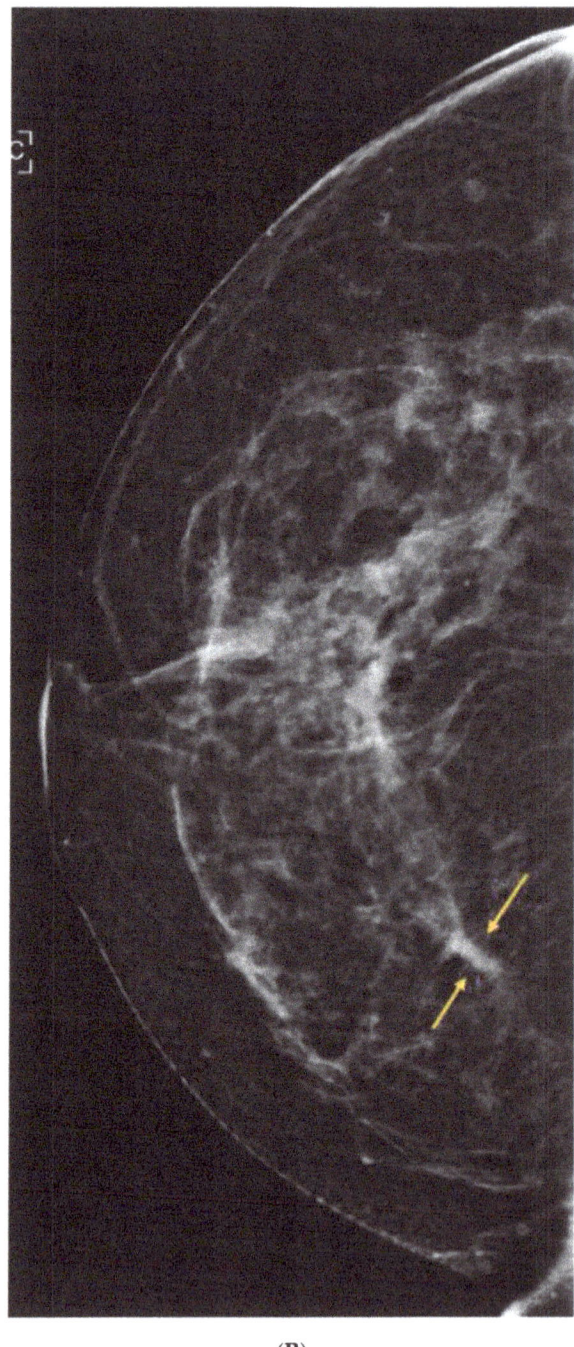

(B)

Figure 5. *Cont.*

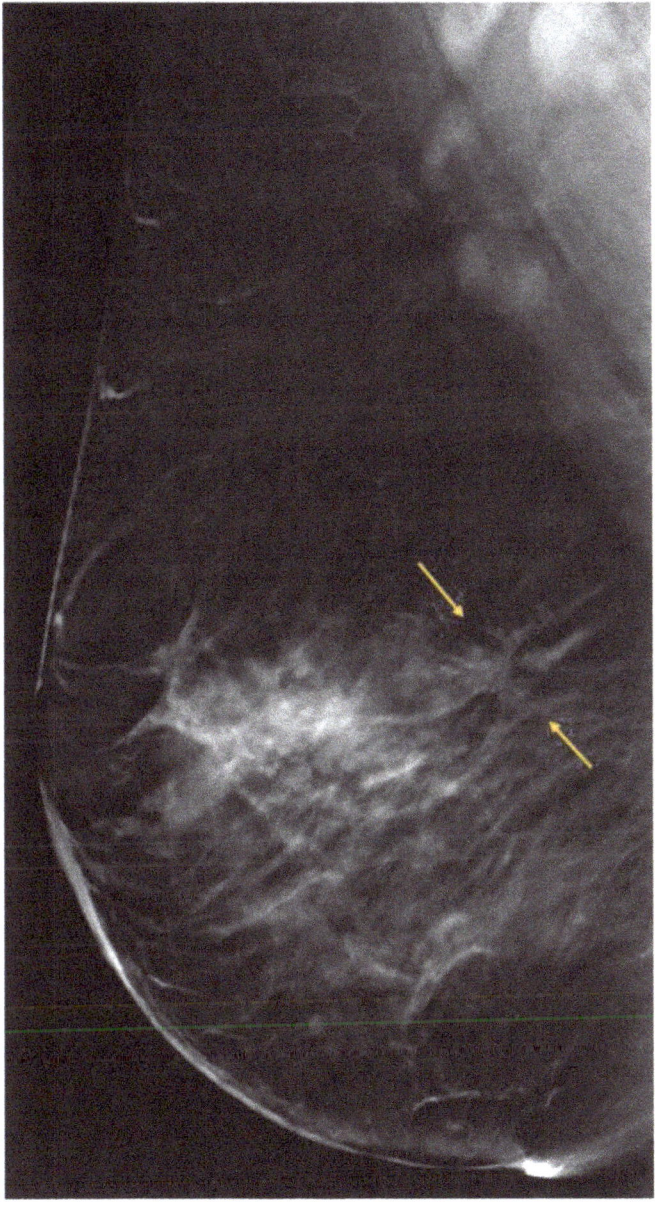

(C)

Figure 5. *Cont.*

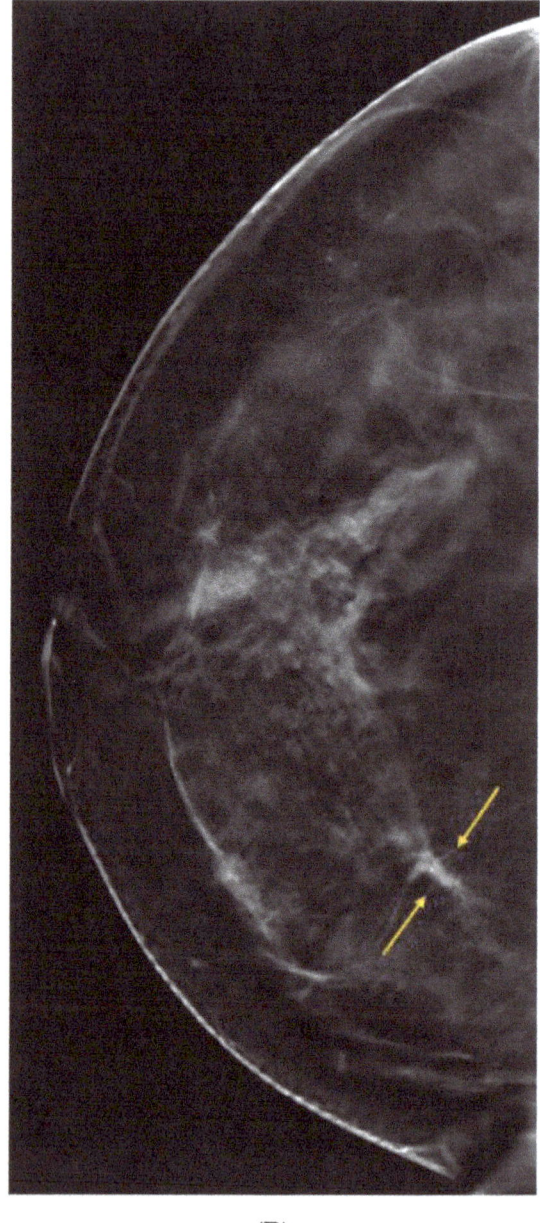

(D)

Figure 5. *Cont.*

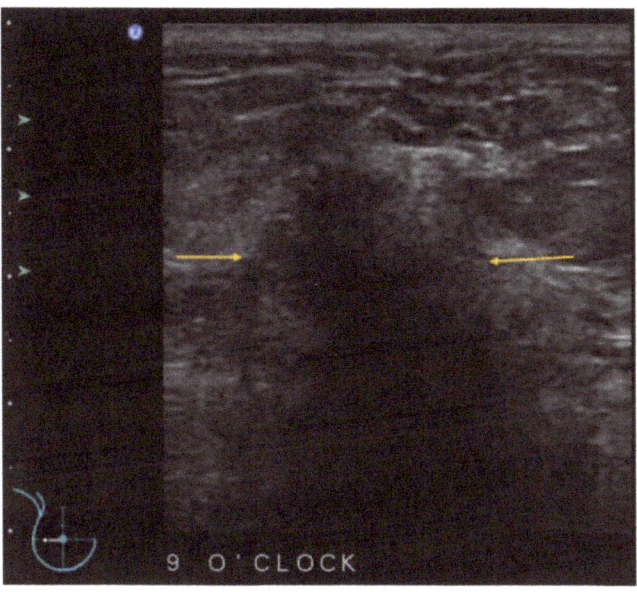

(E)

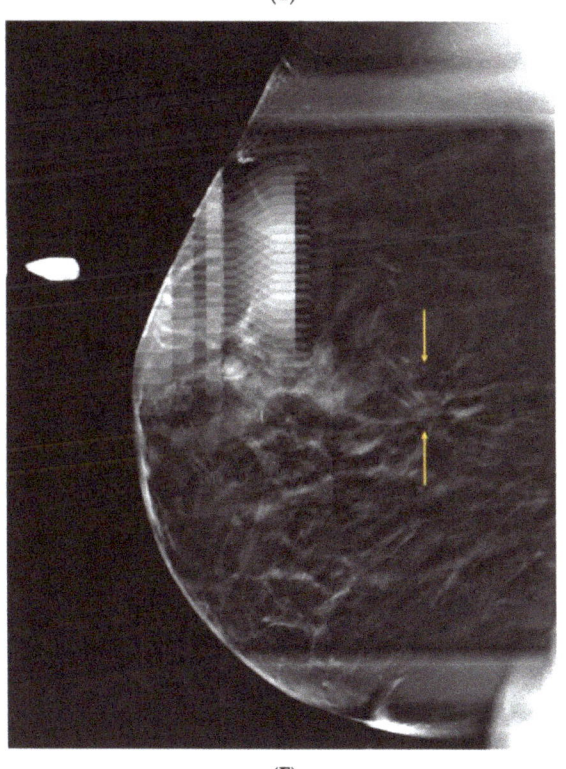

(F)

Figure 5. Fifty-eight-year-old woman with 2 cancers: one seen on DBT but not visible with US, and one seen on US but not on DBT. She presented for screening with DBT. (**A**) Right 2D MLO view was negative, but asymmetry was seen (**B**) medially on the craniocaudal (CC) view. DBT (**C**) MLO and (**D**) CC views show architectural distortion (arrows) in the upper inner quadrant. US was negative in the upper inner quadrant (no image), but showed a suspicious mass in the 9 o'clock position (arrows in (**E**). (**F**) The upper inner quadrant mass was biopsied with DBT-guidance (scout view) and was an invasive lobular carcinoma. The 9 o'clock mass was biopsied with US-guidance and was an invasive ductal carcinoma.

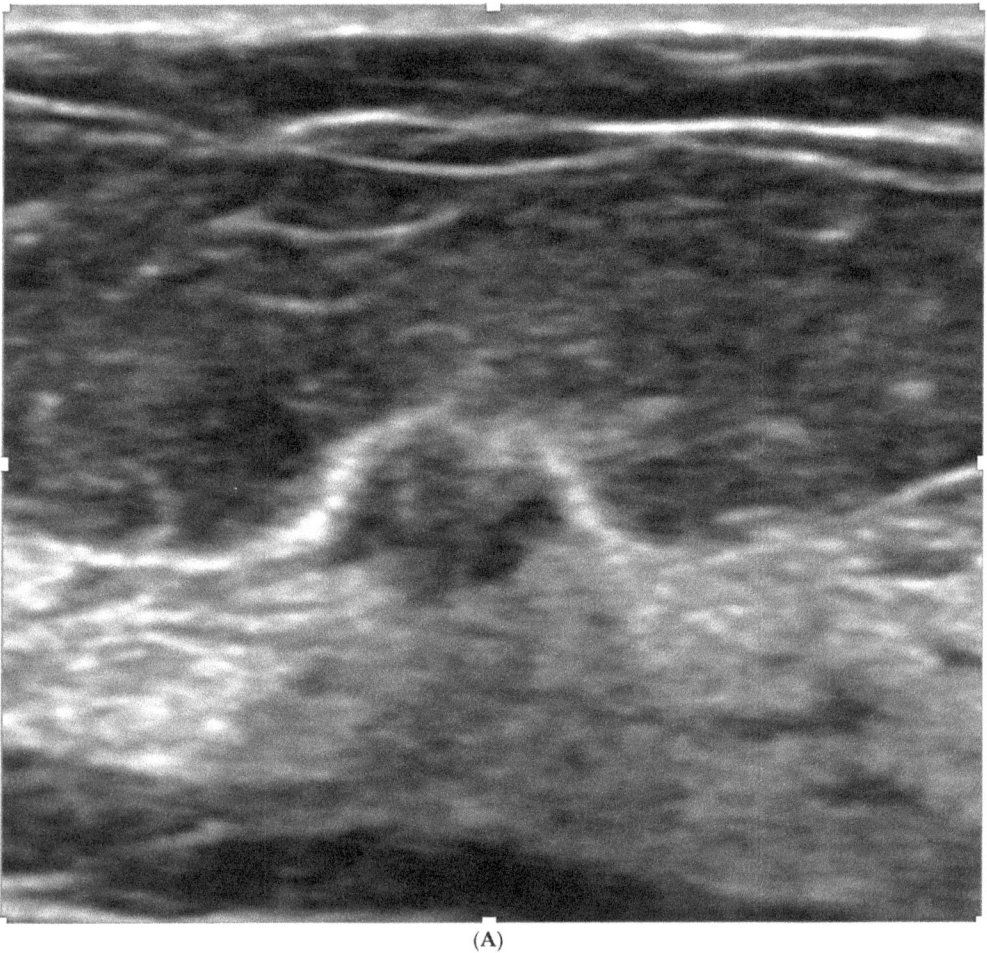

(A)

Figure 6. *Cont.*

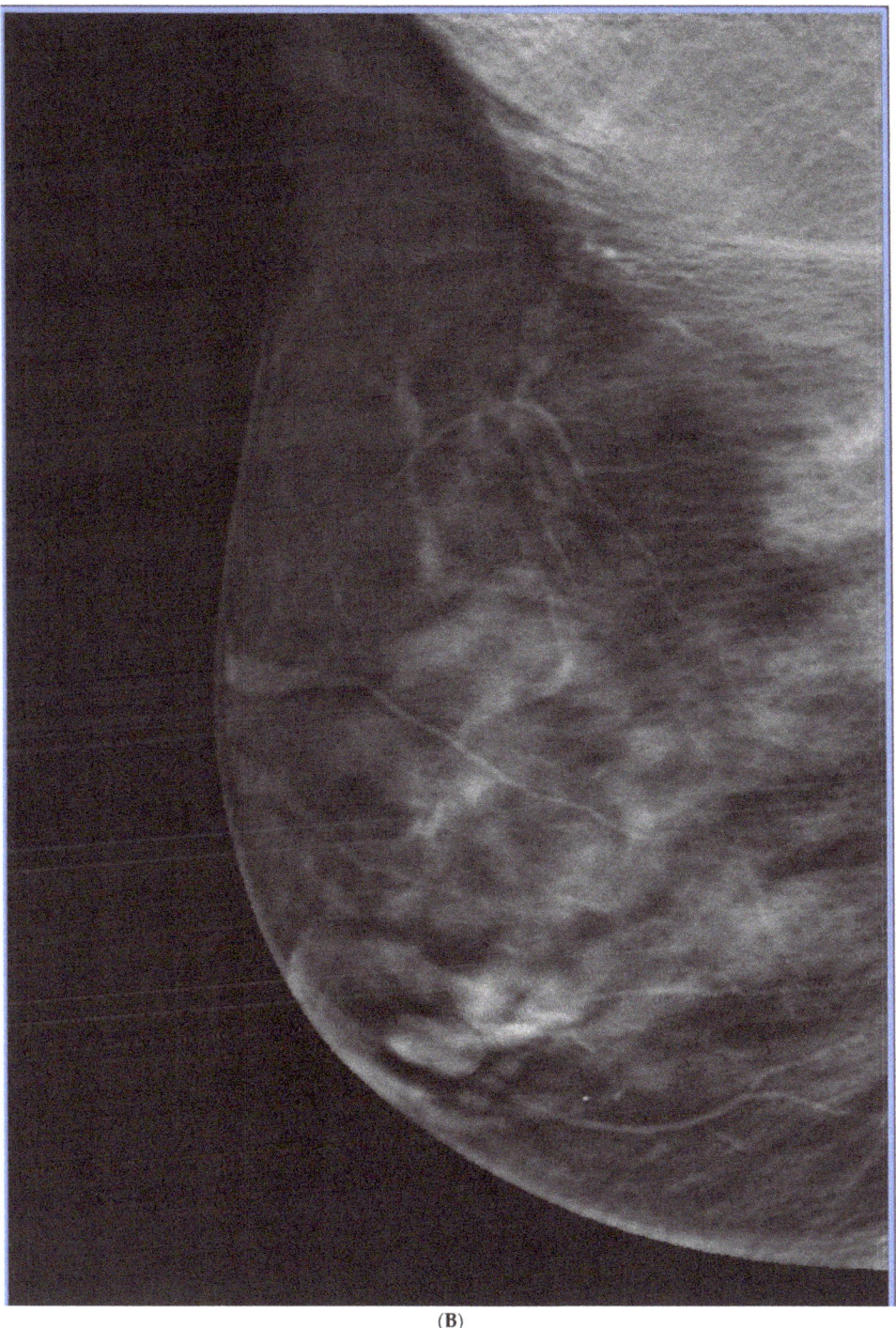

(B)

Figure 6. *Cont.*

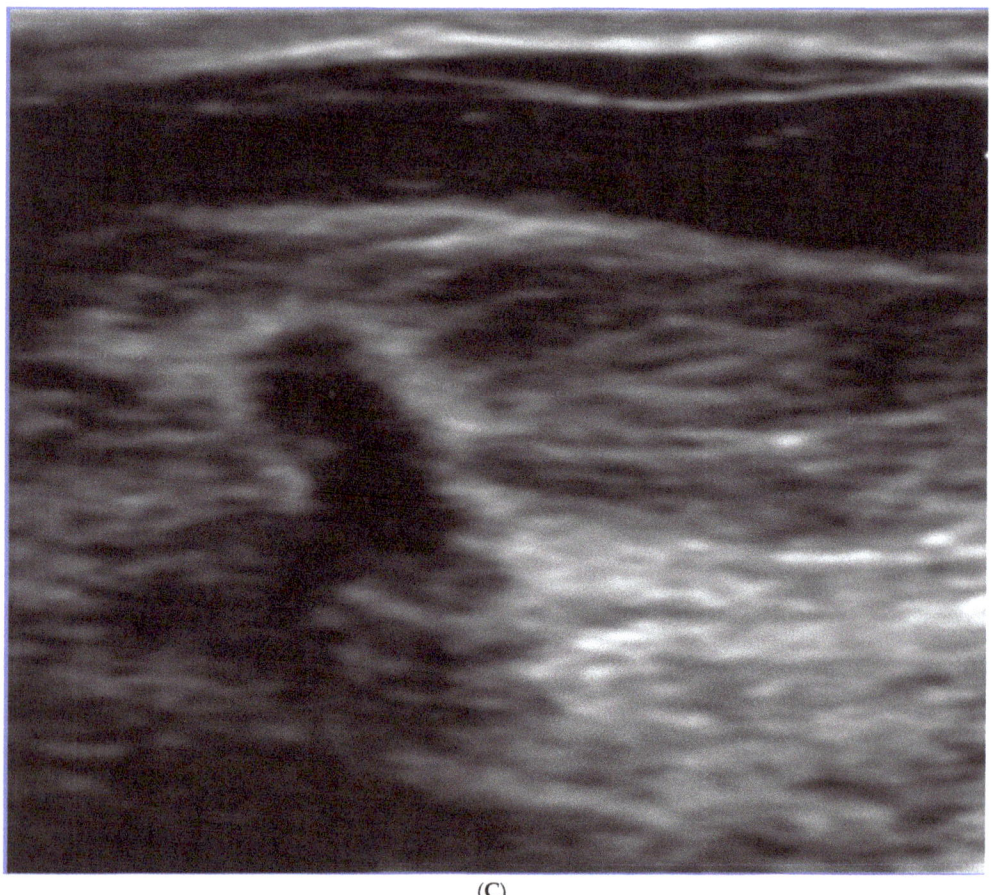

(C)

Figure 6. *Cont.*

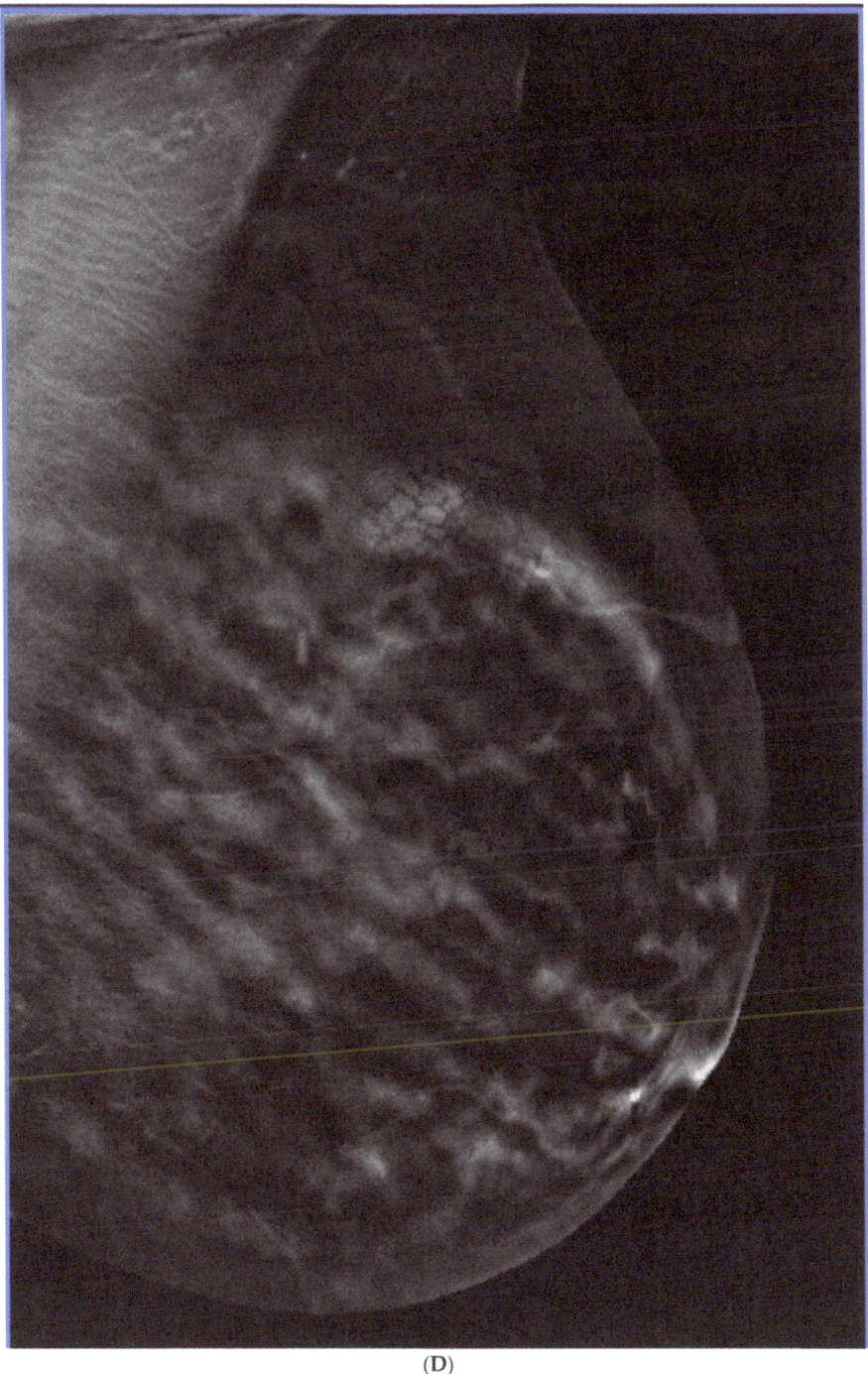

(D)

Figure 6. *Cont.*

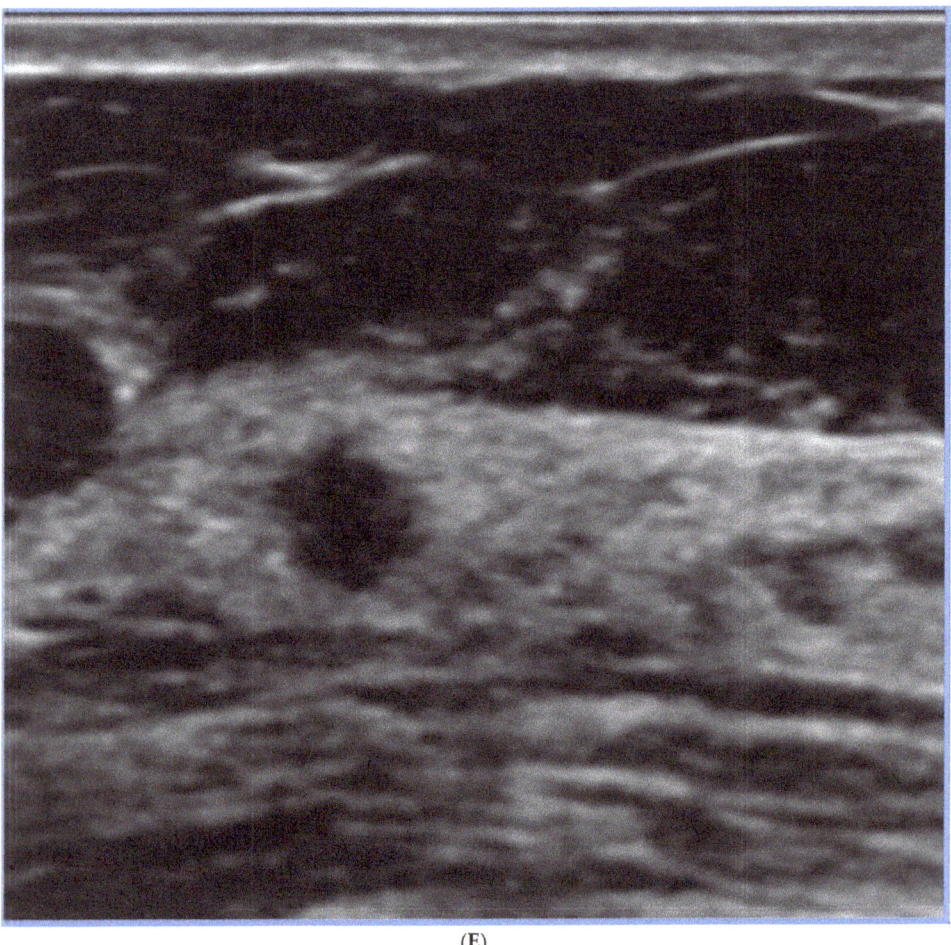

(E)

Figure 6. *Cont.*

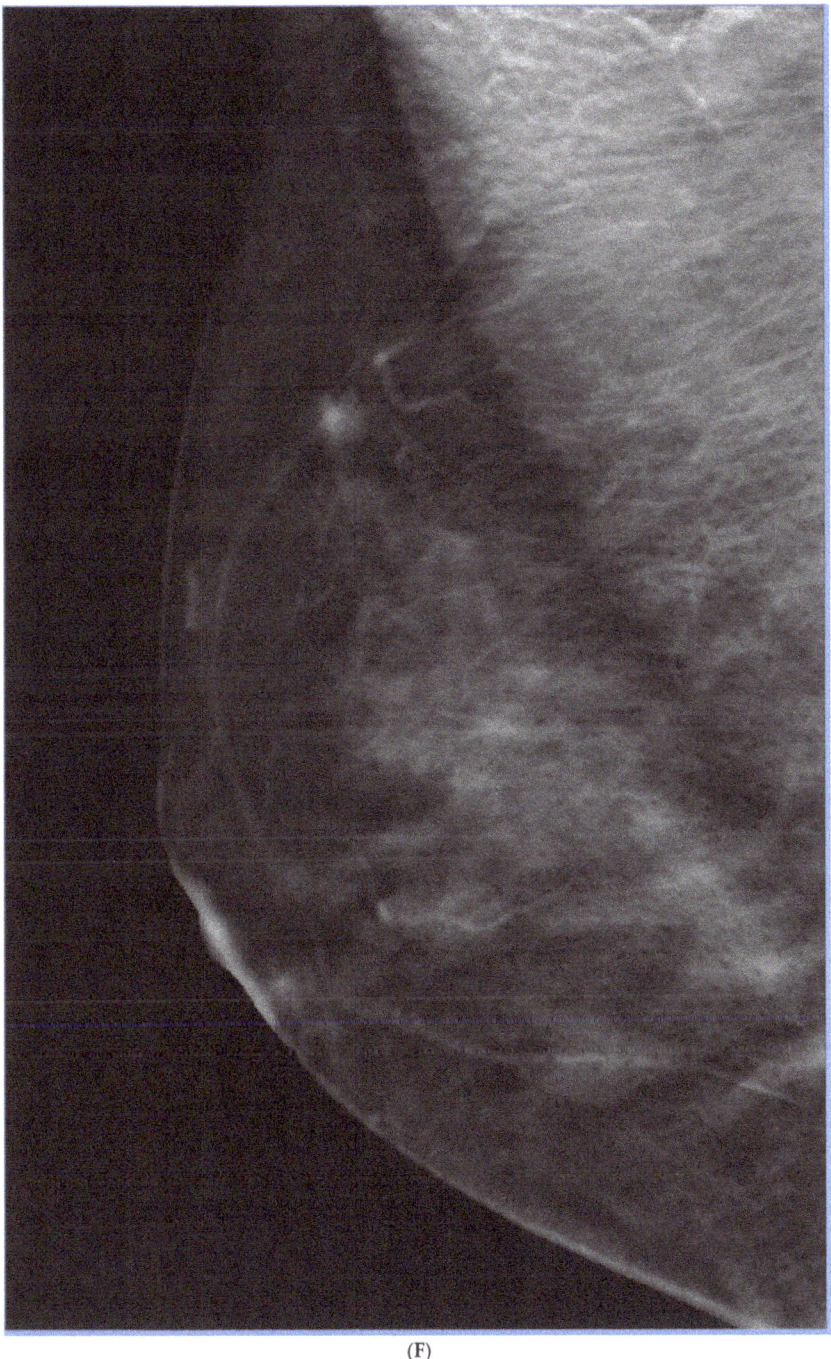

(F)

Figure 6. Courtesy of Dr. Regina Hooley. Three cancers seen on screening US, that were missed on DBT: Mass #1 (**A**) US and (**B**) DBT; Mass #2 (**C**) US and (**D**) DBT; Mass #3 (**E**) US and (**F**) DBT.

7. Magnetic Resonance Imaging (MRI)

Contrast-enhanced MRI (CE MRI) is the most sensitive imaging modality for breast cancer detection, even more so than combined mammography and US [91,92], and when women are being screened with MRI, US finds no additional cancers [92]. Importantly, whereas mammography and DBT are relatively more sensitive to less aggressive cancers, and less sensitive to biologically aggressive cancers, MRI is the opposite. It is arguable that MRI's lower sensitivity to low-grade DCIS is a good thing, leading to reduced "overdiagnosis." Another advantage compared to other modalities is that axillary lymph nodes are included in the scan field. CE MRI uses no ionizing radiation but requires intravenous injection of Gadolinium, which can be classified as linear or macrocyclic. Gadolinium has been shown to accumulate in bone [93,94], skin [95], solid organs [96], and brain tissue [97], albeit with no known long-term effects at the time of writing. Macrocyclic gadolinium is more stable and less likely to accumulate in organs [98].

CE MRI has been shown to be helpful in staging newly-diagnosed breast cancer, guiding surgical planning, and assessing treatment response during/after neoadjuvant chemotherapy [99,100].

Screening MRI was first recommended for women with a lifetime risk $\geq 20\%$ by the American Cancer Society in 2007 [100]. These guidelines were expanded over time, and the American College of Radiology now recommends MRI for women with genetics-based increased risk (and their untested first-degree relatives), with a calculated lifetime risk of 20% or more, women with a history of chest or mantle radiation therapy at a young age, women with dense tissue who have been treated for breast cancer, or those diagnosed by age 50. They recommend consideration of MRI surveillance for women diagnosed with breast cancer or atypia at biopsy, especially if they have other risk factors are. They suggest that ultrasound be considered for those who qualify for but cannot undergo MRI. They recommend that all women, especially black women and those of Ashkenazi Jewish descent, should be evaluated for breast cancer risk no later than age 30, to identify those at higher risk so that they can benefit from supplemental screening [101]. Figure 7 shows a tiny cancer detected on MRI, and subsequently on directed US, in a 52-year-old high risk patient, whose 2D screening mammogram showed BI-RADS C density and was negative. MRI for screening women at high risk is standard in North America. In the USA, there is currently legislation requiring insurance coverage of MRI screening in 10 states and the District of Columbia, although details vary by state. Some specify MRI for high-risk, independent of breast density. Out-of-pocket costs may apply [53].

There is also promising research into the use of MRI for average-risk women with extremely dense breasts. The DENSE trial [102] yielded 16.5 prevalent and 5.9 incident cancers per thousand in women with category D, and ICs were reduced from 4.9/1000 to 0.8/1000 in women who actually had MRI. Kuhl studied average-risk women of all densities, whose conventional screening (mammography +/− US) was negative, and found an ICDR of 22.6 cancers/1000 in the prevalence screen, and 6.9/1000 in the incidence screens. Of the 61 cancers detected over the course of the study (41 invasive, 20 DCIS), 60 were detected only with MRI, and the other was detected with all 3 modalities; no cancer was found with mammography and ultrasound only [63]. The term "prevalence screen" is usually used in the context of a woman's first screening examination, but in that study it refers to the first MRI, since most of the subjects had had conventional screening examinations prior to joining the study. After their last MRI, women were followed for an additional 2 years, and importantly, there were no interval cancers during that time. Reduced interval cancers in both trials suggest future mortality reduction. Of the 61 cancers, 26 (43%) were high-grade, including 46% at incident screening. Twenty of the cancers (33%) were estrogen- and progesterone receptor–negative, so biologically significant, and not over diagnosed.

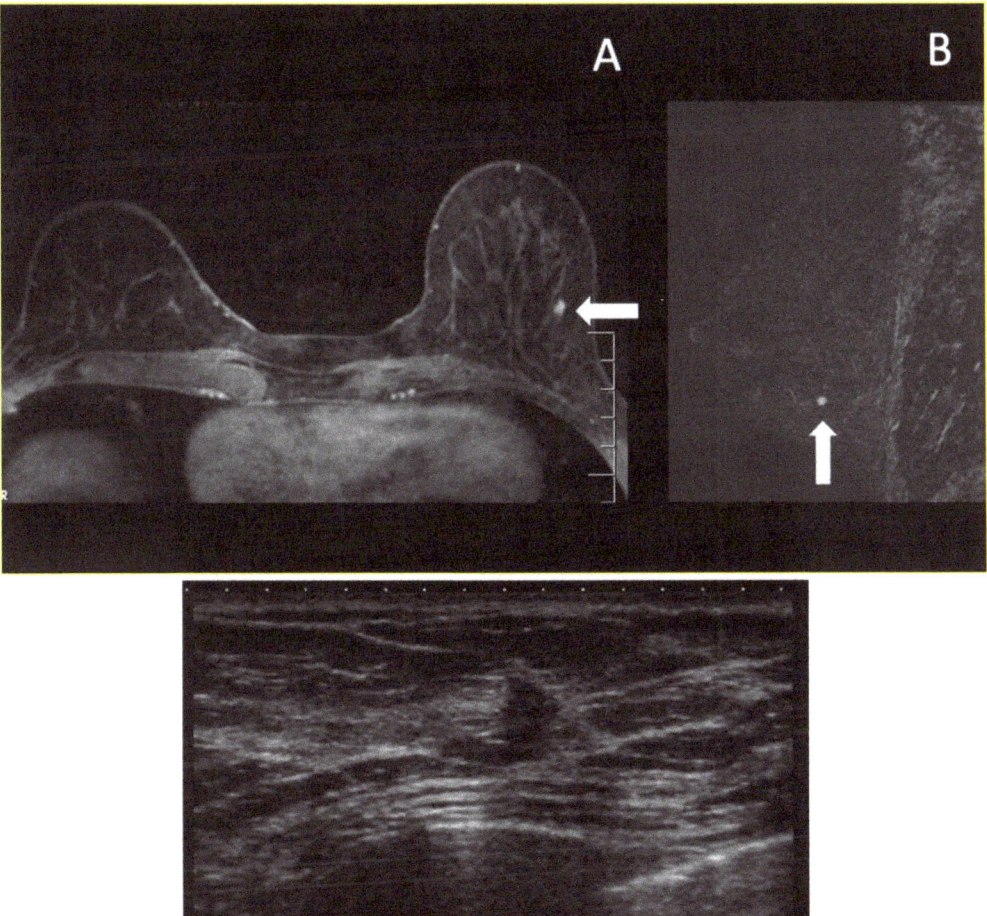

Figure 7. Courtesy of Dr. Anabel Scaranelo. High-risk screening with breast MRI in a 52-year-old woman with a family history of breast cancer in her sister. Screening mammography (not shown) was negative, with category C density. Focus of enhancement (arrow) in the lower outer quadrant of the left breast, (**A**) axial and (**B**) sagittal T1-weighted 3D-gradient echo with fat saturation 2nd minute post contrast. (**C**) The patient was recalled for a second look ultrasound that showed correlation with a suspicious subcentimeter mass lesion at 5 o'clock (arrows). An ultrasound-guided core needle showed grade 2 invasive ductal carcinoma.

Mango performed a Monte Carlo simulation cost–benefit analysis of screening average-risk women with triennial MRI compared to annual mammography beginning at age 40 over 30 years. It was based on Kuhl's study from 2017 which used full-protocol MRI [63]. Using a cost per MRI examination of $549.71, MRI screening is more cost-effective than mammography screening in 24 years. If the cost per MRI is $400, MRI became cost-effective compared to mammography screening in less than 6 years, with over a 22% cost reduction relative to mammography screening in 12 years and reaching a 38% reduction in 30 years [103]. It is not known whether the analysis would have been even more favorable had the model been based on abbreviated MRI, or whether the $400 cost is applicable to it, since at the time of writing, there is no CPT code for abbreviated MRI.

Geuzinge used microsimulation to study the cost-effectiveness of screening MRI for women aged 50–75 in the DENSE trial, taking into consideration numbers of breast cancers, life-years, quality-adjusted life-years (QALYs), breast cancer deaths, and "overdiagnosis," and found that MRI screening for women with extremely dense breasts is cost-effective at 3–4-year intervals compared with biennial mammography [104]. The DENSE trial used full-protocol MRI, and it is not known whether the outcome of the microsimulation would have been even more favorable had abbreviated MRI been studied.

As a result of the favorable metrics in these studies, the European Society of Breast Imaging (EUSOBI) released new recommendations in March 2022 [105]. These include informing women of their breast density, and offering women aged 50–74 with extremely dense breasts supplemental MRI screening every 2–4 years, through a shared decision-making process. They suggest that starting MRI could be adopted at a younger age, if screening is performed younger than age 50. They acknowledge that in areas where access to Breast MRI is limited, that ultrasound in combination with mammography may be used as an alternative.

Not all women accept or tolerate MRI, however. In the Avon-ACRIN 6666 trial, 42% of women offered MRI declined for a variety of reasons including claustrophobia, time constraints, financial concerns and fear of contrast injection [106]. In the DENSE trial, only 59% of the women randomized to the MRI group accepted the invitation [102]. MRI-incompatible pacemakers or cochlear implants are also potential contraindications [107]. Other contraindications include pregnancy and some spinal fixation hardware [108].

Abbreviated MRI (AB-MRI), first introduced by Kuhl et al. in 2014 [109] will reduce cost and improve access to MRI, by reducing both magnet time and interpretation time. It might also be more tolerable for women with claustrophobia. It has been shown to have equivalent diagnostic accuracy to full protocol MRI [110]. Its proven efficiency is established for screening average-risk women at all densities at reduced cost [63].

In the EA1141 study Comstock et al. are comparing AB-MRI with DBT screening in average-risk women with Category C and D densities. The 2020 publication includes data from the baseline studies and one-year follow-up, and additional studies will be obtained for three more years. The invasive cancer detection rate was 11.8/1000 women for abbreviated breast MRI vs. 4.8/1000 women for DBT, and there were no interval cancers [111].

Patel et al. have summarized the current AB-MRI protocols, and the inclusion of ultrafast imaging to provide kinetic information [112].

Because of the demonstrated minimal or zero interval cancer rate, MRI screening can be conducted at longer intervals. MRI could one day replace screening mammography but for the requirement of intravenous gadolinium-based contrast, and the limited number of scanners compared to mammography equipment. There are circumstances when requiring IV gadolinium contrast should not be a deterrent. For high-risk women, the benefits of MRI screening outweigh any potential risks of Gadolinium. It may be some time before we know if this also applies for average-risk women. The alternative functional modalities that potentially have equivalent sensitivity are discussed below.

Diffusion-weighted MRI (DW MRI) is an MRI technique that does not use IV contrast, but measures endogenous water movement within tissue. It has been studied as a supplement to contrast-enhanced MRI to improve differentiation of benign from malignant lesions, and although the combination of DW and CE MRI yielded the best performance, DW MRI alone was comparable to CE MRI for differentiating known suspicious lesions. For screening, its sensitivity has been shown to be intermediate between CE MRI and mammography. DW MRI may be superior to US at detecting mammographically occult cancer, but detects larger cancers than CE MRI. In a study by O'Flynn, the mean size of breast cancers on DW MRI was 29.5 mm [113]. Amornsiripanitch predicts improved performance with optimal acquisition and interpretation protocols, but stresses that standardized approaches in larger patient cohorts are essential prior to widespread implementation [114]. It remains to be seen whether DW MRI can play a role in screening average-risk women, and compete with AB-MRI and contrast-enhanced mammography.

Diffusion Tensor Imaging is a variation of DW MRI with the potential to increase specificity without losing sensitivity [115].

Another potential future application of MRI is the MRI fingerprinting technique, which calculates simultaneous and volumetric T1 and T2 relaxation times for breast tissues, with the goal of being able to distinguish normal tissue from diseased tissue. It can be performed without or with contrast, but its current spatial resolution is lower than that of CE MRI, so whether it ultimately finds a role in screening remains to be seen [116].

An alternate form of non-contrast MRI called luminal water imaging is currently being studied in prostate cancer. It compares favorably with CE MRI and DW MRI [117]. It may be applicable in breast in future, but is not currently the subject of research [118].

8. Contrast-Enhanced Mammography (CEM)

CEM, also known as "contrast-enhanced digital mammography", "contrast-enhanced spectral mammography", or contrast-enhanced dual-energy mammography," is an x-ray subtraction technique.

Iodinated intravenous contrast (the same contrast used for computed tomography (CT) scans is administered, usually via a power injector. After about 2 min, the patient is positioned as for a screening mammogram, and the usual four images are obtained. Further detail about procedure for intravenous (IV) administration and imaging protocol is available from recent reviews [119,120]. At each position, two exposures are obtained simultaneously: One low-energy: 28–33 kilovoltage peak (kVp) and one high energy: 45–49 kVp. These are chosen to be below and above the K-edge of iodine. The low-energy image shows breast tissue and is diagnostically equivalent to a routine digital mammogram image, even though the tissue contains iodine [121]. In a study comparing low-energy with 2D images of 40 biopsy-proven cancers, Konstantopoulos et al. found that cancers may be better visualized on the low energy images compared with the 2D digital mammogram [122].

The high energy image is uninterpretable (Figure 8), but is used to subtract the low-energy from, which subtracts out the normal tissue and leaves just the contrast-containing vessels and vascular tissues visible, including cancers [123]. As with MRI, this is an example of "functional imaging", with demonstration of abnormal "leaky" vessels suggestive of malignancy.

Both the low-energy and subtraction (also known as recombined or iodine) images are required for interpretation. Areas of suspicious calcification on the low-energy images may not have corresponding abnormal vascularity on the subtraction, and conversely, a suspicious finding on the subtraction may not have a correlate on the low-energy image, especially if it is due to a lesion obscured by dense tissue. Amir has shown that a low-energy finding with associated enhancement on the subtraction image, or a finding with a correlate on US or MRI is, predictive of malignancy. Calcifications with associated enhancement had a high malignancy rate. However, 50% of the lesions that enhanced on the subtraction images with no correlate on the low-energy were malignant [124]. Therefore, negative CEM is not sufficient to avoid performing biopsy of suspicious calcifications. Figure 8 shows an example of much more cancer seen on a CEM examination, than was visible on the screening mammogram.

CEM has similar sensitivity to MRI at considerably lower cost. Cheung showed that by using CEM in addition to mammography, sensitivity increased from 71.5% to 92.7% and specificity from 51.8% to 67.9% [125]. Fallenberg reported that 13 of 14 cancers (93%) that were occult on mammography but seen on CEM were in women with dense breasts [126].

The radiation is higher than that of digital mammography or DBT, but is within the allowable range [127–129]. Implementing CEM in a practice requires time for consenting, preparing the injector and starting the IV. IV setup is the same as for MRI, but the CEM examination and interpretation are faster than MRI. Contrast reactions can occur. Most are mild and resolve spontaneously. More moderate reactions occur in less than 1% and personnel must be appropriately trained to manage these. Fatal outcomes are extremely rare with low-osmolality contrast agents [130,131].

CEM has shown potential for screening women eligible for MRI who have a contraindication to it, or choose to avoid or cannot access MRI [132–134]. In addition to the ACR recommendations for screening high-risk women, the National Comprehensive Cancer Network (NCCN) now recommends consideration of contrast-enhanced mammography or whole breast ultrasound for those who qualify for, but cannot undergo MRI [135]. CEM outperforms mammography and US at screening, so women who have CEM do not need supplemental US [135,136].

CEM may be better than MRI at depicting lesions that enhance late because of the longer time after contrast is given before imaging in CEM, and the different structures of Gadolinium and iodinated contrast [126]. CEM-directed biopsy has received FDA and Health Canada approval, but is not yet commercially available [137–139]. For now, if a suspicious lesion is detected. Guidance with either US or MRI is required.

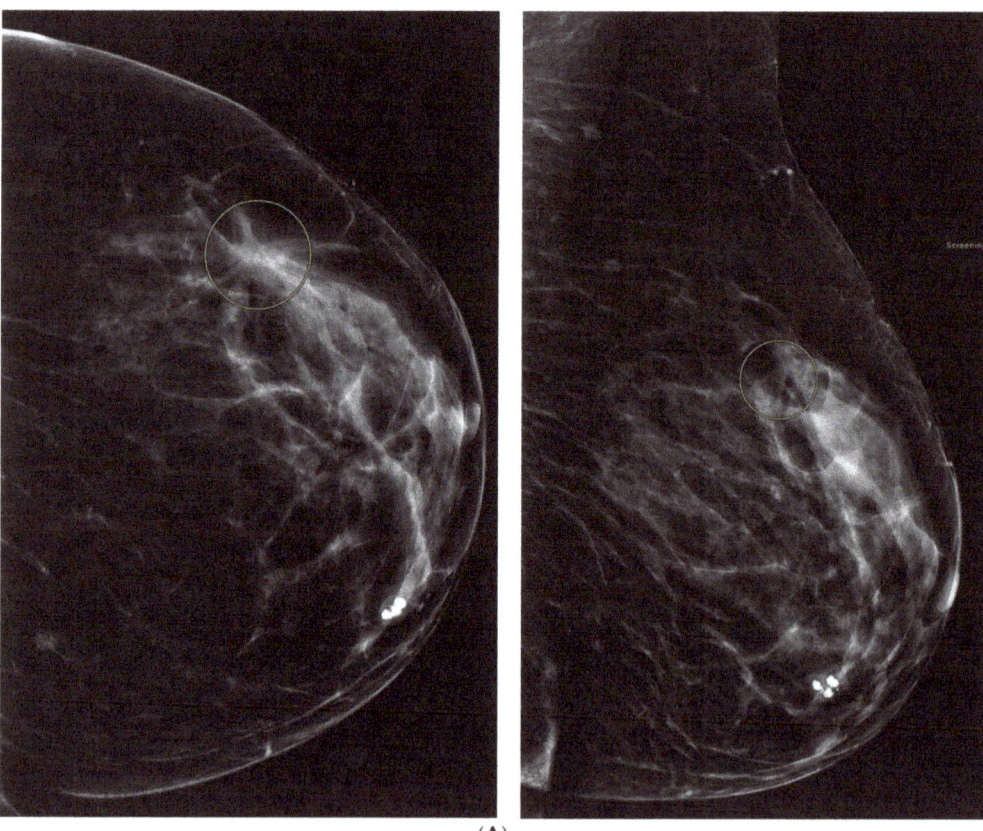

(A)

Figure 8. *Cont.*

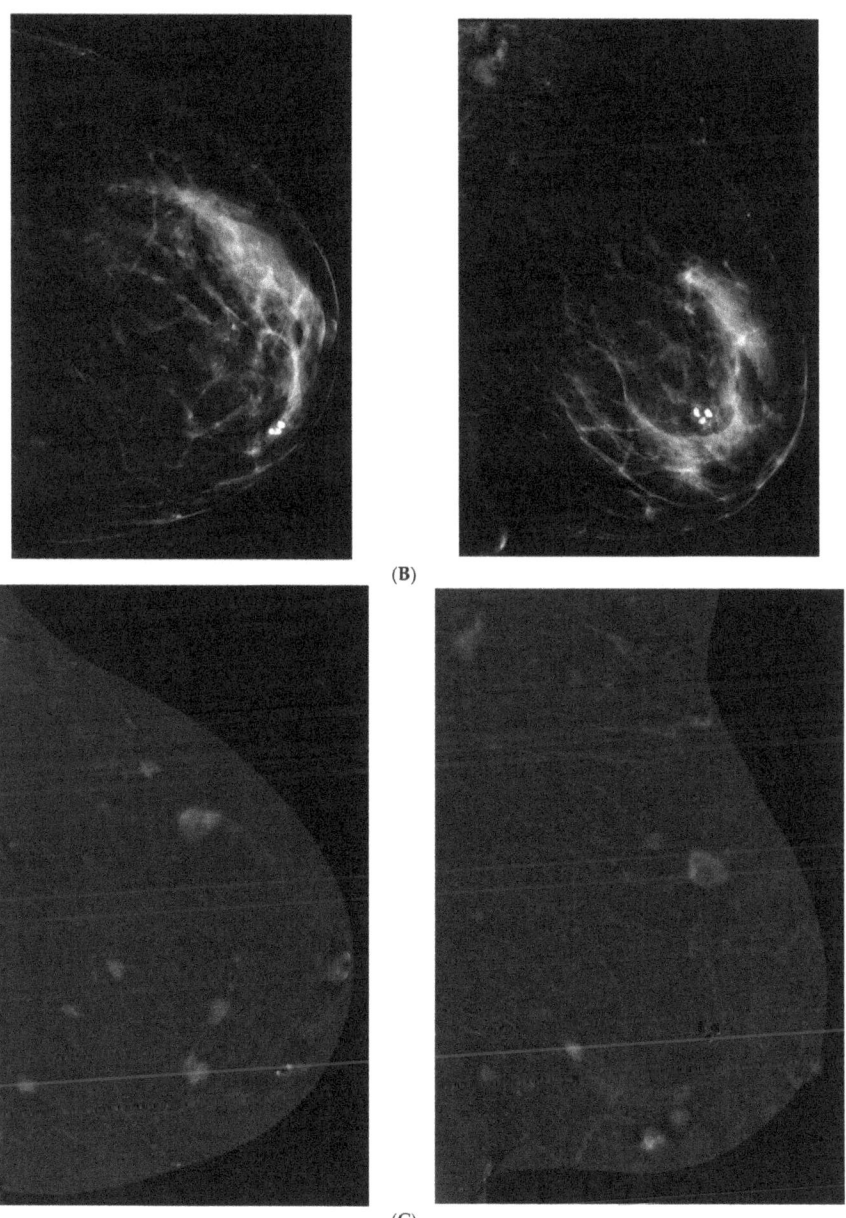

Figure 8. Courtesy of Dr. Anat Kornecki. This 71-year-old woman with BI-RADS C density was recalled from screening because of architectural distortion in the left upper outer quadrant. (**A**) Screening CC and MLO views, with area of distortion circled. (**B**) low-energy CC and MLO views. High-energy views not shown. (**C**) subtraction CC and MLO views, showing multiple areas of enhancement. Note that 5 lesions are in the medial breast, which was not dense mammographically. The two lesions furthest apart were core biopsied, and both confirmed malignant. Mastectomy was performed, and showed 5 foci of invasive lobular carcinoma.

CEM has false alarms, like any other screening test, most commonly fibroadenomas, papillomas, and hyperplasia [140].

A multicenter trial of CEM is in the planning stages. The "Contrast Enhanced Mammography Imaging Screening Trial" (CMIST) will enroll 2500 average-to-intermediate risk women aged 40–75 years for 2 consecutive years of screening with DBT, US and CEM and one year of follow-up. Performance metrics will be compared, in addition to the tumor biologic characteristics of invasive cancers and DCIS detected at CEM and DBT plus screening US [119,141].

The ACR has released a lexicon for CEM as a supplement to the 2013 ACR BI-RADS mammography [142].

9. Molecular Breast Imaging (MBI)

MBI is another functional imaging test. It uses intravenous Tc-99 m sestamibi, which is taken up by cancers more than by normal breast tissue. The dose of intravenous contrast, initially 20 to 30 mCi (740 to 1110 MBq) administered in studies using older breast-specific gamma imaging technology, has been updated to 8 mCi (296 MBq) used with newer semiconductor-based, dedicated systems that allow direct-contact breast positioning, improved spatial resolution, and now biopsy capability [143]. Soon after the injection (within 5 min), the breast is positioned similarly to mammography between two Gamma camera detectors with light compression. Each image takes 10 min, so the total examination time exceeds 40 min. The effective dose is approximately 2 mSv for MBI versus 0.5 for DM or DBT with synthetic reconstructions; 2 mSv is considered to be within safe limits [144]. Unlike low-dose radiation from mammograms, which is limited to the breasts, the radiation from this test is to the whole body, especially the pelvis.

Radionuclide injection is typically performed in a Nuclear Medicine department. Positioning for imaging may be performed by mammography technologists, or by nuclear medicine technologists who have been trained in mammography, and supervised for a minimum 25 cases [145]. Interpretation by radiologists specialized in breast imaging is recommended, to facilitate correlation with other imaging modalities [146].

In single-institution studies, adding MBI to 2D mammography in women with dense breasts detected an additional 6.5–8.8 invasive cancers per 1000 screened, with modest increases in recall rate (6% to 8%) at a lower cost-per-cancer detected than mammography alone, and with a PPV of 33% [146,147].

Density MATTERS (Molecular Breast Imaging and Tomosynthesis to Eliminate the Reservoir of Cancers) is an ongoing multicenter trial comparing DBT to MBI in women aged 40–75 years with dense breasts. It will also assess for change in the advanced cancer rate by performing two consecutive annual MBI scans. Their preliminary report showed cancer detection rates per thousand of 1.9 for DBT vs. 11.2 for MBI (ICDR of 9.3 for MBI). PPV was 8% for DBT, 26% for MBI and 21% for the combination of DBT and MBI [148].

Hruska asserts that concern regarding the radiation dose in MBI has hindered its wider use despite compelling evidence of its benefits [149], and points out that benefit to risk ratios for MBI studied by Brown and Covington [150] and Hendrick [151] are superior to mammography in specific scenarios. Figure 9 shows a cancer seen on MBI that was not detected on FFDM or DBT. She argues that MBI "consistently shows it is doing the task that we wish it to do—finding invasive cancers occult on mammographic screening, at a relatively low false-positive rate and low cost". It is recommended that when used in conjunction with MBI, DBT be performed with synthetic 2D rather than full field digital mammography (FFDM 2D) to reduce dose.

Performance of MBI requires cooperation between nuclear medicine and breast-imaging departments. In the USA, nuclear medicine is part of the radiology residency [152], but this is not the case in Canada. Some radiologists do additional training in Nuclear Medicine, but rarely interpret breast-imaging examinations, so MBI is not currently practiced anywhere in Canada.

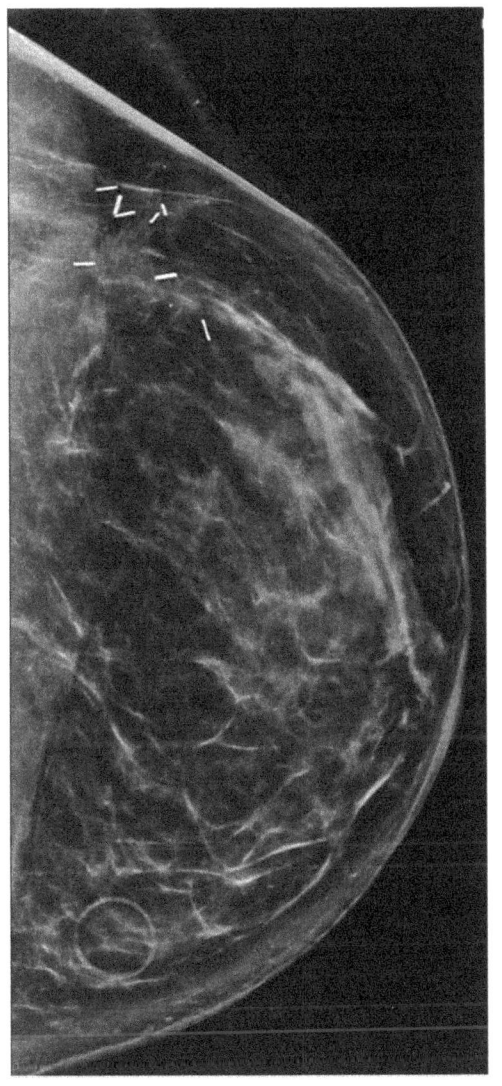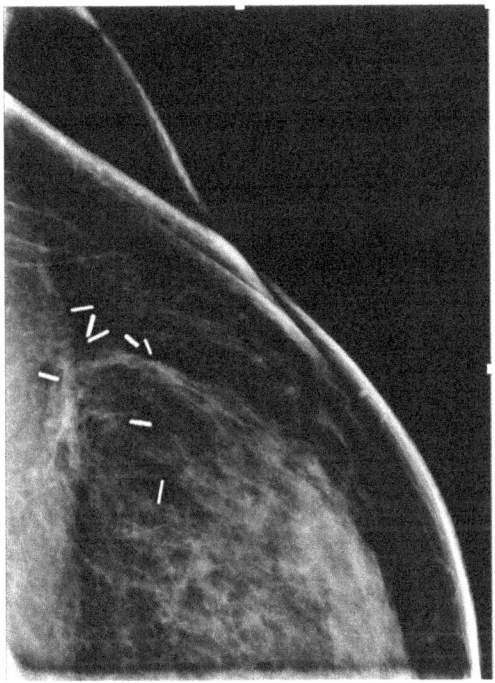

(A)

Figure 9. *Cont.*

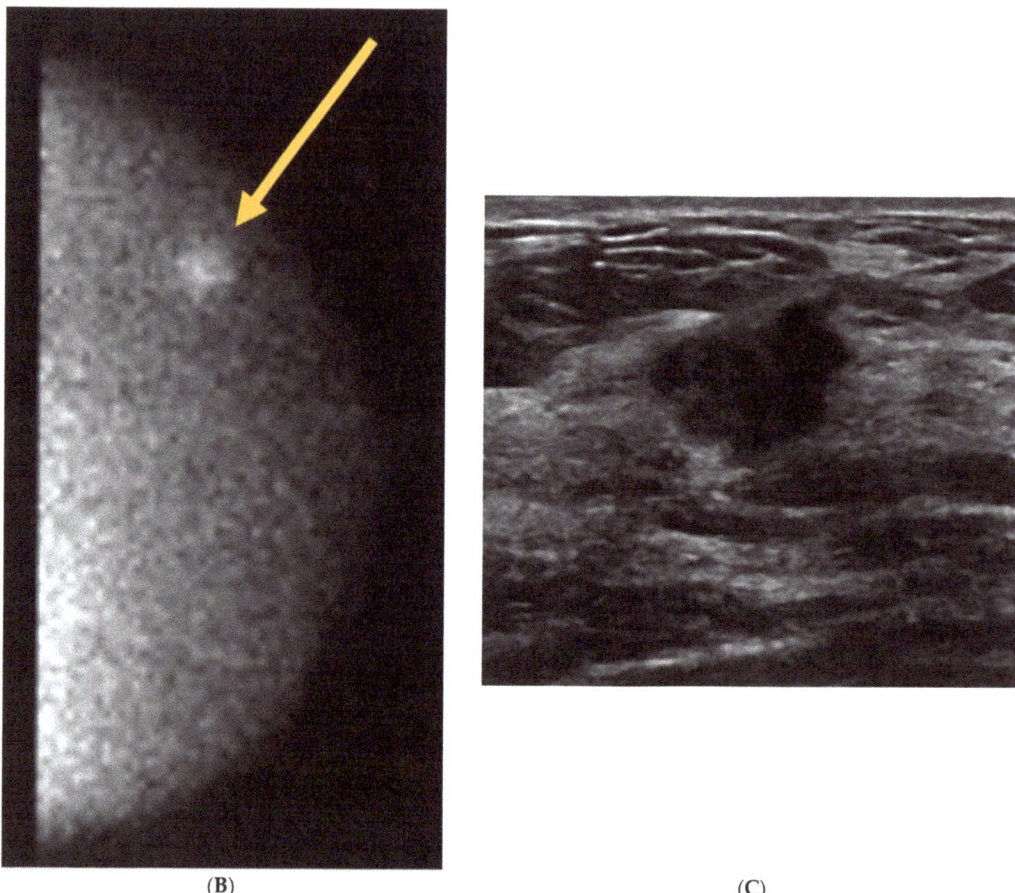

(B) **(C)**

Figure 9. Courtesy of Drs. Deborah Rhodes and Carrie Hruska. Negative mammogram in a woman post lumpectomy. (**A**) cc views, routine and spot magnification. Tomosynthesis (not shown) was also negative. Notably, the breast is category B, not dense. (**B**) Recurrent carcinoma (arrow) detected on MBI (**C**) Targeted US demonstrates the cancer.

10. Artificial Intelligence (AI)

AI shows promise to improve screening in all women, including those with dense breasts. Romero-Martin et al. showed that stand-alone use of AI for digital mammography screening had non-inferior sensitivity and a lower recall rate for 2D mammography than by single or double-reading by dedicated breast radiologists (but not for DBT) [153]. Shoshan et al. tested an AI system for DBT, and showed that it could reduce radiologists' workload by almost 40%, by filtering out negative DBT screening studies with non-inferior sensitivity, and 25% reduction in recalls [154]. However, in the accompanying editorial, Philpotts rightly points out that although "non-inferior", of the 459 detected cancers, 4 detected by the radiologists were missed by the AI. She suggests that false negative AI would not be acceptable to women [155]. Shen et al. described an AI system for breast ultrasound that maintains its sensitivity, while reducing the recall rate by 37% and reduces biopsy recommendations by 28% [156] (Figure 10). As Fuchsjäger points out, "assistance from AI could yield a considerable workload reduction if it could be shown to reliably identify negative mammograms and make US unnecessary". However, prior to AI being implemented without radiologist input, legal issues will have to be addressed, both for medical decision-making and data security [157].

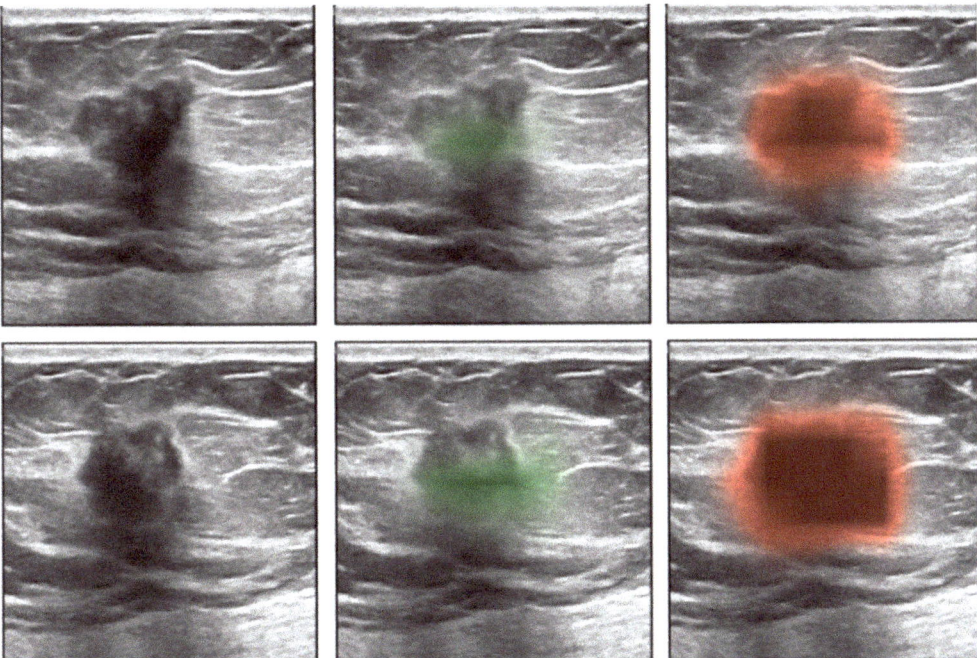

Figure 10. From Shen et al. [156] Case B from their Figure 3. No changes have been made. https://creativecommons.org/licenses/by/4.0/legalcode (accessed 12 March 2022). Sagittal (**top row**) and transverse views (**lower row**) of a biopsy proven-cancer. The images on the (**left**) are the B-mode images. The saliency maps indicate the predicted locations of benign (**middle**) and malignant (**right**) findings.

Mango et al. described a system of AI-based decision support for breast lesion assessment, and showed improved accuracy while reducing inter- and intra-observer variability [158].

All of the modalities discussed are potentially useful in finding cancers missed on mammograms, but it would be helpful to determine which patients are at higher risk of interval cancer. Wanders et al. searched for ICs diagnosed after a normal screening mammogram among 1,163,147 women in the Dutch screening program. There were 2222 women diagnosed with IC within 20 months of a negative mammogram. The control group was 4661 age-matched women who had at least 2 years of normal follow-up findings after negative screening findings. Using software to calculate breast density, combined with an AI cancer detection system based on deep convolutional neural networks, they found a higher proportion of women who subsequently developed IC compared with either one, alone [159]. We can expect to see much more research on AI to refine how to find breast cancer as early as possible for all women.

11. Summary of Benefits vs. Risks

Supplemental screening modalities vary in the degree of associated risks, including cost, anxiety from recalls, including those that lead to negative biopsies, exposure to ionizing radiation, adverse events from injected agents, and "overdiagnosis".

DBT is widely used in the USA, performed most often as part of the screening mammogram rather than as a supplemental screen. It increases cancer detection compared with

2D mammography, but finds more slowly growing cancers than contrast-based techniques, and about half as many additional cancers as US. However, just as important, it reduces recall rate. So its use in initial screening is justified given the equivalency of dose when obtained with synthetic 2D.

Ultrasound is widely available, uses no ionizing radiation or injection, and cost is generally low. Its high initial recall rate increases cost and anxiety, but recalls decrease with experience and availability of priors for comparison. Sensitivity is modest compared to other supplemental modalities. However, the most recent publication showed an impressive ICDR of 7/1000 on the prevalent screen [56].

At the other end of the spectrum, MRI is the most sensitive and expensive, but not as widely available, especially outside the USA [160]. It uses no ionizing radiation but requires IV gadolinium, which accumulates in the bone, skin, solid organs, and brain. Although there are currently no known harmful effects, Neal points out that, "the absence of evidence does not equal the absence of risk" [98]. MRI's longer-term low interval cancer rate may allow less frequent examinations. The cost should drop considerably with wider implementation of abbreviated MRI. Further study with DWI may decrease the need for contrast.

CEM has sensitivity approaching that of MRI, uses standard mammography equipment and is becoming more widely-available. It requires injection, but uses iodinated contrast; not gadolinium.

Molecular breast imaging (MBI) uses injected radioactive material and has an effective dose approximately four times that of digital mammography or DBT. Contrast reactions are rare, but it requires longer exam time and is not widely available.

The choice of supplemental screening should be based on an individual woman's risk profile. In 2010, Kuhl et al. used data from the EVA trial to compare the cancer detection rates of clinical breast examination, mammography, ultrasound, and MRI, either alone or in various combinations, for screening women at ≥20% lifetime risk for breast cancer, irrespective of breast density. Cancer yields were: mammography: 5.4/1000, US: 6/1000, mammography plus US: 7.7/1000, MRI alone: 14.9/1000, MRI plus US: 14.9/1000, and MRI plus mammography 16/1000 (not statistically significantly increased) [92].

More recently, Berg has created a chart summarizing the ICDR in various breast densities, the additional recalls, and the impact on the IC rate of DBT, US, MBI, CEM, MRI and AB MRI, best viewed online at https://densebreast-info.org/screening-technologies/cancer-detection-by-screening-method/ [161].

Panels in North America that create breast cancer screening guidelines [162,163] have traditionally relied exclusively on decades-old RCTs, which did not include considerations of menopausal status, breast density, race/ethnicity, current hormone therapy, and other risk factors. Because they ignore well-performed observational studies and surrogate endpoints, they state that there is insufficient evidence for supplemental screening for breast cancer for women with dense breasts using other imaging modalities.

Guidelines for breast cancer screening in the USA vary considerably, depending on the issuing organization. There is still a moratorium on the United States Preventive Services Task Force guidelines that recommend starting mammography screening at age 50. Most screening in the USA is ad hoc, whereas elsewhere it is largely performed in organized programs. In most Canadian jurisdictions and many European countries, mammography screening is biennial beginning at 50 for women at average risk. Women who are premenopausal after age 50, post-menopausal women on combined hormone therapy, obese women, and women with dense breasts are at increased risk of getting breast cancer, and increased risk of interval cancer [5–14].

Efforts are underway to refine which women are at low, medium or high risk, and whether there is a subset of women who are at such low risk that they can be screened less often. AI may prove effective at discriminating which women are at high risk of IC. Until these studies are completed and to provide equity, organized screening programs that screen less often than annually should consider decreasing the screening interval for mammography for women at higher-than-average risk, and consider issuing recommendations supplemental screening for women at increased risk, and for women with dense breasts.

Funding: This research received no external funding.

Acknowledgments: The author would like to thank Regina Hooley, Anabel Scaranelo, Anat Korneki, Deborah Rhodes and Carrie Hruska for images used in Figures 6–9. Special thanks to Mitchell Goldenberg, who at this late stage in my career, patiently taught me how to use a reference manager.

Conflicts of Interest: The author is a volunteer advisor to Dense Breasts Canada and Dense Breast Info, on the Medical Advisory Board of Besins Healthcare, and a stockholder in Volpara Solutions.

Abbreviations

RCT	Randomized Controlled Trial
ACR	American College of Radiology
BI-RADS	Breast Imaging Reporting and Data System
FFDM	Full Field Digital Mammography
IC	Interval Cancer
ER	Estrogen Receptor
PR	Progesterone Receptor
US	Ultrasound
DBT	Digital Breast Tomosynthesis
MRI	Magnetic Resonance Imaging
CEM	Contrast-Enhanced Mammography
MBI	Molecular Breast Imaging
DCIS	Ductal Carcinoma In-situ
ICDR	Incremental Cancer Detection Rate
ACRIN	American College of Radiology Imaging Network
PPV	Positive Predictive Value
J-START	Japan Strategic Anti-cancer Randomized Trial
FDA	United States Food and Drug Administration
2D	Two Dimensional
MLO	Mediolateral Oblique
CC	Craniocaudal
QUALYs	Quality-Adjusted Life-Years
EUSOBI	European Society of Breast Imaging
DW MRI	Diffusion-Weighted MRI
CE MRI	Contrast-enhanced MRI
AB MRI	Abbreviated MRI
CT	Computed Tomography
IV	Intravenous
kVp	Kilovoltage peak

References

1. Coldman, A.; Phillips, N.; Wilson, C.; Decker, K.; Chiarelli, A.M.; Brisson, J.; Zhang, B.; Payne, J.; Doyle, G.; Ahmad, R. Pan-Canadian study of mammography screening and mortality from breast cancer. *J. Natl. Cancer Inst.* **2014**, *106*, dju261. [CrossRef] [PubMed]
2. Tabár, L.; Dean, P.B.; Chen, T.H.H.; Yen, A.M.; Chen, S.L.; Fann, J.C.; Chiu, S.Y.; Ku, M.M.; Wu, W.Y.; Hsu, C.Y.; et al. The incidence of fatal breast cancer measures the increased effectiveness of therapy in women participating in mammography screening. *Cancer* **2019**, *125*, 515–523. [CrossRef] [PubMed]
3. Broeders, M.; Moss, S.; Nystrom, L.; Njor, S.; Jonsson, H.; Paap, E.; Massat, N.; Duffy, S.; Lynge, E.; Paci, E. The impact of mammographic screening on breast cancer mortality in Europe: A review of observational studies. *J. Med. Screen.* **2012**, *19* (Suppl. S1), 14–25. [CrossRef]
4. Sprague, B.L.; Gangnon, R.E.; Burt, V.; Trentham-Dietz, A.; Hampton, J.M.; Wellman, R.D.; Kerlikowske, K.; Miglioretti, D.L. Prevalence of mammographically dense breasts in the United States. *J. Natl. Cancer Inst.* **2014**, *106*, dju255. [CrossRef]
5. Han, Y.; Moore, J.X.; Colditz, G.A.; Toriola, A.T. Family History of Breast Cancer and Mammographic Breast Density in Premenopausal Women. *JAMA Netw. Open* **2022**, *5*, e2148983. [CrossRef] [PubMed]

6. Boyd, N.F.; Guo, H.; Martin, L.J.; Sun, L.; Stone, J.; Fishell, E.; Jong, R.A.; Hislop, G.; Chiarelli, A.; Minkin, S.; et al. Mammographic density and the risk and detection of breast cancer. *N. Engl. J. Med.* **2007**, *356*, 227–236. [CrossRef] [PubMed]
7. Kerlikowske, K.; Zhu, W.; Tosteson, A.N.A.; Sprague, B.L.; Tice, J.A.; Lehman, C.D.; Miglioretti, D.L.; Breast Cancer Surveillance Consortium. Identifying women with dense breasts at high risk for interval cancer a cohort study. *Ann. Intern. Med.* **2015**, *162*, 673–681. [CrossRef] [PubMed]
8. Weigel, S.; Heindel, W.; Heidrich, J.; Hense, H.W.; Heidinger, O. Digital mammography screening: Sensitivity of the programme dependent on breast density. *Eur. Radiol.* **2017**, *27*, 2744–2751. [CrossRef]
9. Van der Waal, D.; Ripping, T.M.; Verbeek, A.L.M.; Broeders, M.J.M. Breast cancer screening effect across breast density strata: A case–control study. *Int. J. Cancer* **2017**, *140*, 41–49. [CrossRef]
10. Chiu, S.Y.H.; Duffy, S.; Yen, A.M.F.; Tabár, L.; Smith, R.A.; Chen, H.H. Effect of baseline breast density on breast cancer incidence, stage, mortality, and screening parameters: 25-Year follow-up of a Swedish mammographic screening. *Cancer Epidemiol. Biomark. Prev.* **2010**, *19*, 1219–1228. [CrossRef]
11. Engmann, N.J.; Golmakani, M.K.; Miglioretti, D.L.; Sprague, B.L.; Kerlikowske, K. Population-attributable risk proportion of clinical risk factors for breast cancer. *JAMA Oncol.* **2017**, *3*, 1228–1236. [CrossRef] [PubMed]
12. Boyd, N.F.; Dite, G.S.; Stone, J.; Gunasekara, A.; English, D.R.; McCredie, M.R.; Giles, G.G.; Tritchler, D.; Chiarelli, A.; Yaffe, M.J.; et al. Heritability of mammographic density, a risk factor for breast cancer. *N. Engl. J. Med.* **2002**, *347*, 886–894. [CrossRef] [PubMed]
13. McCormack, V.A.; dos Santos Silva, I. Breast density and parenchymal patterns as markers of breast cancer risk: A meta-analysis. *Cancer Epidemiol. Biomark. Prev.* **2006**, *15*, 1159–1169. [CrossRef] [PubMed]
14. Bertrand, K.A.; Tamimi, R.M.; Scott, C.G.; Jensen, M.R.; Pankratz, V.; Visscher, D.; Norman, A.; Couch, F.; Shepherd, J.; Fan, B.; et al. Mammographic Density and Risk of Breast Cancer by Age and Tumor Characteristics. *Breast Cancer Res.* **2013**, *15*, 1–13. [CrossRef] [PubMed]
15. 1Gram, I.T.; Funkhouser, E.; Tabár, L. The Tabár classification of mammographic parenchymal patterns. *Eur. J. Radiol.* **1997**, *24*, 131–136. [CrossRef]
16. Skarping, I.; Förnvik, D.; Sartor, H.; Heide-Jørgensen, U.; Zackrisson, S.; Borgquist, S. Mammographic density is a potential predictive marker of pathological response after neoadjuvant chemotherapy in breast cancer. *BMC Cancer* **2019**, *19*, 1272. [CrossRef]
17. Woodard, G.A.; Ray, K.M.; Joe, B.N.; Price, E.R. Qualitative radiogenomics: Association between oncotype DX test recurrence score and BI-RADS mammographic and breast MR imaging features. *Radiology* **2018**, *286*, 60–70. [CrossRef]
18. Huang, Y.S.; Chen, J.L.Y.; Huang, C.S.; Kuo, S.H.; Jaw, F.S.; Tseng, Y.H.; Ko, W.C.; Chang, Y.C. High mammographic breast density predicts locoregional recurrence after modified radical mastectomy for invasive breast cancer: A case-control study. *Breast Cancer Res.* **2016**, *18*, 1–9. [CrossRef]
19. Eriksson, L.; Czene, K.; Rosenberg, L.; Humphreys, K.; Hall, P. Possible Influence of Mammographic Density on Local and Locoregional Recurrence of Breast Cancer. *Breast Cancer Res.* **2013**, *15*, 1–9. [CrossRef]
20. Porter, P.L.; El-Bastawissi, A.Y.; Mandelson, M.T.; Lin, M.G.; Khalid, N.; Watney, E.A.; Cousens, L.; White, D.; Taplin, S.; White, E. Breast Tumor Character-Istics as Predictors of Mammographic Detection: Comparison of Interval-and Screen-Detected Cancers. *J. Natl. Cancer Inst.* **2022**, *114*, 483–484.
21. Domingo, L.; Salas, D.; Zubizarreta, R.; Baré, M.; Sarriugarte, G.; Barata, T.; Ibáñez, J.; Blanch, J.; Puig-Vives, M.; Fernández, A.; et al. Tumor Phenotype and Breast Density in Distinct Categories of Interval Cancer: Results of Population-Based Mammography Screening in Spain. *Breast Cancer Res.* **2014**, *16*, 1–11. [CrossRef] [PubMed]
22. Houssami, N.; Hunter, K. The epidemiology, radiology and biological characteristics of interval breast cancers in population mammography screening. *Npj Breast Cancer* **2017**, *3*, 1–13. [CrossRef] [PubMed]
23. Gilliland, F.D.; Joste, N.; Stauber, P.M.; Hunt, W.C.; Rosenberg, R.; Redlich, G.; Key, C.R. Biologic Characteristics of Interval and Screen-Detected Breast Cancers. *J. Natl. Cancer Inst.* **2000**, *92*, 743–749. [CrossRef] [PubMed]
24. Kirsh, V.A.; Chiarelli, A.M.; Edwards, S.A.; O'Malley, F.P.; Shumak, R.S.; Yaffe, M.J.; Boyd, N.F. Tumor characteristics associated with mammographic detection of breast cancer in the Ontario breast screening program. *J. Natl. Cancer Inst.* **2011**, *103*, 942–950. [CrossRef]
25. McCarthy, A.M.; Friebel-Klingner, T.; Ehsan, S.; He, W.; Welch, M.; Chen, J.; Kontos, D.; Domchek, S.M.; Conant, E.F.; Semine, A.; et al. Relationship of established risk factors with breast cancer subtypes. *Cancer Med.* **2021**, *10*, 6456–6467. [CrossRef]
26. Lehman, C.D.; Arao, R.F.; Sprague, B.L.; Lee, J.M.; Buist, D.S.; Kerlikowske, K.; Henderson, L.M.; Onega, T.; Tosteson, A.N.; Rauscher, G.H.; et al. National Performance Benchmarks for Modern Screening Digital Mammography: Update from the Breast Cancer Surveillance Consortium. *Radiology* **2017**, *283*, 49–58. [CrossRef]
27. Seely, J.M.; Peddle, S.E.; Yang, H.; Chiarelli, A.M.; McCallum, M.; Narasimhan, G.; Zakaria, D.; Earle, C.C.; Fung, S.; Bryant, H.; et al. Breast Density and Risk of Interval Cancers: The Effect of Annual Versus Biennial Screening Mammography Policies in Canada. *Can. Assoc. Radiol. J. = J. L'association Can. Des Radiol.* **2022**, *73*, 90–100. [CrossRef]
28. Chiarelli, A.M.; Kirsh, V.A.; Klar, N.S.; Shumak, R.; Jong, R.; Fishell, E.; Yaffe, M.J.; Boyd, N.F. Influence of patterns of hormone replacement therapy use and mammographic density on breast cancer detection. *Cancer Epidemiol. Biomark. Prev.* **2006**, *15*, 1856–1862. [CrossRef]

29. Kavanagh, A.M.; Byrnes, G.B.; Nickson, C.; Cawson, J.N.; Giles, G.G.; Hopper, J.L.; Gertig, D.M.; English, D.R. Using mammographic density to improve breast cancer screening outcomes. *Cancer Epidemiol. Biomark. Prev.* **2008**, *17*, 2818–2824. [CrossRef]
30. Ciatto, S.; Visioli, C.; Paci, E.; Zappa, M. Breast density as a determinant of interval cancer at mammographic screening. *Br. J. Cancer* **2004**, *90*, 393–396. [CrossRef]
31. Strand, F.; Azavedo, E.; Hellgren, R.; Humphreys, K.; Eriksson, M.; Shepherd, J.; Hall, P.; Czene, K. Localized mammographic density is associated with interval cancer and large breast cancer: A nested case-control study. *Breast Cancer Res.* **2019**, *21*, 8. [CrossRef] [PubMed]
32. Niraula, S.; Biswanger, N.; Hu, P.Z.; Lambert, P.; Decker, K. Incidence, Characteristics, and Outcomes of Interval Breast Cancers Compared with Screening-Detected Breast Cancers. *JAMA Netw. Open* **2020**, *3*, e2018179. [CrossRef] [PubMed]
33. Kuhl, C.K.; Baltzer, P. You Get What You Pay For: Breast MRI Screening of Women with Dense Breasts Is Cost-effective. *J. Natl. Cancer Inst.* **2021**, *113*, 1439–1441. [CrossRef]
34. Morrison, A.S. Intermediate Determinants of Mortality in the Evaluation of Screening. *Int. J. Epidemiol.* **1991**, *20*, 642–650. Available online: https://academic.oup.com/ije/article/20/3/642/654391 (accessed on 12 March 2022). [CrossRef] [PubMed]
35. Sickles, E.A.; Filly, R.A.; Callen, P.W. Breast cancer detection with sonography and mammography: Comparison using state-of-the-art equipment. *AJR Am. J. Roentgenol.* **1983**, *140*, 843–845. [CrossRef] [PubMed]
36. Bassett, L.W.; Kimme-Smith, C.; Sutherland, L.K.; Gold, R.H.; Sarti, D.; King, W. Automated and hand-held breast US: Effect on patient management. *Radiology* **1987**, *165*, 103–108. [CrossRef]
37. Hilton, S.V.W.; Leopold, G.R.; Olson, L.K.; Wiiison, S.A.; Hilton, S.V.W. Real-Time Breast Sonography: Application in 300 Consecutive Patients. *Am. J. Roentgenol.* **1986**, *147*, 479–486. [CrossRef]
38. Harper, A.P.; Kelly-Fry, E.; Noe, J.S.; Bies, J.R.; Jackson, V.P. Ultrasound in the evaluation of solid breast masses. *Radiology* **1983**, *146*, 731–736. [CrossRef]
39. Stavros, A.T.; Thickman, D.; Rapp, C.L.; Dennis, M.A.; Parker, S.H.; Sisney, G.A. Solid breast nodules: Use of sonography to distinguish between benign and malignant lesions. *Radiology* **1995**, *196*, 123–134. [CrossRef]
40. Gordon, P.B.; Goldenberg, S.L. Malignant breast masses detected only by ultrasound. A retrospective review. *Cancer* **1995**, *76*, 626–630. [CrossRef]
41. Buchberger, W.; Geiger-Gritsch, S.; Knapp, R.; Gautsch, K.; Oberaigner, W. Combined screening with mammography and ultrasound in a population-based screening program. *Eur. J. Radiol.* **2018**, *101*, 24–29. [CrossRef] [PubMed]
42. Kaplan, S.S. Clinical utility of bilateral whole-breast US in the evaluation of women with dense breast tissue. *Radiology* **2001**, *221*, 641–649. [CrossRef] [PubMed]
43. Kolb, T.M.; Lichy, J.; Newhouse, J.H. Comparison of the performance of screening mammography, physical examination, and breast US and evaluation of factors that influence them: An analysis of 27,825 patient evaluations. *Radiology* **2002**, *225*, 165–175. [CrossRef] [PubMed]
44. Crystal, P.; Strano, S.D.; Shcharynski, S.; Koretz, M.J. Using sonography to screen women with mammographically dense breasts. *Am. J. Roentgenol.* **2003**, *181*, 177–182. [CrossRef]
45. Leconte, I.; Feger, C.; Galant, C.; Berlière, M.; Berg, B.V.; D'Hoore, W.; Maldague, B. Mammography and subsequent whole-breast sonography of nonpalpable breast cancers: The importance of radiologic breast density. *Am. J. Roentgenol.* **2003**, *180*, 1675–1679. [CrossRef]
46. Berg, W.A. Supplemental screening sonography in dense breasts. *Radiol. Clin. N. Am.* **2004**, *42*, 845–851. [CrossRef]
47. Berg, W.A.; Zhang, Z.; Lehrer, D.; Jong, R.A.; Pisano, E.D.; Barr, R.G.; Böhm-Vélez, M.; Mahoney, M.C.; Evans, W.P., 3rd; Larsen, L.H.; et al. Detection of breast cancer with addition of annual screening ultrasound or a single screening MRI to mammography in women with elevated breast cancer risk. *JAMA* **2012**, *307*, 1394–1404. [CrossRef]
48. Barr, R.G.; Zhang, Z.; Cormack, J.B.; Mendelson, E.B.; Berg, W.A. Probably Benign Lesions at Screening Breast US in a Population with Elevated Risk: Prevalence and Rate of Malignancy in the ACRIN 6666 Trial 1. *Radiology* **2013**, *269*, 701–712. [CrossRef]
49. Hooley, R.J.; Greenberg, K.L.; Stackhouse, R.M.; Geisel, J.L.; Butler, R.S.; Philpotts, L.E. Screening US in patients with mammographically dense breasts: Initial experience with Connecticut public act 09-41. *Radiology* **2012**, *265*, 59–69. [CrossRef]
50. Philpotts, L.; Raghu, M.; Durand, M.A.; Horvath, L.J.; Butler, R.S.; Levesque, P.H.; Hooley, R.J. Update on Technologist-performed, Screening Breast Ultrasound in Women with Dense Tissue 5 Years after CT Public Act No. 09-41: How Are We Doing Now? In *Radiological Society of North America 2015 Scientific Assembly and Annual Meeting*; RSNA: Oak Brook, IL, USA, 2016.
51. Weigert, J.; Steenbergen, S. The connecticut experiment: The role of ultrasound in the screening of women with dense breasts. *Breast J.* **2012**, *18*, 517–522. [CrossRef]
52. Weigert, J.M. The Connecticut Experiment; The Third Installment: 4 Years of Screening Women with Dense Breasts with Bilateral Ultrasound. *Breast J.* **2017**, *23*, 34–39. [CrossRef]
53. Dense Breast Info. US States with Legislation Mandating Insurance Coverage for Supplemental Screening. Available online: https://densebreast-info.org/wp-content/uploads/2022/03/Table.laws_.insurance.ALPHA_.3.8.22.copyright.pdf (accessed on 12 March 2022).
54. BC Cancer Screening. Breast Density Notification in BC. Available online: http://www.bccancer.bc.ca/screening/Documents/Breast_20191104_BDProviderGuidance_V07_OPT.pdf (accessed on 12 March 2022).
55. Medical Services Plan of BC. Ultrasound for Dense Breast. Available online: https://www2.gov.bc.ca/assets/gov/health/practitioner-pro/medical-services-plan/ultrasound-policy-for-breast-density.pdf (accessed on 12 March 2022).

56. Wu, T.; Warren, L.J. The Added Value of Supplemental Breast Ultrasound Screening for Women with Dense Breasts: A Single Center Canadian Experience. *Can. Assoc. Radiol. J.* **2022**, *73*, 101–106. [CrossRef]
57. Warren, L.J.; University of British Columbia, Vancouver, BC, Canada. Personal communication, 2021.
58. Corsetti, V.; Houssami, N.; Ghirardi, M.; Ferrari, A.; Speziani, M.; Bellarosa, S.; Remida, G.; Gasparotti, C.; Galligioni, E.; Ciatto, S. Evidence of the effect of adjunct ultrasound screening in women with mammography-negative dense breasts: Interval breast cancers at 1 year follow-up. *Eur. J. Cancer* **2011**, *47*, 1021–1026. [CrossRef]
59. Ohuchi, N.; Suzuki, A.; Sobue, T.; Kawai, M.; Yamamoto, S.; Zheng, Y.F.; Shiono, Y.N.; Saito, H.; Kuriyama, S.; Tohno, E.; et al. Sensitivity and specificity of mammography and adjunctive ultrasonography to screen for breast cancer in the Japan Strategic Anti-cancer Randomized Trial (J-START): A randomised controlled trial. *Lancet* **2016**, *387*, 341–348. [CrossRef]
60. Harada-Shoji, N.; Suzuki, A.; Ishida, T.; Zheng, Y.F.; Narikawa-Shiono, Y.; Sato-Tadano, A.; Ohta, R.; Ohuchi, N. Evaluation of Adjunctive Ultrasonography for Breast Cancer Detection among Women Aged 40–49 Years with Varying Breast Density Undergoing Screening Mammography: A Secondary Analysis of a Randomized Clinical Trial. *JAMA Netw. Open* **2021**, *4*, e2121505. [CrossRef] [PubMed]
61. Leong, S.P.L.; Shen, Z.Z.; Liu, T.J.; Agarwal, G.; Tajima, T.; Paik, N.S.; Sandelin, K.; Derossis, A.; Cody, H.; Foulkes, W.D. Is Breast cancer the same disease in Asian and Western countries? *World J. Surg.* **2010**, *34*, 2308–2324. [CrossRef]
62. Kuhl, C.K. A Call for Improved Breast Cancer Screening Strategies, Not only for Women with Dense Breasts. *JAMA Netw. Open* **2021**, *4*, e2121492. [CrossRef]
63. Kuhl, C.K.; Strobel, K.; Bieling, H.; Leutner, C.; Schild, H.H.; Schrading, S. Supplemental breast MR imaging screening of women with average risk of breast cancer. *Radiology* **2017**, *283*, 361–370. [CrossRef]
64. Ohnuki, K.; Tohno, E.; Tsunoda, H.; Uematsu, T.; Nakajima, Y. Overall assessment system of combined mammography and ultrasound for breast cancer screening in Japan. *Breast Cancer* **2021**, *28*, 254–262, Erratum in *Breast Cancer* **2021**, *28*, 263. [CrossRef] [PubMed]
65. Brem, R.F.; Tabár, L.; Duffy, S.W.; Inciardi, M.F.; Guingrich, J.A.; Hashimoto, B.E.; Lander, M.R.; Lapidus, R.L.; Peterson, M.K.; Rapelyea, J.A.; et al. Assessing improvement in detection of breast cancer with three-dimensional automated breast US in women with dense breast tissue: The somoinsight study. *Radiology* **2015**, *274*, 663–673. [CrossRef]
66. Kelly, K.M.; Dean, J.; Comulada, W.S.; Lee, S.J. Breast cancer detection using automated whole breast ultrasound and mammography in radiographically dense breasts. *Eur. Radiol.* **2010**, *20*, 734–742. [CrossRef]
67. Berg, W.A.; Vourtsis, A. Screening Breast Ultrasound Using Handheld or Automated Technique in Women with Dense Breasts. *J. Breast Imaging* **2019**, *1*, 283–296. [CrossRef]
68. Is Optimal Breast Cancer Screening Accessible in Your Province/Territory? Available online: https://mybreastscreening.ca (accessed on 12 March 2022).
69. Dense Breast Info. State Legislation Map. Available online: https://densebreast-info.org/legislative-information/state-legislation-map/ (accessed on 12 March 2022).
70. Dense Breast Info. European Screening Guidelines by Country. Available online: https://densebreast-info.org/europe/european-screening-guidelines/map-screening-guidelines/ (accessed on 12 March 2022).
71. Niklason, L.T.; Christian, B.T.; Niklason, L.E.; Kopans, D.B.; Castleberry, D.E.; Opsahl-Ong, B.H.; Landberg, C.E.; Slanetz, P.J.; Giardino, A.A.; Moore, R.; et al. Digital tomosynthesis in breast imaging. *Radiology* **1997**, *205*, 399–406. [CrossRef] [PubMed]
72. Skaane, P.; Bandos, A.I.; Eben, E.B.; Jebsen, I.N.; Krager, M.; Haakenaasen, U.; Ekseth, U.; Izadi, M.; Hofvind, S.; Gullien, R. Two-view digital breast tomosynthesis screening with synthetically reconstructed projection images: Comparison with digital breast tomosynthesis with full-field digital mammographic images. *Radiology* **2014**, *271*, 655–663. [CrossRef] [PubMed]
73. Friedewald, S.M.; Rafferty, E.A.; Rose, S.L.; Durand, M.A.; Plecha, D.M.; Greenberg, J.S.; Hayes, M.K.; Copit, D.S.; Carlson, K.L.; Cink, T.M.; et al. Breast cancer screening using tomosynthesis in combination with digital mammography. *J. Am. Med. Assoc.* **2014**, *311*, 2499–2507. [CrossRef]
74. Ciatto, S.; Houssami, N.; Bernardi, D.; Caumo, F.; Pellegrini, M.; Brunelli, S.; Tuttobene, P.; Bricolo, P.; Fantò, C.; Valentini, M.; et al. Integration of 3D digital mammography with tomosynthesis for population breast-cancer screening (STORM): A prospective comparison study. *Lancet Oncol.* **2013**, *14*, 583–589. [CrossRef]
75. Skaane, P.; Bandos, A.I.; Niklason, L.T.; Sebuødegård, S.; Østerås, B.H.; Gullien, R.; Gur, D.; Hofvind, S. Digital mammography versus digital mammography plus tomosynthesis in breast cancer screening: The Oslo tomosynthesis screening trial. *Radiology* **2019**, *291*, 23–30. [CrossRef] [PubMed]
76. Conant, E.F.; Zuckerman, S.P.; McDonald, E.S.; Weinstein, S.P.; Korhonen, K.E.; Birnbaum, J.A.; Tobey, J.D.; Schnall, M.D.; Hubbard, R.A. Five consecutive years of screening with digital breast tomosynthesis: Outcomes by screening year and round. *Radiology* **2020**, *295*, 285–293. [CrossRef]
77. Partyka, L.; Lourenco, A.P.; Mainiero, M.B. Detection of mammographically occult architectural distortion on digital breast tomosynthesis screening: Initial clinical experience. *Am. J. Roentgenol.* **2014**, *203*, 216–222. [CrossRef] [PubMed]
78. Rafferty, E.A.; Park, J.M.; Philpotts, L.E.; Poplack, S.P.; Sumkin, J.H.; Halpern, E.F.; Niklason, L.T. Assessing Radiologist Performance Using Combined Digital Mammography and Breast Tomosynthesis Compared with Digital Mammography Alone: Results of a Multicenter, Multireader Trial 1. *Radiology* **2013**, *266*, 104–113. [CrossRef]
79. FDA. MQSA National Statistics. Available online: https://www.fda.gov/radiation-emitting-products/mqsa-insights/mqsa-national-statistics (accessed on 12 March 2022).

80. Digital Tomosynthesis Mammography and Digital Mammography in Screening Patients for Breast Cancer. Available online: https://clinicaltrials.gov/ct2/show/NCT03233191#contacts (accessed on 12 March 2022).
81. Lee, C.; McCaskill-Stevens, W. Tomosynthesis mammographic Imaging Screening Trial (TMIST): An Invitation and Opportunity for the National Medical Association Community to Shape the Future of Precision Screening for Breast Cancer. *J. Natl. Med. Assoc.* 2020, *112*, 613–618. [CrossRef]
82. Conant, E.F.; Beaber, E.F.; Sprague, B.L.; Herschorn, S.D.; Weaver, D.L.; Onega, T.; Tosteson, A.N.; McCarthy, A.M.; Poplack, S.P.; Haas, J.S.; et al. Breast cancer screening using tomosynthesis in combination with digital mammography compared to digital mammography alone: A cohort study within the PROSPR consortium. *Breast Cancer Res. Treat.* 2016, *156*, 109–116. [CrossRef]
83. Bahl, M.; Gaffney, S.; McCarthy, A.M.; Lowry, K.P.; Dang, P.A.; Lehman, C.D. Breast cancer characteristics associated with 2D digital mammography versus digital breast tomosynthesis for screening-detected and interval cancers. *Radiology* 2018, *287*, 49–57. [CrossRef] [PubMed]
84. Rafferty, E.A.; Durand, M.A.; Conant, E.F.; Copit, D.S.; Friedewald, S.M.; Plecha, D.M.; Miller, D.P. Breast Cancer Screening Using Tomosynthesis and Digital Mammography in Dense and Nondense Breasts. *JAMA* 2016, *315*, 1784–1786. [CrossRef] [PubMed]
85. Tagliafico, A.S.; Calabrese, M.; Mariscotti, G.; Durando, M.; Tosto, S.; Monetti, F.; Airaldi, S.; Bignotti, B.; Nori, J.; Bagni, A.; et al. Adjunct screening with tomosynthesis or ultrasound in women with mammography-negative dense breasts: Interim report of a prospective comparative trial. *J. Clin. Oncol.* 2016, *34*, 1882–1888. [CrossRef] [PubMed]
86. Tagliafico, A.S.; Mariscotti, G.; Valdora, F.; Durando, M.; Nori, J.; La Forgia, D.; Rosenberg, I.; Caumo, F.; Gandolfo, N.; Sormani, M.P.; et al. A prospective comparative trial of adjunct screening with tomosynthesis or ultrasound in women with mammography-negative dense breasts (ASTOUND-2). *Eur. J. Cancer* 2018, *104*, 39–46. [CrossRef]
87. Cancer Stat Facts: Cancer Disparities Reports on Cancer Annual Report to the Nation Cancer Stat Facts Breast (Female) Melanoma of the Skin Statistics at a Glance. Available online: https://seer.Cancer.gov/statistics/reports.html (accessed on 12 March 2022).
88. Foy, K.C.; Fisher, J.L.; Lustberg, M.B.; Gray, D.M.; De Graffinreid, C.R.; Paskett, E.D. Disparities in breast cancer tumor characteristics, treatment, time to treatment, and survival probability among African American and white women. *NPJ Breast Cancer* 2018, *4*, 7. [CrossRef]
89. Rochman, S. Study Finds Black Women Have Denser Breast Tissue Than White Women. *J. Natl. Cancer Inst.* 2015, *107*, djv296. [CrossRef]
90. Dietze, E.C.; Sistrunk, C.; Miranda-Carboni, G.; O'regan, R.; Seewaldt, V.L. Triple-Negative Breast Cancer in African-American Women: Disparities Versus Biology. *Nat. Rev. Cancer* 2015, *15*, 248–254. Available online: https://www.nature.com/reviews/cancer (accessed on 12 March 2022). [CrossRef]
91. Berg, W.A. Tailored supplemental screening for breast cancer: What now and what next? *Am. J. Roentgenol.* 2009, *192*, 390–399. [CrossRef]
92. Kuhl, C.; Weigel, S.; Schrading, S.; Arand, B.; Bieling, H.; König, R.; Tombach, B.; Leutner, C.; Rieber-Brambs, A.; Nordhoff, D.; et al. Prospective multicenter cohort study to refine management recommendations for women at elevated familial risk of breast cancer: EVA Trial. *J. Clin. Oncol.* 2010, *28*, 1450–1457. [CrossRef]
93. White, G.W.; Gibby, W.A.; Tweedle, M.F. Comparison of Gd(DTPA-BMA) (Omniscan) versus Gd(HP-DO3A) (ProHance) relative to gadolinium retention in human bone tissue by inductively coupled plasma mass spectroscopy. *Investig. Radiol.* 2006, *41*, 272–278. [CrossRef] [PubMed]
94. Gibby, W.A.; Gibby, K.A.; Gibby, W.A. Comparison of Gd DTPA-BMA (Omniscan) versus Gd HP-DO3A (ProHance) retention in human bone tissue by inductively coupled plasma atomic emission spectroscopy. *Investig. Radiol.* 2004, *39*, 138–142. [CrossRef]
95. Roberts, D.R.; Lindhorst, S.M.; Welsh, C.T.; Maravilla, K.R.; Herring, M.N.; Braun, K.A.; Thiers, B.H.; Davis, W.C. High Levels of Gadolinium Deposition in the Skin of a Patient with Normal Renal Function. *Investig. Radiol.* 2016, *51*, 280–289. [CrossRef] [PubMed]
96. McDonald, R.J.; McDonald, J.S.; Dai, D.; Schroeder, D.; Jentoft, M.E.; Murray, D.L.; Kadirvel, R.; Eckel, L.J.; Kallmes, D.F. Comparison of gadolinium concentrations within multiple rat organs after intravenous administration of linear versus macrocyclic gadolinium chelates. *Radiology* 2017, *285*, 536–545. [CrossRef] [PubMed]
97. McDonald, R.J.; McDonald, J.S.; Kallmes, D.F.; Jentoft, M.E.; Murray, D.L.; Thielen, K.R.; Williamson, E.E.; Eckel, L.J. Intracranial gadolinium deposition after contrast-enhanced MR imaging. *Radiology* 2015, *275*, 772–782. [CrossRef]
98. Neal, C.H. Screening Breast MRI and Gadolinium Deposition: Cause for Concern? *J. Breast Imaging* 2022, *4*, 10–18. [CrossRef]
99. Scheel, J.R.; Kim, E.; Partridge, S.C.; Lehman, C.D.; Rosen, M.A.; Bernreuter, W.K.; Pisano, E.D.; Marques, H.S.; Morris, E.A.; Weatherall, P.T.; et al. MRI, clinical examination, and mammography for preoperative assessment of residual disease and pathologic complete response after neoadjuvant chemotherapy for breast cancer: ACRIN 6657 trial. *Am. J. Roentgenol.* 2018, *210*, 1376–1385. [CrossRef]
100. Saslow, D.; Boetes, C.; Burke, W.; Harms, S.; Leach, M.O.; Lehman, C.D.; Morris, E.; Pisano, E.; Schnall, M.; Sener, S.; et al. American Cancer Society guidelines for breast screening with MRI as an adjunct to mammography. *Cancer J. Clin.* 2007, *57*, 75–89. [CrossRef]
101. Monticciolo, D.L.; Newell, M.S.; Moy, L.; Niell, B.; Monsees, B.; Sickles, E.A. Breast Cancer Screening in Women at Higher-Than-Average Risk: Recommendations From the ACR. *J. Am. Coll. Radiol.* 2018, *15*, 408–414. [CrossRef]

102. Bakker, M.F.; de Lange, S.V.; Pijnappel, R.M.; Mann, R.M.; Peeters, P.H.M.; Monninkhof, E.M.; Emaus, M.J.; Loo, C.E.; Bisschops, R.H.C.; Lobbes, M.B.I.; et al. Supplemental MRI Screening for Women with Extremely Dense Breast Tissue. *N. Engl. J. Med.* **2019**, *381*, 2091–2102. [CrossRef] [PubMed]
103. Mango, V.L.; Goel, A.; Mema, E.; Kwak, E.; Ha, R. Breast MRI screening for average-risk women: A monte carlo simulation cost–benefit analysis. *J. Magn. Reson. Imaging* **2019**, *49*, e216–e221. [CrossRef]
104. Geuzinge, H.A.; Bakker, M.F.; Heijnsdijk, E.A.M.; Ravesteyn, N.T.; Veldhuis, W.B.; Pijnappel, R.M.; de Lange, S.V.; Emaus, M.J.; Mann, R.M.; Monninkhof, E.M.; et al. Cost-Effectiveness of Magnetic Resonance Imaging Screening for Women with Extremely Dense Breast Tissue. *J. Natl. Cancer Inst.* **2021**, *113*, 1476–1483. [CrossRef] [PubMed]
105. Mann, R.M.; Athanasiou, A.; Baltzer, P.A.T.; Camps-Herrero, J.; Clauser, P.; Fallenberg, E.M.; Forrai, G.; Fuchsjäger, M.H.; Helbich, T.H.; Killburn-Toppin, F.; et al. Breast Cancer Screening in Women with Extremely Dense Breasts Recommendations of the European Society of Breast Imaging (EUSOBI). *Eur. Radiol.* **2022**, 1–10. [CrossRef] [PubMed]
106. Berg, W.A.; Blume, J.D.; Adams, A.M.; Jong, R.A.; Barr, R.G.; Lehrer, D.E.; Pisano, E.D.; Evans, W.P., 3rd; Mahoney, M.C.; Hovanessian Larsen, L.; et al. Reasons women at elevated risk of breast cancer refuse breast MR imaging screening: ACRIN 6666. *Radiology* **2010**, *254*, 79–87. [CrossRef] [PubMed]
107. Richter, V.; Hatterman, V.; Preibsch, H.; Bahrs, S.D.; Hahn, M.; Nikolaou, K.; Wiesinger, B. Contrast-enhanced spectral mammography in patients with MRI contraindications. *Acta Radiol.* **2018**, *59*, 798–805. [CrossRef] [PubMed]
108. Ghadimi, M.; Sapra, A. *Magnetic Resonance Imaging Contraindications*; StatPearls Publishing LLC: Bethesda, MD, USA, 2021.
109. Kuhl, C.K.; Schrading, S.; Strobel, K.; Schild, H.H.; Hilgers, R.D.; Bieling, H.B. Abbreviated breast Magnetic Resonance Imaging (MRI): First postcontrast subtracted images and maximum-intensity projection—A novel approach to breast cancer screening with MRI. *J. Clin. Oncol.* **2014**, *32*, 2304–2310. [CrossRef] [PubMed]
110. Kuhl, C.K. Abbreviated Magnetic Resonance Imaging (MRI) for Breast Cancer Screening: Rationale, Concept, and Transfer to Clinical Practice. *Annu. Rev. Med.* **2019**, *70*, 501–519. [CrossRef] [PubMed]
111. Comstock, C.E.; Gatsonis, C.; Newstead, G.M.; Snyder, B.S.; Gareen, I.F.; Bergin, J.T.; Rahbar, H.; Sung, J.S.; Jacobs, C.; Harvey, J.A.; et al. Comparison of Abbreviated Breast MRI vs Digital Breast Tomosynthesis for Breast Cancer Detection among Women with Dense Breasts Undergoing Screening. *J. Am. Med. Assoc.* **2020**, *323*, 746–756. [CrossRef] [PubMed]
112. Patel, S.; Heacock, L.; Gao, Y.; Elias, K.; Moy, L.; Heller, S. Advances in Abbreviated Breast MRI and Ultrafast Imaging. *Semin. Roentgenol.* **2022**. [CrossRef]
113. O'Flynn, E.A.M.; Blackledge, M.; Collins, D.; Downey, K.; Doran, S.; Patel, H.; Dumonteil, S.; Mok, W.; Leach, M.O.; Koh, D.M. Evaluating the diagnostic sensitivity of computed diffusion-weighted MR imaging in the detection of breast cancer. *J. Magn. Reson. Imaging* **2016**, *44*, 130–137. [CrossRef] [PubMed]
114. Amornsiripanitch, N.; Bickelhaupt, S.; Shin, H.J.; Dang, M.; Rahbar, H.; Pinker, K.; Partridge, S.C. Diffusion-weighted MRI for unenhanced breast cancer screening. *Radiology* **2019**, *293*, 504–520. [CrossRef] [PubMed]
115. Luo, J.; Hippe, D.S.; Rahbar, H.; Parsian, S.; Rendi, M.H.; Partridge, S.C. Diffusion tensor imaging for characterizing tumor microstructure and improving diagnostic performance on breast MRI: A prospective observational study. *Breast Cancer Res.* **2019**, *21*, 1–16. [CrossRef]
116. Chen, Y.; Panda, A.; Pahwa, S.; Hamilton, J.I.; Dastmalchian, S.; McGivney, D.F.; Ma, D.; Batesole, J.; Seiberlich, N.; Griswold, M.A.; et al. Three-dimensional MR fingerprinting for quantitative breast imaging. *Radiology* **2019**, *290*, 33–40. [CrossRef] [PubMed]
117. Sabouri, S.; Chang, S.D.; Goldenberg, S.L.; Savdie, R.; Jones, E.C.; Black, P.C.; Fazli, L.; Kozlowski, P. Comparing diagnostic accuracy of luminal water imaging with diffusion-weighted and dynamic contrast-enhanced MRI in prostate cancer: A quantitative MRI study. *NMR Biomed.* **2019**, *32*, e4048. [CrossRef] [PubMed]
118. Retter, A.; Gong, F.; Syer, T.; Singh, S.; Adeleke, S.; Punwani, S. Emerging methods for prostate cancer imaging: Evaluating cancer structure and metabolic alterations more clearly. *Mol. Oncol.* **2021**, *15*, 2565–2579. [CrossRef]
119. Jochelson, M.S.; Lobbes, M.B.I. Contrast-enhanced Mammography: State of the art. *Radiology* **2021**, *299*, 36–48. [CrossRef] [PubMed]
120. Kornecki, A. Current Status of Contrast Enhanced Mammography: A Comprehensive Review. *Can. Assoc. Radiol. J.* **2021**, *73*, 9047. [CrossRef]
121. Francescone, M.A.; Jochelson, M.S.; Dershaw, D.D.; Sung, J.S.; Hughes, M.C.; Zheng, J.; Moskowitz, C.; Morris, E.A. Low energy mammogram obtained in contrast-enhanced digital mammography (CEDM) is comparable to routine full-field digital mammography (FFDM). *Eur. J. Radiol.* **2014**, *83*, 1350–1355. [CrossRef]
122. 1Konstantopoulos, C.; Mehta, T.S.; Brook, A.; Dialani, V.; Mehta, R.; Fein-Zachary, V.; Phillips, J. Cancer Conspicuity on Low-energy Images of Contrast-enhanced Mammography Compared With 2D Mammography. *J. Breast Imaging* **2022**, *4*, 31–38. [CrossRef]
123. Sogani, J.; Mango, V.L.; Keating, D.; Sung, J.S.; Jochelson, M.S. Contrast-enhanced mammography: Past, present, and future. *Clin. Imaging* **2021**, *69*, 269–279. [CrossRef] [PubMed]
124. 1Amir, T.; Hogan, M.P.; Jacobs, S.; Sevilimedu, V.; Sung, J.; Jochelson, M.S. Comparison of False-Positive Versus True-Positive Findings on Contrast-Enhanced Digital Mammography. *Am. J. Roentgenol.* **2022**, *218*, 797–808. [CrossRef]
125. Cheung, Y.C.; Lin, Y.C.; Wan, Y.L.; Yeow, K.M.; Huang, P.C.; Lo, Y.F.; Tsai, H.P.; Ueng, S.H.; Chang, C.J. Diagnostic performance of dual-energy contrast-enhanced subtracted mammography in dense breasts compared to mammography alone: Interobserver blind-reading analysis. *Eur. Radiol.* **2014**, *24*, 2394–2403. [CrossRef] [PubMed]

126. Fallenberg, E.M.; Dromain, C.; Diekmann, F.; Engelken, F.; Krohn, M.; Singh, J.M.; Ingold-Heppner, B.; Winzer, K.J.; Bick, U.; Renz, D.M. Contrast-enhanced spectral mammography versus MRI: Initial results in the detection of breast cancer and assessment of tumour size. *Eur. Radiol.* **2014**, *24*, 256–264. [CrossRef]
127. James, J.R.; Pavlicek, W.; Hanson, J.A.; Boltz, T.F.; Patel, B.K. Breast radiation dose with CESM compared with 2D FFDM and 3D tomosynthesis mammography. *Am. J. Roentgenol.* **2017**, *208*, 362–372. [CrossRef]
128. Phillips, J.; Mihai, G.; Hassonjee, S.E.; Raj, S.D.; Palmer, M.R.; Brook, A.; Zhang, D. Comparative Dose of Contrast-Enhanced Spectral Mammography (CESM), digital mammography, and digital breast tomosynthesis. *Am. J. Roentgenol.* **2018**, *211*, 839–846. [CrossRef]
129. Fusco, R.; Raiano, N.; Raiano, C.; Maio, F.; Vallone, P.; Mattace Raso, M.; Setola, S.V.; Granata, V.; Rubulotta, M.R.; Barretta, M.L.; et al. Evaluation of average glandular dose and investigation of the relationship with compressed breast thickness in dual energy contrast enhanced digital mammography and digital breast tomosynthesis. *Eur. J. Radiol.* **2020**, *126*, 108912. [CrossRef]
130. Zanardo, M.; Cozzi, A.; Trimboli, R.M.; Labaj, O.; Monti, C.B.; Schiaffino, S.; Carbonaro, L.A.; Sardanelli, F. Technique, protocols and adverse reactions for contrast-enhanced spectral mammography (CESM): A systematic review. *Insights Imaging* **2019**, *10*, 1–15. [CrossRef]
131. Lobbes, M.B.I.; Smidt, M.L.; Houwers, J.; Tjan-Heijnen, V.C.; Wildberger, J.E. Contrast enhanced mammography: Techniques, current results, and potential indications. *Clin. Radiol.* **2013**, *68*, 935–944. [CrossRef]
132. Jochelson, M.S.; Pinker, K.; Dershaw, D.D.; Hughes, M.; Gibbons, G.F.; Rahbar, K.; Robson, M.E.; Mangino, D.A.; Goldman, D.; Moskowitz, C.S.; et al. Comparison of screening CEDM and MRI for women at increased risk for breast cancer: A pilot study. *Eur. J. Radiol.* **2017**, *97*, 37–43. [CrossRef]
133. NCCN Guidelines Version 1. 2021 Breast Cancer Screening and Diagnosis. Available online: https://www.nccn.org/professionals/physician_gls/pdf/breast-screening.pdf (accessed on 16 April 2022).
134. Sung, J.S.; Lebron, L.; Keating, D.; D'Alessio, D.; Comstock, C.E.; Lee, C.H.; Pike, M.C.; Ayhan, M.; Moskowitz, C.S.; Morris, E.A.; et al. Performance of dual-energy contrast-enhanced digital mammography for screening women at increased risk of breast cancer. *Radiology* **2019**, *293*, 81–88. [CrossRef] [PubMed]
135. Klang, E.; Krosser, A.; Amitai, M.M.; Sorin, V.; Halshtok Neiman, O.; Shalmon, A.; Gotlieb, M.; Sklair-Levy, M. Utility of routine use of breast ultrasound following contrast-enhanced spectral mammography. *Clin. Radiol.* **2018**, *73*, 908.e11–908.e16. [CrossRef] [PubMed]
136. Sorin, V.; Yagil, Y.; Yosepovich, A.; Shalmon, A.; Gotlieb, M.; Neiman, O.H.; Sklair-Levy, M. Contrast-enhanced spectral mammography in women with intermediate breast cancer risk and dense breasts. *Am. J. Roentgenol.* **2018**, *211*, W267–W274. [CrossRef]
137. Health Canada, F. Active Licence Search Results. 2017. Available online: https://health-products.canada.ca/mdall-limh/ (accessed on 12 March 2022).
138. GE Press Release. GE Healthcare Receives FDA Clearance of the Industry's First Contrast-Enhanced Mammography Solution for Biopsy. Available online: https://health-products.canada.ca/mdall-limh/dispatch-repartition.do?type=active.HealthCanadaApproval (accessed on 12 March 2022).
139. FDA. FDA Approval Letter. Available online: https://www.accessdata.fda.gov/cdrh_docs/pdf19/K193334.pdf (accessed on 12 March 2022).
140. Houben, I.P.L.; van de Voorde, P.; Jeukens, C.R.L.P.N.; Wildberger, J.E.; Kooreman, L.F.; Smidt, M.L.; Lobbes, M.B.I. Contrast-enhanced spectral mammography as work-up tool in patients recalled from breast cancer screening has low risks and might hold clinical benefits. *Eur. J. Radiol.* **2017**, *94*, 31–37. [CrossRef] [PubMed]
141. ACR announcement. CMIST Clinical Trial. Available online: https://www.acr.org/-/media/ACR/Files/Breast-Imaging-Resources/GEHC_CMIST_2020_01_113019---Post-Card.pdf (accessed on 12 March 2022).
142. Contrast Enhanced Mammography (CEM) (A Supplement to ACR BI-RADS® Mammography 2013). Available online: https://www.acr.org/-/media/ACR/Files/RADS/BI-RADS/BIRADS_CEM_2022.pdf (accessed on 16 April 2022).
143. Hruska, C.B. Molecular breast imaging for screening in dense breasts: State of the art and future directions. *Am. J. Roentgenol.* **2017**, *208*, 275–283. [CrossRef]
144. Berg, W.A.; Rafferty, E.A.; Friedewald, S.M.; Hruska, C.B.; Rahbar, H. Screening algorithms in dense breasts: AJR expert panel narrative review. *Am. J. Roentgenol.* **2021**, *216*, 275–294. [CrossRef]
145. Berg, W.A. Nuclear breast imaging: Clinical results and future directions. *J. Nucl. Med.* **2016**, *57*, 46S–52S. [CrossRef]
146. Rhodes, D.J.; Hruska, C.B.; Conners, A.L.; Tortorelli, C.L.; Maxwell, R.W.; Jones, K.N.; Toledano, A.Y.; O'Connor, M.K. Molecular breast imaging at reduced radiation dose for supplemental screening in mammographically dense breasts. *Am. J. Roentgenol.* **2015**, *204*, 241–251. [CrossRef]
147. Shermis, R.B.; Wilson, K.D.; Doyle, M.T.; Martin, T.S.; Merryman, D.; Kudrolli, H.; Brenner, R.J. Supplemental breast cancer screening with molecular breast imaging for women with dense breast tissue. *Am. J. Roentgenol.* **2016**, *207*, 450–457. [CrossRef]
148. Rhodes, D.; Hunt, K.; Conners, A.; Zingula, S.; Whaley, D.; Ellis, R.; Gasal Spilde, J.; Mehta, R.; Polley, M.-Y.; O'Connor, M.; et al. Abstract PD4-05: Molecular breast imaging and tomosynthesis to eliminate the reservoir of undetected cancer in dense breasts: The Density MATTERS trial. *Am. Assoc. Cancer Res.* **2019**, *79*, PD4-05. [CrossRef]
149. Hruska, C.B. Let's Get Real about Molecular Breast Imaging and Radiation Risk. *Radiol. Imaging Cancer* **2019**, *1*, e190070. [CrossRef] [PubMed]

150. Brown, M.; Covington, M.F. Comparative Benefit-to-Radiation Risk Ratio of Molecular Breast Imaging, Two-Dimensional Full-Field Digital Mammography with and without Tomosynthesis, and Synthetic Mammography with Tomosynthesis. *Radiol. Imaging Cancer* **2019**, *1*, e190005. [CrossRef] [PubMed]
151. Hendrick, R.E.; Tredennick, T. Benefit to radiation risk of breast-specific gamma imaging compared with mammography in screening asymptomatic women with dense breasts. *Radiology* **2016**, *281*, 583–588. [CrossRef] [PubMed]
152. Initial Certification for Diagnostic Radiology Certification Requirements. Available online: https://www.theabr.org/diagnostic-radiology/initial-certification/core-exam (accessed on 12 March 2022).
153. Romero-Martín, S.; Elías-Cabot, E.; Raya-Povedano, J.L.; Gubern-Mérida, A.; Rodríguez-Ruiz, A.; Álvarez-Benito, M. Stand-Alone Use of Artificial Intelligence for Digital Mammography and Digital Breast Tomosynthesis Screening: A Retrospective Evaluation. *Radiology* **2021**, *302*, 211590. [CrossRef] [PubMed]
154. Shoshan, Y.; Bakalo, R.; Gilboa-Solomon, F.; Ratner, V.; Barkan, E.; Ozery-Flato, M.; Amit, M.; Khapun, D.; Ambinder, E.B.; Oluyemi, E.T.; et al. Artificial Intelligence for Reducing Workload in Breast Cancer Screening with Digital Breast Tomosynthesis. *Radiology* **2022**, *303*, 211105. [CrossRef]
155. Philpotts, L.E. Advancing Artificial Intelligence to Meet Breast Imaging Needs. *Radiology* **2022**, *303*, 78–79. [CrossRef]
156. Shen, Y.; Shamout, F.E.; Oliver, J.R.; Witowski, J.; Kannan, K.; Park, J.; Wu, N.; Huddleston, C.; Wolfson, S.; Millet, A.; et al. Artificial intelligence system reduces false-positive findings in the interpretation of breast ultrasound exams. *Nat. Commun.* **2021**, *12*, 5645. [CrossRef]
157. Fuchsjäger, M.H.; Adelsmayr, G. Artificial Intelligence as an Assistant in Breast Cancer Screening. *Radiology* **2021**, *302*, 212675. [CrossRef]
158. Mango, V.L.; Sun, M.; Wynn, R.T.; Ha, R. Should we ignore, follow, or biopsy? Impact of artificial intelligence decision support on breast ultrasound lesion assessment. *Am. J. Roentgenol.* **2020**, *214*, 1445–1452. [CrossRef]
159. Wanders, A.J.T.; Mees, W.; Bun, P.A.M.; Janssen, N.; Rodríguez-Ruiz, A.; Dalmış, M.U.; Karssemeijer, N.; van Gils, C.H.; Sechopoulos, I.; Mann, R.M.; et al. Interval Cancer Detection Using a Neural Network and Breast Density in Women with Negative Screening Mammograms. *Radiology* **2022**, *303*, 269–275. [CrossRef]
160. Organisation for Economic Co-Operation and Development (OECD) Data on MRI Units. Available online: https://data.oecd.org/healtheqt/magnetic-resonance-imaging-mri-units.htm (accessed on 16 April 2022).
161. Cancer Detection by Screening Method. Available online: https://densebreast-info.org/screening-technologies/cancer-detection-by-screening-method/ (accessed on 15 April 2022).
162. Klarenbach, S.; Sims-Jones, N.; Lewin, G.; Singh, H.; Thériault, G.; Tonelli, M.; Doull, M.; Courage, S.; Garcia, A.J.; Thombs, B.D.; et al. Recommendations on screening for breast cancer in women aged 40-74 years who are not at increased risk for breast cancer. *CMAJ* **2018**, *190*, E1441–E1451. [CrossRef] [PubMed]
163. Siu, A.L. Screening for breast cancer: U.S. Preventive services task force recommendation statement. *Ann. Intern. Med.* **2016**, *164*, 279–296. [CrossRef] [PubMed]

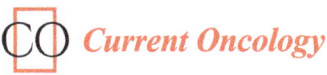

Commentary

Misinformation and Facts about Breast Cancer Screening

Daniel B. Kopans

Harvard Medical School, Boston, MA 02114, USA; dkopans@verizon.net; Tel.: +1-617-584-4584

Abstract: Quality medical practice is based on science and evidence. For over a half-century, the efficacy of breast cancer screening has been challenged, particularly for women aged 40–49. As each false claim has been raised, it has been addressed and refuted based on science and evidence. Nevertheless, misinformation continues to be promoted, resulting in confusion for women and their physicians. Early detection has been proven to save lives for women aged 40–74 in randomized controlled trials of mammography screening. Observational studies, failure analyses, and incidence of death studies have provided evidence that there is a major benefit when screening is introduced to the general population. In large part due to screening, there has been an over 40% decline in deaths from breast cancer since 1990. Nevertheless, misinformation about screening continues to be promoted, adding to the confusion. Despite claims to the contrary, a careful reading of the guidelines issued by major groups such as the U.S. Preventive Services Task Force and the American College of Physicians shows that they all agree that most lives are saved by screening starting at the age of 40. There is no scientific support for using the age of 50 as a threshold for screening. All women should be provided with the facts and not false information about breast cancer screening so that they can make "informed decisions" for themselves about whether to participate.

Keywords: breast; cancer; screening

1. Introduction

The deaths from the COVID pandemic that could have been avoided have emphasized the tragic consequences resulting from the promulgation of inaccurate information and ignoring science. Unfortunately, "alternative facts" have been generated about breast cancer screening that go back decades. Confusion has resulted from the misinformation that has been published due to poor peer review in some of the most prestigious journals [1–4]. These erroneous analyses are then reported to the public by the media, which is unable to understand some of the complexities of the claims being made, resulting in confusing messages. The following reviews just a few of the many false issues that have been raised over the years that are not supported by science. These have been used in an effort to reduce access to screening and to distract from the scientific evidence that supports the fact that annual screening starting at the age of 40 saves the most lives.

Early detection has secondary benefits such as a reduced need for mastectomies, less need for axillary dissection with the attendant reduced risk of lymphedema, and less toxic systemic therapy [5–7], but the following discussion will concentrate on the main benefit, which is mortality reduction and the fact that randomized controlled trials have proven that early detection saves lives for women aged 40–74.

2. The Decades-Long Effort to Reduce Access to Breast Cancer Screening

I suspect that most are unaware of the fact that there has been an almost continuous effort, dating back to the 1950s, to limit access to breast cancer screening. This is probably, and primarily, an effort to save money, but opponents know that if they told women they did not want to pay to save their lives, there would be "a discussion" that they would lose. Consequently, numerous scientifically unsupportable claims have been made to limit access.

As long ago as the 1950s, it was claimed that breast cancer was systemic before it could be found so that earlier detection would have no advantage. This was the origin of the effort to develop systemic treatments.

In the 1960s, based on the standardization of the mammographic technique, the first randomized controlled trial (RCT) of screening was conducted by the Health Insurance Plan of New York (HIP). HIP proved that lives could be saved by earlier detection [8]. Since HIP, the importance of early detection has been reinforced by multiple RCTs of breast cancer screening [9].

In the 1970s, the Breast Cancer Detection Demonstration Project (BCDDP)) was conducted to challenge the claim that it was not possible to screen large numbers of women efficiently and effectively. More than 275,000 women had annual mammography and clinical breast examinations over a 5-year period. In the BCDDP, 40% of the cancers were found only by mammography [10], proving the feasibility of population-based early detection.

In the mid-1970s, while the BCDDP was underway, it was claimed that the low doses of radiation needed for mammography might cause more cancers than would be cured [11]. This "radiation scare" resulted in the BCDDP stopping screening for women aged 40–49. It is now known that radiation risk to the breast is primarily for teenage women and those in their early twenties, likely related to incomplete terminal differentiation of the lobules. This risk falls rapidly with increasing age so that by the time women are in their 40s, there is no measurable risk. It is impossible to prove that there is "no risk," but even extrapolating the risk from younger women, it is far below even the smallest benefit [12,13]. Based on the evidence, even those groups that are trying to reduce access to screening have stopped raising radiation risk as a major concern.

The debate continued as to what age screening should begin. In 1989, major medical groups, including the U.S. National Cancer Institute (NCI), reached a "consensus" and advised that women aged 40–49 be screened every 1 to 2 years and women aged 50 and over be screened annually [14]. However, there were those at the NCI who did not support screening, particularly for women in their forties, so that in 1993, with a change in leadership, the NCI ignored the science and reversed its initial advice by deciding that women should wait until the age of 50 and be screened every 2 years [15].

Statistical power is critical for scientific validity. If a trial does not include sufficient numbers of women, there may be a reduction in deaths, but it will be ignored since it does not reach "statistical significance." In 1993, as a supposedly science-based organization, the NCI used an inappropriate statistical approach by analyzing the data for women aged 40–49 separately from older women in randomized controlled trials. They ignored the fact that the trials had not been planned to evaluate age subgroups and were not designed with sufficient power to permit legitimate "subgroup" analyses. As we showed, and the NCI ignored, it was impossible for the trials to show a significant mortality reduction of the expected 25% within 5 years of the start of the trials that the NCI was requiring [16]. Based on an unplanned retrospective subgroup analysis of trials lacking statistical power for this analysis to be legitimate and, for the first time in history, ignoring the advice of their main advisory group known as the National Cancer Advisory Board (NCAB), the NCI dropped support for screening women aged 40–49 and advised women aged 50 and over to be screened every 2 years despite having no data to support reducing the interval between screens from one year to two [17].

Due to concerns raised about the NCI decision in 1993, and under new leadership, the NCI agreed, in 1997, to a consensus development conference (CDC) to examine the value of screening women in their forties [18]. Despite reassurances that the CDC would be a neutral review and would be conducted without NCI influence (it was the NCI's guidelines that were under review), the CDC was organized by a declared opponent of screening working at the NCI and a review panel with several members having a conflict of interest (undisclosed NCI funding) was convened. The CDC was provided with a longer follow-up of the RCTs that showed an unambiguous, statistically significant decline in breast cancer deaths for women aged 40–49 even when analyzed separately [19]. Despite the fact that the CDC had been organized to evaluate these latest data, they were ignored (not even mentioned), and the CDC falsely claimed that there was insufficient support for screening women in their forties [20] and that the misinformation was spread by the media [21]. The updated information was subsequently reviewed by the NCAB, and recognizing that they provided scientific proof and based on NCAB advice, the NCI once again supported screening starting at the age of 40 [22]. Soon after, the NCI decided it would no longer issue guidelines.

In 2007, the American College of Physicians (ACP), having supported screening, suddenly changed course and advised women to wait until the age of 50 and be screened every 2 years [23]. The ACP and the United States Preventive Services Task Force (USPSTF) are closely allied, and the USPSTF followed suit with the same recommendations in 2009 [24].

In 2015, the American Cancer Society, a previously staunch supporter of annual mammography starting at the age of 40, submitted to political pressure and developed very strange recommendations. They initially stated that "women should have the opportunity to begin annual screening between the ages of 40 and 44 years (qualified recommendation)," but went on to recommend a scientifically unjustified hybrid recommendation stating that women might want to delay screening until the age of 45 and be screened annually until the age of 55 and then biennially after that [25].

In 2016, the USPSTF reaffirmed its advice to delay screening [26].

All three groups (USPSTF, ACP, and ACS) agree that most lives are saved by screening starting at the age of 40 [25–27], but in 2019, the ACP reaffirmed their support for the USPSTF and advised women that they should wait until the age of 50 and be screened every 2 years [28].

The USPSTF and the ACP advised delaying participation because of the "harms" of screening, which they claimed were "false positives" (a misnomer for women recalled for a few extra pictures and an ultrasound); "overdiagnosis" of cancers that would never harm a woman in her lifetime and, if left alone, would regress and disappear; and "overtreatment," which is the unnecessary treatment of "overdiagnosed" cancers.

Of course, if it even occurs, "overdiagnosis" is the fault of pathologists and not screening, and oncologists, not screening, are responsible for deciding treatment. Blaming screening for these is analogous to blaming the engines in our cars for traffic accidents. Regardless, the claims of "overdiagnosis" are based on the incredibly rare cases of clinically evident cancer that have disappeared without treatment. These are so rare that they can be considered true "miracles." In fact, the relative handful that has been reported has all been clinically evident. No one has ever observed a mammographically detected invasive breast cancer disappear on its own [29]. Since this never happens, it is misleading to advise women that they should delay screening until age 50 to reduce "overdiagnosis" since these cancers, if they even exist, will still be detected at age 50. Delaying screening will not avoid "overdiagnosed" cancers, but women will die unnecessarily if screening is delayed.

Unfortunately, although the USPSTF, ACS, and ACP all agree that delaying screening will result in avoidable deaths, they stress their claims of "harms." They have not directly stated to women and their physicians the actual number of lives that will be lost. They have not told women that, if their guidelines are followed, it is predicted that thousands will die unnecessarily that could be saved by annual screening starting at the age of 40.

The groups that advise waiting until age 50 (or 45 as per the ACS) and then screening every 2 years instead of annually have not made it clear that the only "harm" that is affected by delaying screening is the "false positive rate." The term "false positive" is a misleading, pejorative choice of words. Women are not being told (falsely) that they have breast cancer. Instead, based on the findings of their screening study, these women are simply being asked to return for a few extra pictures and sometimes an ultrasound to be careful, and, contrary to the "false positive" terminology used, most are reassured that there is no evidence of cancer.

Approximately 2% of the women screened are advised to have a very safe, image-guided needle biopsy using local anesthesia in an outpatient setting, and 20–40% of these are found to have breast cancer.

3. How Frequently Should Women Be Advised to Be Screened?

Despite the fact that there has never been an RCT to evaluate the optimum time interval between screens (annual vs. biennial or longer), there is a large amount of inferential data [30–32] supporting annual screening. Not surprisingly, the shorter the time between screens, the greater the likely benefit [33].

The NCI supports CISNET (the Cancer Intervention and Surveillance and Modeling Network), which includes six groups that have developed separate computer models to predict the result of interventions. All six agree that the most lives are saved by annual screening starting at the age of 40 [34]. The CISNET models show that if the ACS, ACP, or USPSTF guidelines are followed, thousands of lives will be lost that could be saved by annual screening starting at the age of 40 [35].

4. The RCTs Proved That Screening Saves Lives for Women Aged 40–74

RCTs are the only way to eliminate biases such as "lead time," "length bias," "selection bias," etc., which can make it difficult to evaluate the benefit of an intervention such as screening for breast cancers. The RCTs of screening proved that early detection reduces deaths among women aged 40–74, which are the ages of the women who participated in the trials [36]. This does not mean that women under age 40 and over age 74 may not also benefit from screening, but we have clear scientific proof for women aged 40–74 [19].

It is important to understand that RCTs underestimate the benefit. Once a woman is allocated to a study arm or a control arm, whatever happens to her is attributed to that assignment. Some of the women who are invited to be screened refuse the invitation. This is termed "noncompliance." In order to avoid selection bias, if they should die from breast cancer, they are still counted as a death among the screened women and dilute the benefit from screening. If a woman is assigned to a control arm, she is not prevented from obtaining a mammogram on her own outside the trial (called "contamination"). If her life is saved by the mammogram, she is still counted as an unscreened control. Since there was "noncompliance" and "contamination" in all of the trials, the RCTs likely underestimated the benefit. Although the RCTs proved that screening reduces deaths, because of noncompliance and contamination, they do not provide an accurate measure of the absolute mortality reduction. Observational studies suggest that if all women participate in screening, deaths may be reduced by over 50%.

5. There Is No Scientific Support for Using the Age of 50 as a Threshold for Screening

This cannot be stated too emphatically. There is no scientific support for using the age of 50 as a threshold for screening. It originated because investigators in the HIP trial were interested in identifying whether menopause had any influence on their results. Since they had not collected any menopausal data on their participants, they chose the age of 50 as a surrogate for menopause and, retrospectively, evaluated women aged 40–49 separately from those aged 50–64. Ignoring the fact that this subgroup analysis of the younger women lacked statistical power, they misinterpreted their results and claimed that screening was more robust for women aged 50–64 because there appeared to be an immediate decrease in deaths (likely statistical fluctuation with early small numbers), while the decline in deaths among the younger women did not begin to appear for 5–7 years. In fact, periodic screening is unlikely to produce an immediate reduction in deaths, while the "delayed benefit" is exactly what would have been expected [37]. Based on that faulty analysis, it was falsely claimed that screening was more robust for older women, and the age of 50 continues to be falsely claimed as a legitimate threshold for starting screening.

Not only was the HIP analysis not scientifically supported, but, in fact, there are no data that have not been grouped and averaged that show that any of the parameters of screening change abruptly at menopause, age 50, or any other age [38]. False claims of a sudden change at age 50 [39] have arisen by taking factors such as breast cancer detection and deaths and by grouping ages together and then taking the average of women aged 40–49 compared with the average for women aged 50–74, rather than examining rates by individual age. This takes a variable that actually changes steadily with increasing age and makes it appear to change suddenly when there is no such sudden change [40]. The only starting age for screening based on science and evidence is the age of 40.

6. The Benefit of Screening, Proven by RCTs, Is Confirmed by Observational Studies in the General Population

RCTs have proven that screening and early detection reduce deaths. As noted above, differences in death rates between study and control groups prove the benefit, but because of noncompliance and contamination, their results are diluted and do not provide absolute measures. The reduction in deaths has been confirmed when screening is introduced into the general population, in which women who have access to screening have much better survival than those who do not [34,41–55]. In these observational studies, it has been found that women aged 40 and over who actually participate in screening have a greater than 40% reduction in deaths.

7. Failure Analyses Add More Support for Screening

Another way to evaluate the benefit of early detection is using "failure analysis." What is different about women who die from breast cancer than those who do not? In a study of women who died from breast cancer in the Harvard teaching hospitals, 71% of the deaths were among the 20% of women who were not participating in screening despite all the women having access to modern therapy [56]. In an analysis by Spencer et al., the results were similar [57]. Among women who die from breast cancer, despite access to modern therapy, most deaths were among the smaller percentage of women who had not participated in screening.

8. "Incidence of Death" Is Another Way to Evaluate the Effects of Screening

A very large study of more than 500,000 women in Sweden provides additional evidence of the benefit of screening. The risk of dying from breast cancer was reduced by 41% within 10 years of diagnosis for women who participated in screening compared with those who did not [58].

9. Data from the U.S. Strongly Support the Benefits of Screening

It has never been explained why, in the U.S., our National Cancer Institute's Surveillance Epidemiology and End Results (SEER) National database has never included the method by which breast cancers are detected (MOD). This has led to numerous claims opposing mammography screening that cannot be challenged using SEER data. Unfortunately, I suspect that this is not accidental. History shows that the NCI has not been a supporter of screening, particularly for women aged 40–49, so it may well be that failing to collect data on MOD has been a conscious decision. Thus, in the U.S., we have no direct data on the results of mammography screening.

Nevertheless, by examining the data that have been collected (incidence numbers), it can be estimated that screening began in the mid-1980s in large enough numbers to influence national statistics. At this time, there was a relatively sudden increase in breast cancer incidence [59] that likely signaled the beginning of screening at a population level with sufficient numbers to be seen in national incidence estimates. Since there is no nationally organized screening program in the U.S., screening did not begin suddenly for all women. Perhaps 20% of women had at least one mammogram in the mid-1980s. It appears that participation in screening gradually increased in the 1980s and 1990s and then plateaued at the end of the 1990s when it is estimated that approximately 70% of women had had at least one mammogram [60]. I would speculate that these data support a prolonged "prevalence peak" as more and more women began to participate in screening in the late 1980s and 1990s. Prevalence screening likely ended by 1999 and explains why there was a fairly abrupt decline in "incidence" that began in 1999.

The participation in screening in the mid-1980s suggested by the data is likely the reason for the sudden decline in deaths from breast cancer that began in 1990. Data from the Connecticut Tumor Registry [61] dating back to the 1940s (SEER only began in 1974) show that the death rate from breast cancer had been unchanged for decades. As the rate of local breast cancers increased fairly abruptly and the relative rate of advanced cancers began to fall, the death rate from breast cancer began to fall in 1990, 5–7 years after the start of screening, as has been the case in the RCTs. As more and more women have participated in screening and cancer detection has improved, the death rate has continued to decline. A recent review of the SEER data shows that there are now more than 40% fewer women dying each year from breast cancer, saving an estimated 600,000 lives since 1990 [59]. There is no question that therapy has improved. Lives are being prolonged, but there is still no cure for metastatic breast cancers. Curing breast cancer is only possible when it is treated earlier. We do not know why 40,000 women still die each year despite advances in treatment because SEER does not collect MOD. What we can say is that they were not cured by therapy. The failure analyses noted earlier suggest that many of those who die are likely not participating in screening.

10. Men with Breast Cancer Have Worse Outcomes than Women

There are not many other ways to evaluate the benefit of screening. One is to compare deaths from breast cancer among men to deaths among women. The death rate from breast cancer for women has fallen dramatically since 1990 and continues to fall. Over the same time period, deaths among men with breast cancer actually increased for several years and then fell back to 1990 levels and have stayed at that level [62]. Treatment for breast cancer in men is similar to treatment for women. Men, however, generally present with more advanced cancers than women. This would suggest that the differences in deaths are likely due to the fact that women are being screened and men are not.

There is no doubt that therapy for breast cancer has improved, but treating these cancers earlier saves the most lives.

11. Most Recently, Fundamental Errors in the Canadian National Breast Screening Studies Have Been Confirmed

The Canadian National Breast Screening Studies (CNBSS) have been major outliers among the RCTs of breast cancer screening. Unlike other trials, they failed to show any benefit from mammography and clinical breast examination screening for women aged 40–49 and no benefit from mammography screening for women aged 50–59. The CNBSS results have been used to reduce access to screening for women in their 40s in Canada and around the world.

The only way to "prove" that medical intervention is efficacious is an RCT. RCTs are designed to produce identical groups. In an RCT of screening, if conducted properly, the same number of women in both groups will develop breast cancer, and the same number of women will die from breast cancer if nothing else is done. If one of the groups is offered screening and the other is not, and statistically, significantly fewer women die in the screening arm compared with the controls, then this is proof that screening saves lives.

In order for the groups to be identical, it is critical that the participants be divided randomly. Say I performed an RCT for treating breast cancer in which I chose to test an obsolete chemotherapeutic agent (similar to the outdated mammography used in the Canadian National Breast Screening Studies) to determine whether it was superior to no treatment at all, but I first examined all the women who volunteered for the trial, allowing me to identify the women with advanced cancer prior to assigning them to the treatment or control arm. Then I assigned them on open lists so that I could, undetectably, assign women to whichever arm I wanted out of random order, and I placed more women with advanced cancers in the treatment arm than the control arm, and it turned out that there were more deaths among the treated women than among controls in the early years of the trial, and, at the end of the trial, there was no difference in survival between both groups, and I concluded that there was no benefit from ANY form of systemic therapy. You would, legitimately, wonder how my trial passed a human studies review since I had violated the main "rules" for RCTs. I would likely be cited for ethics violations, and you would ask how I was able to publish the results from my flawed trial, and you would be correct in arguing that my publications should be withdrawn.

This would, in fact, be the correct response to such a compromised trial, yet similar violations of the rules for RCTs took place in the Canadian National Breast Screening Studies (CNBSS). For inexplicable reasons, these trials passed institutional reviews, peer reviews in journals, and subsequent reviews by various other panels. Instead of being ignored as having unreliable results, these trials have been praised by supposed trial experts [63], and their negative results have been used for decades to deny women access to screening [64].

In other RCTs of screening, a general population was first identified, and then, without knowing anything about the women, they were randomly assigned to the study or the control arms. The women allocated to the study arms were invited to participate in screening. The women allocated to the control arms had their "usual care." The CNBSS was different. Volunteers were first recruited. This means that there was a likelihood that women "self-selected." Perhaps women who were more health conscious agreed to participate. They tend to have better outcomes. Regardless, they were likely not representative of a general population, so the results would not be "generalizable," yet they have been applied to all women.

In order to be certain that assignment to study or control arms is random, "blinded allocation" is required. Nothing can be known about the participants prior to allocation that could be used to inadvertently or intentionally "load" one side or the other. This fundamental rule was violated in the CNBSS. The investigators have admitted, and an independent review has verified, that most of the women in the CNBSS underwent a clinical breast examination (CBE) by highly trained nurses [65] prior to allocation. These CBEs identified women with suspicious clinical findings before they were assigned to the study or control arm. Of course, you might ask why these women, many of whom had clinically evident cancers and could not benefit from mammography screening, were not excluded from a trial testing the value of mammography screening.

The preallocation CBE was a major violation, but this was compounded by the fact that the CBE results were provided to the coordinators, who determined to which group the women would be assigned. Had this still been a blinded assignment, then it is likely that the women with signs or symptoms of breast cancer would have been assigned equally to both arms, and their participation would have only diluted the benefit. However, the CNBSS violated another basic rule. Instead of blinded assignment, the women were assigned on open lists. The coordinators knew which lists would result in mammography screening and could assign women, out of random order, to either group in a process that could not be traced.

A problem was first recognized [66] when the trialists reported 19 women with advanced cancers allocated to the screening arm while only 5 were assigned to the control arm in CNBSS1. This proved to be a "statistically significant" difference [67]. The trialists have falsely argued that this was because "mammography finds more of everything." They ignored the fact that 17 of the 19 advanced cancers were evident on the preallocation CBE.

Numerous other published facts have indicated that assignments were not all random and that the screening arm was "loaded," but the unsupportable denials by the investigators have always been accepted by various reviewers. No one has ever suggested that the imbalances were intended by the trialists, but the trials' designs and executions made imbalances possible. The coordinators were not experienced in RCTs and may well have, naively, wanted to be certain that a woman with probable cancer had a mammogram and assigned her out of random order to be certain that she had a mammogram.

It seemed that the facts would never be known. I personally wrote to MacMahon and Bailar, who were brought in to review the trials [68]. I cited the obvious need to interview the coordinators (with protection from any retribution) [69] to determine whether they had assigned women out of random order as the data suggested, but the CNBSS investigators would never permit them to be interviewed to find out what actually took place.

In March of 2021, I presented a talk virtually to the Toronto Society of Breast Imaging, in which I outlined the concerns raised by the published data about the CNBSS and, in particular, the indications of nonrandom allocation. Soon after, I received an email from an attendee who had been an X-ray technologist in the CNBSS. She attested to the fact that she had witnessed nonrandom allocation of women with clinical evidence of breast cancer who were assigned out of random order to the mammography arms [70]. An extensive effort to interview any remaining workers in the CNBSS has confirmed the fact that not only were women with signs or symptoms assigned out of random order but that, in fact, many were actually recruited into these trials of screening despite the fact that they could not benefit from screening [71–73].

You would also think that trials of mammography screening would use state-of-the-art systems. What has also been ignored over the years is the well-documented fact that the CNBSS used some inferior, obsolete mammography systems. The technologists had no special training in obtaining mammograms and used obsolete positioning that did not image the axillary tail of the breast where many cancers develop. Grids to reduce scatter X-rays were not employed, likely causing some small cancers to be obscured. Their own reference physicist cited problems with their imaging [74]. I was one of three radiologists whom the investigators chose to conduct a blinded review of their mammograms [75]. This review confirmed the poor quality of the images. It showed that for much of the studies, the images were poor to unacceptable [76]. Evidence of the poor quality of the images is suggested by the fact that in the CNBSS, fewer cancers were detected by mammography alone (30%) than with older techniques used 10 years earlier in the BCDDP (40%). These and other problems also worked against the demonstration of the benefit of mammography. Most reviews of these trials that have been undertaken over the years have excluded experts in mammography screening. It is likely that the inexpert reviewers have made the false assumption that "a mammogram is a mammogram."

There are numerous reasons to withdraw the results from these trials. Assigning women with more advanced cancers in nonrandom order to the screening arms, imaging using obsolete systems by technologists who had no training, and radiologists who had minimal if any training in interpreting mammograms—the CNBSS results were clearly imbalanced against screening. It is not surprising that these trials are major outliers among the other RCTs by not showing a benefit of mammography for women at any age from 40–59.

The data have long shown, and an eyewitness has now verified, that there were fundamental flaws in the execution of the CNBSS, rendering their results unreliable. They should not be used to advise women on screening guidelines, and the publication of their results should be withdrawn.

12. Conclusions

The most rigorous medical studies have proven that mammography screening reduces deaths from breast cancer for women aged 40–74. This has been confirmed by observational studies, failure analyses, and incidence of death studies. Mammography is far from perfect. It does not find all cancers, and even earlier detection does not guarantee a cure. Therapy has improved, but there is still no cure for advanced cancers, and screening has helped cut the death rate from breast cancer in half. Computer models all show that annual screening saves the most lives. The age of 50 has no scientific support as a threshold for screening.

The promulgation of misinformation needs to stop. All women and their physicians need to be provided with scientifically valid information to make "informed decisions." Women should be advised that annual screening starting at the age of 40 saves the most lives.

Funding: This research received no external funding.

Institutional Review Board Statement: Not applicable.

Informed Consent Statement: Not applicable.

Data Availability Statement: Not applicable.

Conflicts of Interest: D.B.K. receives royalties from IZI Medical and is a consultant to DART Imaging, which makes mammography devices for China.

References

1. Kopans, D. Breast Cancer Screening Panels Continue to Confuse the Facts and Inject Their Own Biases. *Curr. Oncol.* **2015**, *22*, 376–379. [CrossRef]
2. Kopans, D.B. Bias in the Medical Journals: A Commentary. *Am. J. Roentgenol.* **2005**, *185*, 176–182. [CrossRef]
3. Kopans, D.B. More misinformation on breast cancer screening. *Gland Surg.* **2017**, *6*, 125–129. [CrossRef] [PubMed]
4. Kopans, D.B. Informed decision making: Age of 50 is arbitrary and has no demonstrated influence on breast cancer screening in women. *Am. J. Roentgenol.* **2005**, *185*, 177–182.
5. Ahn, S.; Wooster, M.; Valente, C.; Moshier, E.; Meng, R.; Pisapati, K.; Couri, R.; Margolies, L.; Schmidt, H.; Port, E. Impact of Screening Mammography on Treatment in Women Diagnosed with Breast Cancer. *Ann. Surg. Oncol.* **2018**, *25*, 2979–2986. [CrossRef] [PubMed]
6. Coldman, A.J.; Phillips, N.; Speers, C. A retrospective study of the effect of participation in screening mammography on the use of chemotherapy and breast conserving surgery. *Int. J. Cancer* **2007**, *120*, 2185–2190. [CrossRef] [PubMed]
7. Yaffe, M.J.; Jong, R.A.; I Pritchard, K. Breast Cancer Screening: Beyond Mortality. *J. Breast Imaging* **2019**, *1*, 161–165. [CrossRef]
8. Shapiro, S. Evidence on screening for breast cancer from a randomized trial. *Cancer* **1977**, *39*, 2772–2782. [CrossRef]
9. Smith, R.A.; Duffy, S.W.; Gabe, R.; Tabár, L.; Yen, A.M.; Chen, T.H. The randomized trials of breast cancer screening: What have we learned? *Radiol. Clin. N. Am.* **2004**, *42*, 793–806. [CrossRef] [PubMed]
10. Smart, C.R.; Byrne, C.; Smith, R.A.; Garfinkel, L.; Letton, A.H.; Dodd, G.D.; Beahrs, O.H. Twenty-year follow-up of the breast cancers diagnosed during the Breast Cancer Detection Demonstration Project. *CA A Cancer J. Clin.* **1997**, *47*, 134–149. [CrossRef] [PubMed]
11. Bailar, J.C. Mammography: A Contrary View. *Ann. Intern. Med.* **1976**, *84*, 77–84. [CrossRef]
12. Mettler, F.A.; Upton, A.C.; Kelsey, C.A.; Rosenberg, R.D.; Linver, M.N. Benefits versus Risks from Mammography: A Critical Assessment. *Cancer* **1996**, *77*, 903–909. [CrossRef]
13. Yaffe, M.J.; Mainprize, J.G. Risk of Radiation-induced Breast Cancer from Mammographic Screening. *Radiology* **2011**, *258*, 98–105. [CrossRef] [PubMed]
14. Press release from the National Medical Roundtable on Mammography Screening Guidelines. 27 June 1989.
15. Fletcher, S.W.; Black, W.; Harris, R.; Rimer, B.K.; Shapiro, S. Report of the International Workshop on Screening for Breast Cancer. *JNCI J. Natl. Cancer Inst.* **1993**, *85*, 1644–1656. [CrossRef] [PubMed]
16. Kopans, D.B.; Halpern, E.; Hulka, C.A. Statistical power in breast cancer screening trials and mortality reduction among Women 40–49 years of age with particular emphasis on the national breast screening study of Canada. *Cancer* **1994**, *74*, 1196–1203. [CrossRef]
17. House Committee on Government Operations. *Misused Science: The National Cancer Institutes Elimination of Mammography Guidelines for Women in Their Forties*; Union Calendar No. 480. House Report 103–863; National Cancer Institute: Bethesda, MD, USA, 1994.
18. Available online: https://consensus.nih.gov/1997/1997BreastCancerScreening103html.htm (accessed on 2 August 2022).
19. Hendrick, R.E.; Smith, R.A.; Rutledge, J.H.; Smart, C.R. Benefit of Screening Mammography in Women Aged 40–49: A New Meta-Analysis of Randomized Controlled Trials. *J. Natl. Cancer Inst. Monogr.* **1997**, *1997*, 87–92. [CrossRef] [PubMed]
20. NCI Adopts New Mammography Screening Guidelines For Women. *JNCI J. Natl. Cancer Inst.* **1997**, *89*, 538–540. [CrossRef] [PubMed]
21. Kolata, G. Stand on Mammograms Greeted by Outrage. *New York Times*, 28 January 1997.
22. NCI Moves to Resolve Controversy over Mammography Screening in 40 s. 1997. Diagnostic Imaging. Available online: http://www.diagnosticimaging.com/practice-management/nci-moves-resolve-controversy-over-mammography-screening-40s (accessed on 2 August 2022).
23. Armstrong, K.; Moye, E.; Williams, S.; Berlin, J.A.; Reynolds, E.E. Screening Mammography in Women 40 to 49 Years of Age: A Systematic Review for the American College of Physicians. *Ann. Intern. Med.* **2007**, *146*, 516–526. [CrossRef] [PubMed]
24. US Preventive Services Task Force. Screening for breast cancer: U.S. Preventive Services Task Force recommendation statement. *Ann. Intern. Med.* **2009**, *151*, 716–726. [CrossRef]

25. Oeffinger, K.C.; Fontham, E.T.; Etzioni, R.; Herzig, A.; Michaelson, J.S.; Shih, Y.C.; Walter, L.C.; Church, T.R.; Flowers, C.R.; LaMonte, S.J.; et al. Breast Cancer Screening for Women at Average Risk: 2015 Guideline Update From the American Cancer Society. *JAMA* **2015**, *314*, 1599–1614. [CrossRef]
26. Siu, A.L.; U.S. Preventive Services Task Force. Screening for Breast Cancer: U.S. Preventive Services Task Force Recommendation Statement. *Ann. Intern. Med.* **2016**, *164*, 279–296. [CrossRef]
27. Screening Mammography in Women Aged 40–49: A Report of the American College of Physicians and American College of Radiology Consensus Meeting. 2012. ACP Internist. Available online: http://www.acpinternist.org/archives/2012/05/policy.htm (accessed on 15 July 2022).
28. Qaseem, A.; Lin, J.S.; Mustafa, R.A.; Horwitch, C.A.; Wilt, T.J.; For the Clinical Guidelines Committee of the American College of Physicians. Screening for Breast Cancer in Average-Risk Women: A Guidance Statement From the American College of Physicians. *Ann. Intern. Med.* **2019**, *170*, 547–560. [CrossRef]
29. Arleo, E.K.; Monticciolo, D.L.; Monsees, B.; McGinty, G.; Sickles, E.A. Persistent Untreated Screening-Detected Breast Cancer: An Argument Against Delaying Screening or Increasing the Interval Between Screenings. *J. Am. Coll. Radiol.* **2017**, *14*, 863–867. [CrossRef]
30. Hunt, K.A.; Rosen, E.L.; Sickles, E.A. Outcome analysis for women undergoing annual versus biennial screening mammography: A review of 24,211 examinations. *Am. J. Roentgenol.* **1999**, *173*, 285–289. [CrossRef]
31. Anderson, T.J.; Waller, M.; Ellis, I.O.; Bobrow, L.; Moss, S. Influence of annual mammography from age 40 on breast cancer pathology. *Hum. Pathol.* **2004**, *35*, 1252–1259. [CrossRef]
32. Miglioretti, D.L.; Zhu, W.; Kerlikowske, K.; Sprague, B.L.; Onega, T.; Buist, D.S.M.; Henderson, L.M.; Smith, R.A. Breast Cancer Surveillance Consortium Breast Tumor Prognostic Characteristics and Biennial vs Annual Mammography, Age, and Menopausal Status. *JAMA Oncol.* **2015**, *1*, 1069–1077. [CrossRef]
33. Michaelson, J.S.; Halpern, E.; Kopans, D.B. Breast Cancer: Computer Simulation Method for Estimating Optimal Intervals for Screening. *Radiology* **1999**, *212*, 551–560. [CrossRef]
34. Mandelblatt, J.S.; Cronin, K.A.; Bailey, S.; Berry, D.A.; De Koning, H.J.; Draisma, G.; Huang, M.H.; Lee, D.S.J.; Munsell, M.M.; Plevritis, S.K.; et al. Effects of Mammography Screening Under Different Screening Schedules: Model Estimates of Potential Benefits and Harms. *Ann. Intern. Med.* **2009**, *151*, 738–747. [CrossRef]
35. Hendrick, R.E.; Helvie, M.A. USPSTF Guidelines on Screening Mammography Recommendations: Science Ignored. *Am. J. Roentgenol.* **2011**, *196*, W112–W116. [CrossRef]
36. Tabár, L.; Yen, A.M.; Wu, W.Y.; Chen, S.L.; Chiu, S.Y.; Fann, J.C.; Ku, M.M.; Smith, R.A.; Duffy, S.W.; Chen, T.H. Insights from the breast cancer screening trials: How screening affects the natural history of breast cancer and implications for evaluating service screening programs. *Breast J.* **2015**, *21*, 13–20. [CrossRef]
37. Kopans, D.B. Screening for breast cancer and mortality reduction among women 40–49 years of age. *Cancer* **1994**, *74*, 311–322. [CrossRef] [PubMed]
38. Kopans, D.B.; Moore, R.H.; McCarthy, K.A.; Hall, D.A.; Hulka, C.; Whitman, G.J.; Slanetz, P.J.; Halpern, E.F. Biasing the Interpretation of Mammography Screening Data by Age Grouping: Nothing Changes Abruptly at Age 50. *Breast J.* **1998**, *4*, 139–145. [CrossRef]
39. Kerlikowske, K.; Grady, D.; Barclay, J.; Sickles, E.A.; Eaton, A.; Ernster, V. Positive Predictive Value of Screening Mammography by Age and Family History of Breast Cancer. *JAMA* **1993**, *270*, 2444–2450. [CrossRef] [PubMed]
40. Sox, H.C. Screening Mammography in Women Younger than 50 Years of Age. *Ann. Intern. Med.* **1995**, *122*, 550–552. [CrossRef]
41. Tabar, L.; Vitak, B.; Tony, H.H.; Yen, M.F.; Duffy, S.W.; Smith, R.A. Beyond randomized controlled trials: Organized mammographic screening substantially reduces breast carcinoma mortality. *Cancer* **2001**, *91*, 1724–1731. [CrossRef]
42. Duffy, S.W.; Tabár, L.; Chen, H.-H.; Holmqvist, M.; Yen, M.-F.; Abdsalah, S.; Epstein, B.; Frodis, E.; Ljungberg, E.; Hedborg-Melander, C.; et al. The impact of organized mammography service screening on breast carcinoma mortality in seven Swedish counties. *Cancer* **2002**, *95*, 458–469. [CrossRef]
43. Otto, S.J.; Fracheboud, J.; Looman, C.W.N.; Broeders, M.J.M.; Boer, R.; Hendriks, J.N.H.C.L.; Verbeek, A.L.M.; de Koning, H.J.; The National Evaluation Team for Breast Cancer Screening. Initiation of population-based mammography screening in Dutch municipalities and effect on breast-cancer mortality: A systematic review. *Lancet* **2003**, *361*, 411–417.
44. The Swedish Organised Service Screening Evaluation Group. Reduction in Breast Cancer Mortality from Organized Service Screening with Mammography: 1. Further Confirmation with Extended Data. *Cancer Epidemiol. Biomark. Prev.* **2006**, *15*, 45–51. [CrossRef]
45. Coldman, A.; Phillips, N.; Warren, L.; Kan, L. Breast cancer mortality after screening mammography in British Columbia women. *Int. J. Cancer* **2006**, *120*, 1076–1080. [CrossRef]
46. Jonsson, H.; Bordás, P.; Wallin, H.; Nyström, L.; Lenner, P. Service screening with mammography in Northern Sweden: Effects on breast cancer mortality—An update. *J. Med. Screen.* **2007**, *14*, 87–93. [CrossRef] [PubMed]
47. Paap, E.; Holland, R.; Heeten, G.J.D.; Van Schoor, G.; Botterweck, A.A.M.; Verbeek, A.L.M.; Broeders, M.J.M. A remarkable reduction of breast cancer deaths in screened versus unscreened women: A case-referent study. *Cancer Causes Control* **2010**, *21*, 1569–1573. [CrossRef] [PubMed]

48. Otto, S.J.; Fracheboud, J.; Verbeek, A.L.M.; Boer, R.; Reijerink-Verheij, J.C.I.Y.; Otten, J.D.M.; Broeders, M.J.M.; de Koning, H.J.; The National Evaluation Team for Breast Cancer Screening. Mammography Screening and Risk of Breast Cancer Death: A Population-Based Case–Control Study. *Cancer Epidemiol Biomark. Prev.* **2011**, *21*, 66–73. [CrossRef] [PubMed]
49. van Schoor, G.; Moss, S.M.; Otten, J.D.; Donders, R.; Paap, E.; den Heeten, G.J.; Holland, R.; Broeders, M.J.; Verbeek, A.L. Increasingly strong reduction in breast cancer mortality due to screening. *Br. J. Cancer.* **2011**. [CrossRef] [PubMed]
50. Hellquist, B.N.; Duffy, S.W.; Abdsaleh, S.; Björneld, L.; Bordás, P.; Tabár, L.; Viták, B.; Zackrisson, S.; Nyström, L.; Jonsson, H. Effectiveness of population-based service screening with mammography for women ages 40 to 49 years: Evaluation of the Swedish Mammography Screening in Young Women (SCRY) cohort. *Cancer* **2011**, *117*, 714–722. [CrossRef]
51. Broeders, M.; Moss, S.; Nyström, L.; Njor, S.; Jonsson, H.; Paap, E.; Massat, N.; Duffy, S.; Lynge, E.; Paci, E. The Impact of Mammographic Screening on Breast Cancer Mortality in Europe: A Review of Observational Studies. *J. Med. Screen.* **2012**, *19*, 14–25. [CrossRef]
52. Hofvind, S.; Ursin, G.; Tretli, S.; Sebuødegård, S.; Møller, B. Breast cancer mortality in participants of the Norwegian Breast Cancer Screening Program. *Cancer* **2013**, *119*, 3106–3112. [CrossRef] [PubMed]
53. Sigurdsson, K.; Ólafsdóttir, E.J. Population-based service mammography screening: The Icelandic experience. *Breast Cancer Targets Ther.* **2013**, *5*, 17–25. [CrossRef] [PubMed]
54. Coldman, A.; Phillips, N.; Wilson, C.; Decker, K.; Chiarelli, A.M.; Brisson, J.; Zhang, B.; Payne, J.; Doyle, G.; Ahmad, R. Pan-Canadian Study of Mammography Screening and Mortality from Breast Cancer. *JNCI J. Natl. Cancer Inst.* **2014**, *106*. [CrossRef]
55. Puliti, D.; Bucchi, L.; Mancini, S.; Paci, E.; Baracco, S.; Campari, C.; Canuti, D.; Cirilli, C.; Collina, N.; Conti, G.M.; et al. Advanced breast cancer rates in the epoch of service screening: The 400,000 women cohort study from Italy. *Eur. J. Cancer* **2017**, *75*, 109–116. [CrossRef]
56. AB, M.L.W.; Cady, B.; Michaelson, J.S.; Bush, D.M.; Calvillo, K.Z.; Kopans, D.B.; Smith, B.L. A failure analysis of invasive breast cancer: Most deaths from disease occur in women not regularly screened. *Cancer* **2013**, *120*, 2839–2846. [CrossRef]
57. Spencer, D.B.; Potter, J.E.; Chung, M.A.; Fulton, J.; Hebert, W.; Cady, B. Mammographic Screening and Disease Presentation of Breast Cancer Patients Who Die of Disease. *Breast J.* **2004**, *10*, 298–303. [CrossRef] [PubMed]
58. Duffy, S.W.; Tabár, L.; Yen, A.M.; Dean, P.B.; Smith, R.A.; Jonsson, H.; Törnberg, S.; Chen, S.L.-S.; Chiu, S.Y.; Fann, J.C.; et al. Mammography screening reduces rates of advanced and fatal breast cancers: Results in 549,091 women. *Cancer* **2020**, *126*, 2971–2979. [CrossRef]
59. Hendrick, R.E.; Baker, J.A.; Helvie, M.A. Breast cancer deaths averted over 3 decades. *Cancer* **2019**, *125*, 1482–1488. [CrossRef] [PubMed]
60. Available online: http://www.cdc.gov/nchs/data/hus/2010/086.pdf (accessed on 2 August 2022).
61. Anderson, W.F.; Jatoi, I.; Devesa, S.S. Assessing the impact of screening mammography: Breast cancer incidence and mortality rates in Connecticut (1943–2002). *Breast Cancer Res. Treat.* **2006**, *99*, 333–340. [CrossRef] [PubMed]
62. Available online: http://seer.cancer.gov/csr/1975_2010/results_merged/sect_04_breast.pdfTable4.6 (accessed on 15 July 2022).
63. Olsen, O. Screening for breast cancer with mammography. *Cochrane Database Syst. Rev.* **2001**, CD001877. [CrossRef]
64. Nelson, H.D.; Cantor, A.; Humphrey, L.; Fu, R.; Pappas, M.; Daeges, M.; Griffin, J. *Screening for Breast Cancer: A Systematic Review to Update the 2009 U.S. Preventive Services Task Force Recommendation [Internet]*; Report No.: 14–05201-EF-1; Agency for Healthcare Research and Quality (US): Rockville, MD, USA, 2016.
65. Miller, A.B.; Baines, C.J.; Turnbull, C. The role of the nurse-examiner in the National Breast Screening Study. *Can. J. Public Health* **1991**, *82*, 162–167.
66. Kopans, D.B.; Feig, S.A. The Canadian National Breast Screening Study: A critical review. *Am. J. Roentgenol.* **1993**, *161*, 755–760. [CrossRef]
67. Tarone, R.E. The excess of patients with advanced breast cancer in young women screened with mammography in the Canadian National Breast Screening Study. *Cancer* **1995**, *75*, 997–1003. [CrossRef]
68. Bailar, J.C.; MacMahon, B. Randomization in the Canadian National Breast Screening Study: A review for evidence of subversion. *Can. Med. Assoc. J.* **1997**, *156*, 193–199.
69. Kopans, D.B. NBSS: Opportunity to compromise the process. *Can. Med. Assoc. J.* **1997**, *157*, 247–248.
70. Yaffe, M.J.; Seely, J.M.; Gordon, P.B.; Appavoo, S.; Kopans, D.B. The randomized trial of mammography screening that was not—A cautionary tale. *J. Med. Screen.* **2021**, *29*, 7–11. [CrossRef]
71. Seely, J.M.; Eby, P.R.; Yaffe, M.J. The Fundamental Flaws of the CNBSS Trials: A Scientific Review. *J. Breast Imaging* **2022**, *4*, 108–119. [CrossRef]
72. Duffy, S.W. Problems With the Canadian National Breast Screening Studies. *J. Breast Imaging* **2022**, *4*, 120–121. [CrossRef]
73. Seely, J.M.; Eby, P.R.; Gordon, P.B.; Appavoo, S.; Yaffe, M.J. Errors in Conduct of the CNBSS Trials of Breast Cancer Screening Observed by Research Personnel. *J. Breast Imaging* **2022**, *4*, 135–143. [CrossRef]
74. Yaffe, M.J. Correction: Canada Study. *Lett. Ed. JNCI* **1993**, *85*, 94.
75. Baines, C.J.; Miller, A.B.; Kopans, D.B.; Moskowitz, M.; Sanders, D.E.; Sickles, E.A.; To, T.; Wall, C. Canadian National Breast Screening Study: Assessment of technical quality by external review. *Am. J. Roentgenol.* **1990**, *155*, 743–747. [CrossRef]
76. Kopans, D.B. The Canadian Screening Program: A Different Perspective. *Am. J. Roentgenol.* **1990**, *155*, 748–749. [CrossRef]

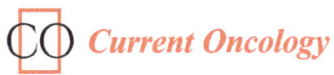

Commentary

How Did CNBSS Influence Guidelines for So Long and What Can That Teach Us?

Shushiela Appavoo

Department of Radiology and Diagnostic Imaging, University of Alberta, 2A2.41 WMC 8440-112 Street, Edmonton, Alberta, AB T6G 2B7, Canada; sappavoo@ualberta.ca

Abstract: The biased randomization and other quality concerns about the Canadian National Breast Screening Studies (CNBSS) were documented and criticized for decades, even by several individuals very close to the research. CNBSS were the outlier studies among several RCTs of the era and yet were given equal weighting and occasionally higher importance than the remainder of the canon of mammography RCTs. These studies have had an ongoing influence on subsequent evidence review, guideline formation, and, ultimately, patient access to screening. This article explores possible reasons for the ongoing inclusion of CNBSS in the body of mammography screening evidence, discusses the lack of expertise in critical healthcare guideline processes, and, ultimately, suggests several actions and reforms.

Keywords: mammography; mammographic screening; randomization; expertise; guidelines; evidenc; epistemic trespassing; evidence-based medicine

Citation: Appavoo, S. How Did CNBSS Influence Guidelines for So Long and What Can That Teach Us? *Curr. Oncol.* **2022**, *29*, 3922–3932. https://doi.org/10.3390/curroncol29060313

Received: 27 March 2022
Accepted: 25 May 2022
Published: 30 May 2022

Publisher's Note: MDPI stays neutral with regard to jurisdictional claims in published maps and institutional affiliations.

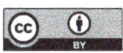

Copyright: © 2022 by the author. Licensee MDPI, Basel, Switzerland. This article is an open access article distributed under the terms and conditions of the Creative Commons Attribution (CC BY) license (https://creativecommons.org/licenses/by/4.0/).

1. Introduction

People talk about evidence as if it could really be weighed in scales by a blind Justice. No man can judge what is good evidence on any particular subject, unless he knows that subject well. George Eliot (Mary Ann Evans), Middlemarch

Recent eyewitness accounts [1–3] of the Canadian National Breast Screening Studies (CNBSS) have finally confirmed what was long suspected about the biased allocation of symptomatic women in the screening arm of the trials. Clinical breast examination was performed before allocation at 14 out of 15 study sites, and witnesses confirm that in at least some of those sites, symptomatic women were preferentially placed in the mammography arm of the study. Additionally, symptomatic patients were recruited for mammographic assessment within the screening arm of the studies. This skewed the data, resulting in more late-stage cancers and deaths for women undergoing mammography than for women allocated to the non-mammography arm.

The results of CNBSS have created ongoing doubt about the benefit of screening mammography, particularly in the 40–49 age group, where there was little other research at the time. CNBSS have been used in the formulation of guidelines worldwide for decades, including the Canadian Task Force on Preventive Health Care (CTFPHC) [4], the US Preventive Services Task Force (USPSTF) [5], European Commission [6], World Health Organization (WHO) [7], and more. Yet, early on, CNBSS received extensive criticism about many aspects of implementation.

The volunteer-based recruitment for CNBSS was fundamentally different from the remainder of the mammography randomized controlled trials (RCTs), which were population-based. As a result of the volunteer recruitment, there were high levels of contamination in CNBSS. Women allocated to the control arm of the trial, but who had volunteered because they were motivated to screen, were more likely to seek mammography outside the trial [8,9]. Difficulties in recruitment were even acknowledged by one of the studies' authors [10], lending plausibility to the eyewitness accounts of CNBSS accepting referrals of symptomatic patients.

The study data also pointed to non-random allocation of women between the mammography and usual care arms. In CNBSS1 [11], equal numbers of women were randomized to either mammography or usual care. Twenty-four late-stage cancers were noted in total. Of these, 19 were allocated to mammography, and 5 were allocated to usual care, a 380% difference. As an expected consequence of this overwhelming imbalance, the 7-year follow-up study demonstrated that 38 women had died in the mammography arm, and 28 women had died in the usual care arm. A study of enrollees at the Winnipeg study site demonstrated that eight out of nine enrolled women, who had prior billing records for breast cancer (an exclusion criterion), were allocated to the mammography arm of the trial, further suggesting non-random allocation [12].

Several articles were published criticizing the allocation and skewed statistics, including a calculation that the imbalance of late-stage cancers between the mammography and non-mammography arms could have occurred randomly only 3.3 times out of 1000 [13–15]. The eyewitness accounts of flawed randomization confirm that which has been evident in the data since early in the studies.

Unfortunately, very few RCTs specifically addressed the 40–49 age group, and, therefore, CNBSS1 has had a large influence on breast screening recommendations for women in this age range. The statistical problems are obvious, so why was this study not excluded by the statistics and epidemiology experts writing guidelines? Several factors may be at play and point to a larger problem with the practical application of evidence-based medicine.

2. The Flaws in CNBSS Ignored

CNBSS were criticized long before the results were published. The problematic implementation was questioned by external reviewers [16] and the studies' own physicists [17]. There were even attempts to explain away the implausible and unprecedented early finding of excess deaths in the screening arm of the trial [18]. No other study among the eight mammography RCTs ever demonstrated this finding. This lack of reproducibility, alone, should have resulted in skepticism about the results.

Early criticism of CNBSS was so widespread that a forensic assessment was published in 1997. This review was limited. Only 3 of 15 sites were assessed, and, importantly, the study staff was not interviewed at that time, despite this step being mandated in the study design [19]. In fact, the authors of this assessment suggested a confirmation bias in their own article, stating that, "We believe that there would be two advantages to publishing the 7-year follow-up data ... First, this criticism of the study would end ... ". Unfortunately, the quality of the forensic assessment was not questioned, and this study appeased those who would use CNBSS for future guidelines [20,21].

Interestingly, a recent modelling study used only CNBSS as the source material, choosing to focus on the outlier study and ignoring the remaining body of RCTs that converged on a significant benefit to screening [22]. The 2016 USPSTF guideline article went so far as to state, "[Malmo Mammographic Screening Trial I and the Canadian National Breast Screening Study 1 and 2] provided the least-biased estimates" [5].

Despite problematic recruitment and glaring statistical imbalances, recognized decades ago, CNBSS continue to influence research, guidelines, and worldwide guideline-based policy around breast screening. In Canada, CTFPHC guidelines strongly influence many provincial Clinical Practice Guidelines, which may, in turn, define patient access to screening through physician referral practices, programmatic screening structure, and billing restrictions.

How does a study that has been plagued by extensive international criticism over its design and skewed data manage to continue influencing recommendations for decades?

3. Evidence-Based Medicine, Evidence Review, and Guidelines Methodology

As a result of the evidence-based medicine movement, modern guidelines hinge on evidence review. This is performed by specialized bodies that conduct systematic searches for literature, decide which evidence is appropriate to include in the review, and then synthesize the data, often building upon older evidence reviews of the same topic. While this appears to be an ideal and objective way to expertly handle large amounts of research and perform the complicated statistical and epidemiological calculations involved, evidence review has some limitations.

Content experts have little to no substantial influence on evidence review. For example, no radiologist is included on the list of contributors for the 2018 CTFPHC breast screening evidence review [23].

Many members and frequently the chairs of evidence review and guideline bodies are non-physicians, and, thus, clinical experience and context are minimized. The continued inclusion of CNBSS in guideline evidence reviews is a stark example of the peril of minimizing content expert input. Had content experts been allowed appropriate input into the guideline processes, the well-documented imbalance in late-stage cancers and other significant problems with implementation could have been made clear to the reviewers.

Evidence review is expensive, and evidence reviews are built upon older reviews to save time and money. Once an error has been made, however, it may be perpetuated by copying that error into future versions of the review. This is what is known in radiology as "alliterative error", which is the tendency to perpetuate prior errors, particularly when the previous report has been viewed before assessment of the images—or evidence—one has been tasked with assessing [24].

In addition to the evidence review process, guideline methodology and guideline oversight are problematic. While the evidence review tool, GRADE [25], recommends including observational data, the evidence review team and guideline bodies may choose to ignore this, as seen in the 2018 CTFPHC breast screening recommendations [4]. In this guideline, the evidence review included only randomized controlled trials, largely performed between the 1960s and the 1980s, for the calculation of benefits. Decades of more recent screening program data were ignored. The largest observational study of screening program data in the world is known as the Pan Canadian Study, published in 2014 [26]. This demonstrates an overall mortality benefit of 40% for women attending the screening. In the 40–49 age group, this mortality benefit is even higher at 44%. This study is missing from the 2018 CTFPHC breast screening guideline references, and it is even absent from the list of excluded evidence [27]. It is difficult to explain the fact that landmark Canadian evidence is missing from a Canadian evidence review, but the near-complete absence of content experts from the evidence review process may contribute to this oversight.

The AGREEII [28] guideline development and appraisal instrument recommends the inclusion of content experts and patients as advisors on guideline panels, as do many other guideline methodology recommendations [29,30]. Again, however, oversight into the actual guideline process is lacking, and the systematic exclusion of content experts and patients from panels such as CTFPHC's has largely gone unnoticed.

4. Epistemic Trespassing

When is an expert not an expert? Perhaps the answer to this lies in the concept of epistemic trespassing [31,32]. This term was coined by philosopher Nathan Ballantyne and describes the intrusion of experts into fields outside their own expertise. We have seen many examples of this during the COVID-19 pandemic. Particularly embarrassing to radiologists, Scott Atlas, a neuroradiologist, acted as COVID-19 advisor to Donald Trump during his presidency. Dr. Mehmet Oz, a cardiovascular surgeon and TV host, challenged Dr. Anthony Fauci, an accomplished expert in infectious disease and immunology, to a debate on COVID-19 "doctor to doctor". A well-known anti-vaccine "doctor" in Australia has her doctorate in geology [33].

The composition of evidence review teams and some guideline panels suggests that epistemic trespassing is a factor in current guideline formulation. For example, the CTFPHC produces guidelines largely intended for use by primary care providers, predominantly physicians and nurses. Until recently, however, it was chaired by a psychologist. The CTFPHC breast screening guideline panel was chaired by nephrologists in both 2011 and 2018, and a chiropractor was on the knowledge tools team for the 2018 guideline. There was, however, no breast surgeon, radiologist, technologist, physicist, pathologist, oncologist, or patient on these teams. The main opportunity for input from content experts was an emailed form, similar to that provided to all external stakeholders. There was no opportunity for dialogue or teaching by content experts. The urologists involved with the 2014 CTFPHC prostate guideline were so dismayed at the CTFPHC consultation process that they resigned in protest.

In my conversations, with patients and even referrers, almost all of them are surprised to learn that the panels that form guidelines exclude the very experts they trust with their specialized healthcare. I suspect most people make the natural and trusting assumption that content experts make significant contributions to their healthcare guidelines. While the credentials of the authors of the CTFPHC guidelines are not hidden, they are not openly disclosed. The names of the authors of each guideline are provided, but their areas of expertise are not visible unless one specifically searches for their credentials. One could say that the lack of content expertise is hidden in plain sight.

5. Conflict of Interest (COI)

What is the reason for this counterintuitive guideline panel composition and lack of fulsome expert consultation? The stated reason seems to be an avoidance of conflict of interest (COI) [34,35]. There is an assumption that content specialists would try to boost their own incomes by influencing guidelines. When asked about the experts' signatures on an open letter rebutting the 2018 breast screening guideline, the then-chair of the CTFPHC said, "They earn a living carrying out imaging services, and some also earn income through their work with companies that produce imaging equipment." [36]. The news report did not mention any evidence-based rebuttal to the many points made in opposition to the breast screening guideline, however. This is an example of a logical fallacy known as *ad hominem*, in this case attacking the motivation of the speaker and ignoring the substance of the argument.

While COI is an important concern, particularly in the case of industry-sponsored research, it is far less pertinent to practising Canadian medical specialists. Many, if not most, Canadian medical specialists are overwhelmed with waitlists [37] throughout their careers and are unlikely to boost income with screening. In some cases, such as serologic screening for prostate and liver disease, the specialist physician has no direct financial COI at all.

Unfortunately, these unsubstantiated accusations of specialist physician COI lead to exclusion of content expertise. As we have seen with the continued use of CNBSS for guidelines, however, this is detrimental to the appropriate determination of scientific rigour. In fact, the implication of COI has specifically been used to dismiss valid concerns by experts, such as the excess deaths in the CNBSS screening arm [18].

I posit that in a single-payor healthcare system, the largest financial COI is that of the payor. In Canada, this is the government, which also happens to fund the CTFPHC via the Public Health Agency of Canada (PHAC). Screening programs are expensive and create further downstream expenses. It is understandable that minimizing screening recommendations would be a desirable guideline outcome for the healthcare payor.

6. Lack of Accountability

In April 2019, when asked by NDP Health Critic, Don Davies, to halt the use of the 2018 CTFPHC breast screening guideline, the federal Health Minister at the time, Ginette Petitpas Taylor, absolved the ministry of any responsibility, stating, "While the government provides its support to the Task Force to the breast cancer screening work group [sic] its decision was totally done independently. As such these are not official government guidelines" [38]. This statement was repeated almost verbatim by the Health Minister's Parliamentary Secretary a few weeks later [39].

When asked about the news regarding the eyewitness accounts of misallocation of patients during randomization of CNBSS, PHAC issued a statement indicating that it provides funding to the Task Force and referred to the body as being an "arms-length from the government" [40], but took no further responsibility for the CTFPHC recommendations.

The current co-chair of the CTFPHC, when asked about the same eyewitness accounts, indicated that the group conducts "rigorous, detailed evidence reviews to formulate guidelines" and did not indicate that any further reviews would be performed, even in light of the new information [40].

The CTFPHC claims that its guidelines are ranked among the best in the world [40], but this warrants a closer inspection. A guidance statement and quality review of breast screening guidelines, authored by a group of guideline methodologists [41], failed to acknowledge that GRADE and AGREEII were not appropriately applied to the CTFPHC guideline. Despite completely excluding all modern observational evidence from the analysis of screening benefits and excluding any genuine consultation with content experts, the CTFPHC guideline scored well in this analysis. Guideline methodologists assess the quality of guidelines without the benefit of content expert input nor outcomes analyses, much like "marking each others' homework".

To whom is this publicly funded government agency accountable? It would appear that CTFPHC answers to no one.

Why might the government have set up an unusually unaccountable body to develop healthcare guidelines? As mentioned above, there is a large financial cost to screening, both directly and indirectly. Guidelines can be used to help control healthcare costs, and, ideally, good guideline recommendations will balance appropriate safe health care and judicious use of resources. Structuring a guideline body to be unaccountable, however, removes this balance and allows its recommendations to stand for years without correction of errors. There is another benefit to the arm's-length status, however. According to National Cancer Institute Cancer Intervention and Surveillance Modeling Network (CISNET) modelling, 400 women may die each year as a result of the CTFPHC recommendation against screening women in the 40–49 age group [42]. Arm's-length status may protect both PHAC and the Health Ministry from responsibility for these avoidable deaths.

7. Casting Doubt

When the rest of the evidence converges on the conclusion that screening saves lives, even for women aged 40–49, why continue to include the poorly performed outlier study in evidence analyses? One can certainly speculate that there is strong motivation to perpetuate the use of studies such as CNBSS. The outlier creates doubt around the benefit of screening women 40–49 and keeps the mammography screening controversy alive. In fact, the various techniques used to challenge the benefits of mammographic screening have been extensively discussed by Dr. Daniel Kopans in his analyses [43,44].

Have we seen this pattern of perpetuating doubt for financial benefit in the past? In fact, this strategy is known as "manufactured doubt" and has been employed for decades by large organizations [45,46]. In its typical form, it is used by industry to delay regulation by creating doubt about whether evidence converges on a particular outcome. It was famously used by the tobacco industry to delay regulation for decades, while the industry continued to reap billions of dollars of profits. Other examples include the opiate, silicates, talc, diesel, alcohol, and sugar industries. Doubt is manufactured by stressing outlier studies (such as CNBSS), cherry-picking data (such as excluding all observational data), and many other methods.

Strategies for manufacturing doubt are well documented [47], as many of the above-mentioned industries have undergone scrutiny and even litigation for these practices. The following is a selection of known strategies employed to manufacture doubt, listed in the linked article https://ehjournal.biomedcentral.com/articles/10.1186/s12940-021-00723-0 (accessed on 26 May 2022). These have been correlated to examples of their use by the CTFPHC and other critics of screening. Keep in mind that the strategies were written with large commercial industries in mind, and the wording may not be fully applicable to government and screening scenarios. Additionally, I limit most of my examples to breast screening recommendations.

1. **Attack study design**—Characterization of any studies that favour screening as flawed, frequently using CNBSS study as a comparator [48,49].

2. **Misrepresent data**—Cherry-picking or diluting the evidence by pooling poor- and good-quality studies in meta-analyses and evidence review [23,50,51]. Continuing to include CNBSS is an example of this. Another example is also noted in the prostate screening literature, mentioned later. Overestimations of overdiagnosis [4,51,52] are also used to create fear and discourage screening.

3. **Suppress incriminating information**—Observational studies, many of which are more modern than the RCTs, demonstrate a large degree of effectiveness. These are, however, excluded from the evaluation of the benefits of screening mammography in CTFPHC analysis [23]. Despite this, observational studies and even questionnaires are permitted in the evaluation of harms.

4. **Contribute misleading literature**—The CTFPHC performed a review of women's values questionnaires [53], interpreted to suggest women would not want to screen, even though the questionnaire review demonstrates that women do desire screening

5. **Host conferences or seminars**—In 1997, the National Cancer Institute held a Consensus Development Conference of the National Institutes of Health on "Breast Cancer Screening for Women Ages 40–49". Minority opinion was ignored, and the decision not to recommend screening for this age group was called "unanimous" [54].

6. **Blame other causes**—In the case of screening, rather than blame, benefits are attributed to other causes, particularly modern treatment [4,49,51].

7. **Invoke liberties/censorship/overregulation**—The recommendation not to screen women aged 40-49 is couched as "shared decision-making" [4], even though the CTFPHC recommendations result in limitation of the option to screen women aged 40-49 in many jurisdictions.

8. **Define how to measure outcome/exposure**—The CTFPHC assesses mortality benefits only, ignoring well-documented non-mortality benefits associated with earlier diagnosis, such as decreased severity of treatments, as well as lower incidence of long-term complications, such as lymphedema in screened populations [55].

9. **Pose as a defender of health or truth**—The CTFPHC emphasizes harms and minimizes benefits, stressing anxiety, biopsies, and exaggerated overdiagnosis rates. While the recommendations appear to put the patient's emotional health first, they are paternalistic and represent a false equivalency in comparison with unnecessarily delayed diagnoses.

10. **Obscure involvement**—The unaccountable structure of the CTFPHC falls into this category.

11. **Normalize negative outcomes**—The CTFPHC stresses a lack of evidence of improvement in all-cause mortality (difficult to prove considering a relatively small proportion of the population dies of breast cancer [49,56]), minimizing the mortality benefits. This implies that excess deaths among non-screened women are acceptable. Additionally, the false equivalency of the potential harms (anxiety, biopsy, overdiagnosis) over the potential benefits of screening (lower likelihood of dying of breast cancer among those screened) normalizes avoidable breast cancer deaths.

12. **Attack Opponents (scientifically/personally)**—*Ad hominem* attacks on the motivation of dissenters, discussed earlier.

13. **Abuse of credentials**—Epistemic trespassing by non-content-experts, discussed earlier.

8. Broader Problems

I have largely emphasized the problems with the 2018 CTFPHC breast cancer screening recommendations, but similar problems exist within many of the other major extant CTFPHC guidelines. In a personal correspondence, a prominent urologist mentioned inappropriate handling of prostate screening evidence for the 2014 guideline.

"There is a precise analogy [to CNBSS] in the prostate cancer field, the PLCO study [57] of PSA screening. 85% contamination in the control arm and 15% non-compliance in the study arm (this is documented and published) resulted in no difference in the proportion tested, and therefore no mortality difference between the 2 arms. The other large scale study, ERSPC (European Randomised Study of Screening for Prostate Cancer) [58], was strongly positive. The task force looked at the 2 studies, noted one was positive and one negative, and concluded that therefore no convincing evidence of benefit.

We pointed out the flaw in their reasoning with our 'stakeholders comments' in 2014 and we received no response from the task force, and no evidence that they took our comments into account.

Dr. Laurence Klotz, MD, FRCSC, CM
Professor of Surgery, University of Toronto
Sunnybrook Chair of Prostate Cancer Research
Chairman, World Urologic Oncology Federation
Chairman, SI (Stability Index) UCare Research Office9
Chairman, Canadian Urology Research Consortium
Sunnybrook Health Sciences Centre"

Again, this indicates the pooling of poorly performed and well-performed research, creating doubt. Additionally, this demonstrates the lack of meaningful dialogue with highly qualified content experts. The use of the term "stakeholder" [59] is prejudicial, implying a material interest, or "stake", in the guidelines, rather than professional interest and a role as expert advisors. The term "topic advisor" is preferable and is used in the NICE UK methodology [60].

In fact, multiple other prominent specialists and specialist societies have written rebuttals to the CTFPHC guidelines, many of which are evidence-based [61–69] (Supplementary Materials).

9. CTFPHC and the Suppression of Science

Is there any evidence that the government would deliberately suppress science? In fact, the Harper government did exactly that in the late 2000s. Climate change and environmental scientists were muzzled, and environmental research was inhibited, culminating in a 2012 protest on Parliament Hill, nicknamed the Death of Evidence March [70,71]. Climate change and environmental science have an impact on development of fossil fuels and thus the Canadian economy. During approximately the same time period and under the same federal government, the current structure of CTFPHC was initiated in 2010 [72].

10. Suggestions for Reform

The lack of expert guidance in the performance of evidence review and the formation of guidelines is problematic. This requires urgent reform, but CTFPHC requires a robust accountability structure for any reforms to take place. As it currently stands, the lack of expert guidance constitutes a breach of the public trust. The public should insist on fundamental reform to the structure of the CTFPHC. A new national guidelines body should be formed with appropriate oversight and accountability built in.

While COI is of serious concern, practising Canadian healthcare practitioners should not be conflated with "product defence" and other industry-funded experts. COI should be acknowledged for both content experts and for government agencies' funding guidelines. COI should not, however, outweigh expertise and clinical experience. Ad hominem attacks on motivation should be avoided.

Any CTFPHC guidelines formed without fulsome expert guidance, particularly if Canadian content experts have provided evidence-based rebuttals, should be suspended from use pending content expert review and, if necessary, revision. In the interim, many national specialty societies have their own guidelines, which can be substituted for suspended CTFPHC recommendations.

Full disclosure of the credentials of personnel involved in evidence review and guideline formation is required for rebuilding trust in the processes.

Process transparency should be emphasized, and satisfaction surveys of panel members should be a mandatory element of guideline quality assessment. A tool such as PANELVIEW [73] could be adapted to this purpose.

Guideline quality should not only be evaluated based on adherence to guideline methodology, but also by outcomes. Following the USPSTF recommendation against PSA screening in 2012, metastatic prostate cancer increased, as predicted by modelling [74]. Outcomes follow-up should be mandatory following guideline recommendations, and this should be used to define guideline quality, rather than self-referential adherence to methodologies, which, as we have seen, may be misapplied or misrepresented.

Ethicists should be involved in the restructuring process of the CTFPHC, the formation of guidelines, and ongoing oversight of methodological processes. The Precautionary Principle [75] should be employed in all decisions that impact the well-being and lives of the population.

Where costs and other resource limitations are factored into guideline recommendations, this should be clearly disclosed. Science should not be manipulated to accommodate budgetary concerns.

11. Conclusions

The ongoing use of the flawed CNBSS is the natural consequence of significant systemic problems with the application of guideline methodology and, in Canada, with the unaccountable structure of the CTFPHC. While the practice of medicine requires close adherence to evidence, common sense and clinical judgment are the lenses through which evidence must be filtered. The evidence-based movement has been criticized, even by its proponents, calling for a "return to real evidence based medicine", including "increasing depth of knowledge and sensitivity to context when applying rules" [76].

Making medical recommendations outside one's area of specialty training is not accepted in clinical practice and should not be accepted in the formation of guidelines. Guideline oversight and methodology reform are required to provide appropriate expertise in guideline formulation. As a result of specialists' career-long waitlists and resultant minimal COI, Canada is well positioned to produce excellent guidelines. To achieve these improvements, however, clinicians and patients must advocate for fundamental reform to guideline practices.

Supplementary Materials: The following supporting information can be downloaded at: https://www.mdpi.com/article/10.3390/curroncol29060313/s1. References [77–81] are cited in the Supplementary Materials.

Funding: The author received no external funding.

Acknowledgments: Many thanks for ongoing advice and historical context provided by Daniel Kopans, Martin Yaffe, Paula Gordon, Jean Seely, and Laurence Klotz, and Jennie Dale.

Conflicts of Interest: The author declares no conflict of interest.

References

1. Yaffe, M.J.; Seely, J.M.; Gordon, P.B.; Appavoo, S.; Kopans, D.B. The randomized trial of mammography screening that was not—A cautionary tale. *J. Med. Screen.* **2021**, *29*, 7–11. [CrossRef] [PubMed]
2. Seely, J.M.; Eby, P.R.; Gordon, P.B.; Appovoo, S.; Yaffe, M.J. Errors in conduct of the CNBSS trials of breast cancer screening observed by research personnel. *J. Breast Imag.* **2022**, *4*, 135–143. [CrossRef]
3. Seely, J.M.; Eby, P.R.; Yaffe, M.J. The fundamental flaws of the CNBSS trials. *J. Breast Imag.* **2022**, *4*, 108–119. [CrossRef]

4. Klarenbach, S.; Sims-Jones, N.; Lewin, G.; Singh, H.; Thériault, G.; Tonelli, M.; Doull, M.; Courage, S.; Garcia, A.J.; Thombs, B.D.; et al. Recommendations on screening for breast cancer in women aged 40–74 years who are not at increased risk for breast cancer. *CMAJ* **2018**, *190*, E1441–E1451. [CrossRef] [PubMed]
5. Siu, A.L.; U.S. Preventive Services Task Force. Screening for Breast Cancer: U.S. Preventive Services Task Force Recommendation Statement. *Ann. Intern. Med.* **2016**, *164*, 279–296. [CrossRef] [PubMed]
6. Deandrea, S.; Molina-Barceló, A.; Uluturk, A.; Moreno, J.; Neamtiu, L.; Peiró-Pérez, P.; Saz-Parkinson, Z.; Lopez-Alcalde, J.; Lerda, D.; Salas, D. Presence, characteristics and equity of access to breast cancer screening programmes in 27 European countries in 2010 and 2014. Results from an international survey. *Prev. Med.* **2016**, *91*, 250–263. [CrossRef]
7. Geneva: World Health Organization. WHO Position Paper on Mammography Screening. Annex B, Evidence Summary: Benefits and Harms of Mammography Screening: Umbrella Systematic Review. 2014. Available online: https://www.ncbi.nlm.nih.gov/books/NBK269537/ (accessed on 26 May 2022).
8. Baines, C.J. The Canadian National Breast Screening Study: A perspective on criticisms. *Ann. Intern. Med.* **1994**, *120*, 326–334. [CrossRef]
9. Tabár, L.; Yen, A.M.-F.; Wu, W.Y.-Y.; Chen, S.L.-S.; Chiu, S.Y.-H.; Fann, J.C.-Y.; Ku, M.M.-S.; Smith, R.A.; Duffy, S.W.; Chen, T.H.-H. Insights from the Breast Cancer Screening Trials: How Screening Affects the Natural History of Breast Cancer and Implications for Evaluating Service Screening Programs. *Breast J.* **2015**, *21*, 13–20. [CrossRef]
10. Baines, C.J. Impediments to recruitment in the Canadian National Breast Screening Study: Response and resolution. *Control. Clin. Trials* **1984**, *5*, 129–140. [CrossRef]
11. Miller, A.B.; Baines, C.J.; To, T.; Wall, C. Canadian National Breast Screening Study: 1. Breast cancer detection and death rates among women aged 40 to 49 years. *Can. Med. Assoc. J.* **1993**, *148*, 718, reprinted in *Can. Med. Assoc. J.* **1992**, *147*, 1459–1476.
12. Cohen, M.M.; Kaufert, P.A.; MacWilliam, L.; Tate, R.B. Using an alternative data source to examine randomization in the Canadian national breast screening study. *J. Clin. Epidemiol.* **1996**, *49*, 1039–1044. [CrossRef]
13. Burhenne, L.J.; Burhenne, H.J. The Canadian National Breast Screening Study: A Canadian critique. *Am. J. Roentgenol.* **1993**, *161*, 761–763. [CrossRef] [PubMed]
14. Boyd, N.F.; Jong, R.A.; Yaffe, M.J.; Tritchler, D.; Lockwood, G.; Zylak, C.J. A critical appraisal of the Canadian National Breast Cancer Screening Study. *Radiology* **1993**, *189*, 661–663. [CrossRef] [PubMed]
15. Tarone, R.E. The excess of patients with advanced breast cancer in young women screened with mammography in the Canadian National Breast Screening Study. *Cancer* **1995**, *75*, 997–1003. [CrossRef]
16. Kopans, D. The Canadian Screening Program: A Different Perspective. *Am. J. Roentgenol.* **1990**, *155*, 748–749. [CrossRef]
17. Yaffe, M.J. Correction: Canada Study. *Lett. Ed. JNCI* **1993**, *85*, 94.
18. Cassidy, J.; Rayment, T. *Breast Scans Boost Risk of Cancer Death*; Sunday Times: London, UK, 2 June 1991.
19. Bailar, J.C.; MacMahon, B. Randomization in the Canadian National Breast Screening Study: A review for evidence of subversion. *CMAJ* **1997**, *156*, 193–199.
20. Ringash, J.; the Canadian Task Force on Preventive Health Care. Preventive health care, 2001 update: Screening mammography among women aged 40–49 years at average risk of breast cancer. *CMAJ* **2001**, *164*, 469–476.
21. Brackstone, M.; Latosinsky, S.; Saettler, E.; George, R. CJS debate: Is mammography useful in average-risk screening for breast cancer? *Can. J. Surg.* **2016**, *59*, 62–66. [CrossRef]
22. Le, T.T.T.; Adler, F.R. Is mammography screening beneficial: An individual-based stochastic model for breast cancer incidence and mortality. *PLoS Comput. Biol.* **2020**, *16*, e1008036. [CrossRef]
23. Available online: https://canadiantaskforce.ca/wp-content/uploads/2019/02/Systematic-Review-Evidence-Report_v2_FINAL.pdf (accessed on 26 May 2022).
24. Kim, Y.W.; Mansfield, L.T. Fool me twice: Delayed diagnoses in radiology with emphasis on perpetuated errors. *Am. J. Roentgenol.* **2014**, *202*, 465–470. [CrossRef] [PubMed]
25. Guyatt, G.H.; Oxman, A.D.; Vist, G.E.; Kunz, R.; Falck-Ytter, Y.; Alonso-Coello, P.; Schünemann, H.J. GRADE: An emerging consensus on rating quality of evidence and strength of recommendations. *BMJ* **2008**, *336*, 924. [CrossRef] [PubMed]
26. Coldman, A.; Phillips, N.; Wilson, C.; Decker, K.; Chiarelli, A.M.; Brisson, J.; Zhang, B.; Payne, J.; Doyle, G.; Ahmad, R. Pan-Canadian study of mammography screening and mortality from breast cancer. *J. Natl. Cancer. Inst.* **2014**, *106*, 261, Erratum in *J. Natl. Cancer. Inst.* **2015**, *107*, 404. [CrossRef] [PubMed]
27. Available online: https://canadiantaskforce.ca/wp-content/uploads/2018/11/Excluded-Studies-List-Evidence-Report-Breast-Cancer-Screening_Final.pdf (accessed on 26 May 2022).
28. Available online: https://www.agreetrust.org/wp-content/uploads/2017/12/AGREE-II-Users-Manual-and-23-item-Instrument-2009-Update-2017.pdf (accessed on 26 May 2022).
29. Available online: https://www.nice.org.uk/process/pmg20/chapter/decision-making-committees#topic-specific-committees (accessed on 26 May 2022).
30. Schünemann, H.J.; Wiercioch, W.; Etxeandia, I.; Falavigna, M.; Santesso, N.; Mustafa, R.; Ventresca, M.; Brignardello-Petersen, R.; Laisaar, K.; Kowalski, S.; et al. Guidelines 2.0: Systematic development of a comprehensive checklist for a successful guideline enterprise. *CMAJ* **2014**, *186*, E123–E142. [CrossRef]
31. Ballantyne, N. Epistemic trespassing. *Mind* **2019**, *128*, 510. [CrossRef]

32. Available online: https://blogs.scientificamerican.com/observations/which-experts-should-you-listen-to-during-the-pandemic/ (accessed on 26 May 2022).
33. Leask, J.; McIntyre, P. Public opponents of vaccination: A case study. *Vaccine* **2003**, *21*, 4700–4703. [CrossRef]
34. Kelsall, D. New *CMAJ* policy on competing interests in guidelines. *CMAJ* **2019**, *191*, E350–E351. [CrossRef]
35. Jatoi, I.; Sah, S. Clinical practice guidelines and the overuse of health care services: Need for reform. *CMAJ* **2019**, *191*, E297–E298. [CrossRef]
36. Available online: https://globalnews.ca/video/rd/1440815171884/?jwsource=cl (accessed on 26 May 2022).
37. Available online: https://www.fraserinstitute.org/studies/waiting-your-turn-wait-times-for-health-care-in-canada-2020 (accessed on 26 May 2022).
38. Available online: https://youtu.be/62yyMjgVclQ (accessed on 26 May 2022).
39. Available online: https://youtu.be/QQgXtRDKTVQ (accessed on 26 May 2022).
40. Available online: https://www.stcatharinesstandard.ca/ts/life/health_wellness/2021/11/25/canadas-breast-cancer-screening-policy-based-off-flawed-study-researchers.html (accessed on 26 May 2022).
41. Qaseem, A.; Lin, J.S.; Mustafa, R.A.; Horwitch, C.A.; Wilt, T.J. Screening for Breast Cancer in Average-Risk Women: A Guidance Statement From the American College of Physicians. *Ann. Intern. Med.* **2019**, *170*, 547–560. [CrossRef]
42. Yaffe, M.J.; Mittmann, N.; Lee, P.; Tosteson, A.N.; Trentham-Dietz, A.; Alagoz, O.; Stout, N.K. Clinical outcomes of modelling mammography screening strategies. *Health Rep.* **2015**, *26*, 9–15.
43. Kopans, D.B.; Webb, M.L.; Cady, B. The 20-year effort to reduce access to mammography screening: Historical facts dispute a commentary in *Cancer*. *Cancer* **2014**, *120*, 2792–2799. [CrossRef] [PubMed]
44. Kopans, D.B. The Breast Cancer Screening "Arcade" and the "Whack-A-Mole" Efforts to Reduce Access to Screening. *Semin Ultrasound CT MRI* **2018**, *39*, 2–15. [CrossRef] [PubMed]
45. Michaels, D. *Doubt Is Their Product: How Industry's Assault on Science Threatens Your Health*; Oxford University Press: New York, NY, USA, 2008; pp. 3–4. ISBN 978-0-19-530067-3.8.
46. Michaels, D. *The Triumph of Doubt: Dark Money and the Science of Deception*; Oxford University Press: New York, NY, USA, 2020; ISBN 978-0-19-092266-5.
47. Goldberg, R.F.; Vandenberg, L.N. The science of spin: Targeted strategies to manufacture doubt with detrimental effects on environmental and public health. *Environ. Health* **2021**, *20*, 33. [CrossRef] [PubMed]
48. Berry, D.A. Failure of researchers, reviewers, editors, and the media to understand flaws in cancer screening studies: Application to an article in *Cancer*. *Cancer* **2014**, *120*, 2784–2791. [CrossRef] [PubMed]
49. Gotzsche, P.C.; Olsen, O. Is screening for breast cancer with mammography justifiable? *Lancet* **2000**, *355*, 129–134. [CrossRef]
50. Fletcher, S.W.; Black, W.; Harris, R.; Rimer, B.K.; Shapiro, S. Report of the International Workshop on Screening for Breast Cancer. *J. Natl. Cancer Inst.* **1993**, *85*, 1644–1656. [CrossRef]
51. Welch, H.G. Cancer Screening—The Good, the Bad, and the Ugly. *JAMA Surg.* **2022**. [CrossRef]
52. Puliti, D.; Duffy, S.W.; Miccinesi, G.; de Koning, H.; Lynge, E.; Zappa, M.; Paci, E.; EUROSCREEN Working Group. Overdiagnosis in mammographic screening for breast cancer in Europe: A literature review. *J. Med. Screen.* **2012**, *19*, 42–56. [CrossRef]
53. Available online: https://canadiantaskforce.ca/wp-content/uploads/2018/11/Womens-Values-and-Preferences-on-Breast-Cancer-Screening_FINAL.pdf (accessed on 26 May 2022).
54. National Institutes of Health Consensus Development Panel. The National Institutes of Health (NIH) Consensus Development Program: >Breast Cancer Screening for Women Ages 40–49. *J. Natl. Cancer Inst.* **1997**, *89*, 960–965.
55. Ahn, S.; Wooster, M.; Valente, C.; Moshier, E.; Meng, R.; Pisapati, K.; Couri, R.; Margolies, L.; Schmidt, H.; Port, E. Impact of Screening Mammography on Treatment in Women Diagnosed with Breast Cancer. *Ann. Surg. Oncol.* **2018**, *25*, 2979–2986. [CrossRef]
56. Tabar, L.; Duffy, S.W.; Yen, M.F.; Warwick, J.; Vitak, B.; Chen, H.H.; Smith, R.A. All-cause mortality among breast cancer patients in a screening trial: Support for breast cancer mortality as an end point. *J. Med. Screen.* **2002**, *9*, 159–162. [CrossRef] [PubMed]
57. Gulati, R.; Tsodikov, A.; Wever, E.M.; Mariotto, A.B.; Heijnsdijk, E.A.M.; Katcher, J.; de Koning, H.J.; Etzioni, R. The impact of PLCO control arm contamination on perceived PSA screening efficacy. *Cancer Causes Control.* **2012**, *23*, 827. [CrossRef] [PubMed]
58. Schröder, F.H.; Hugosson, J.; Roobol, M.J.; Tammela, T.L.J.; Zappa, M.; Nelen, V.; Kwiatkowski, M.; Lujan, M.; Määttänen, L.; Lilja, H.; et al. Screening and prostate cancer mortality: Results of the European Randomised Study of Screening for Prostate Cancer (ERSPC) at 13 years of follow-up. *Lancet* **2014**, *384*, 2027–2035. [CrossRef]
59. Available online: https://canadiantaskforce.ca/about/#:~{}:text=Stakeholder%20Engagement,into%20guideline%20topics%20and%20materials. (accessed on 26 May 2022).
60. Available online: https://www.nice.org.uk/process/pmg20/resources/developing-nice-guidelines-the-manual-pdf-72286708 7008691 (accessed on 26 May 2022).
61. Cervix Screening: Cervical Screening Guidelines-Discordance Discussed. Available online: https://www.cmaj.ca/content/185/1/35/tab-e-letters#cervical-screening-guidelines--discordance-discussed (accessed on 26 May 2022).
62. Colorectal Screening: Colonoscopy is Probably the Best Colon Cancer Screening Test, It's Not Proven Yet. Available online: https://www.cmaj.ca/content/188/5/340/tab-e-letters#colonoscopy-is-probably-the-best-colon-cancer-screening-test-its-not-proven-yet (accessed on 26 May 2022).

63. Developmental Delay Screening: Take Home Message of Task Force Report: NOT the Strong Recommendation against Developmental Screening, but the Need for Rigorous Research and Practice. Available online: https://www.cmaj.ca/content/188/8/579/tab-e-letters#take-home-message-of-task-force-report-not-the-strong-recommendation-against-developmental-screening-but-the-need-for-rigorous-research-and-practice (accessed on 26 May 2022).
64. Canadian Task Force on Preventive Health Care. Recommendations on Hepatitis C Screening for Adults. *CMAJ* **2017**, *189*, E594–E604. Available online: https://www.cmaj.ca/content/189/16/E594/tab-e-letters#recommendations-on-hepatitis-c-screening-for-adults-cmaj-2017-april-24189e594-604-doi-101503-cmaj161521 (accessed on 26 May 2022). [CrossRef]
65. RE: Screening for Impaired Vision in Community-Dwelling Adults Aged 65 Years and Older in Primary Care Settings. Available online: https://www.cmaj.ca/content/190/19/E588/tab-e-letters#re-screening-for-impaired-vision-in-community-dwelling-adults-aged-65-years-and-older-in-primary-care-settings (accessed on 26 March 2022).
66. Lung Cancer Screening: The Consequences of A Short Duration of Lung Cancer Screening. Available online: https://www.cmaj.ca/content/188/6/425/tab-e-letters#the-consequences-of-a-short-duration-of-lung-cancer-screening (accessed on 26 May 2022).
67. Canadian Task Force on Preventive Health Care* Recommendations for Prevention of Weight Gain and Use of Behavioural and Pharmacologic Interventions to Manage Overweight and Obesity in Adults in Primary Care. Available online: https://www.cmaj.ca/content/187/3/184/tab-e-letters#canadian-task-force-on-preventive-health-care-recommendations-for-prevention-of-weight-gain-and-use-of-behavioural-and-pharmacologic-interventions-to-manage-overweight-and-obesity-in-adults-in-primary-care (accessed on 26 May 2022).
68. Canadian Society of Breast Imaging Position Statement on CTFPHC Breast Screening Recommendations. Available online: https://csbi.ca/wp-content/uploads/2019/05/CSBI_Statement_CTFPHC_Dec_2018_FINAL.pdf#:~||:text=The%20Canadian%20Society%20of%20Breast%20Imaging%20response%20to,on%20Preventive%20Health%20Care%20%28CTFPHC%29%20guidelines%20are%20outdated. (accessed on 26 May 2022).
69. Canadian Association of Radiologists position statement on CTFPHC Breast Screening Recommendations. Available online: https://car.ca/news/statement-on-the-canadian-task-force-on-preventative-health-care-ctfphc-2018-updated-guidelines-for-breast-cancer-screening/ (accessed on 26 May 2022).
70. Available online: https://www.smithsonianmag.com/science-nature/canadian-scientists-open-about-how-their-government-silenced-science-180961942/ (accessed on 26 May 2022).
71. Available online: https://academicmatters.ca/harpers-attack-on-science-no-science-no-evidence-no-truth-no-democracy/ (accessed on 26 May 2022).
72. Available online: https://canadiantaskforce.ca/about/history/ (accessed on 26 May 2022).
73. Wiercioch, W.; Akl, E.A.; Santesso, N.; Zhang, Y.; Morgan, R.L.; Yepes-Nuñez, J.J.; Kowalski, S.; Baldeh, T.; Mustafa, R.A.; Laisaar, K.; et al. Assessing the process and outcome of the development of practice guidelines and recommendations: PANELVIEW instrument development. *CMAJ* **2020**, *192*, E1138–E1145. [CrossRef]
74. Nyame, Y.A.; Gulati, R.; Tsodikov, A.; Gore, J.L.; Etzioni, R. Prostate-Specific Antigen Screening and Recent Increases in Advanced Prostate Cancer. *JNCI Cancer Spectr.* **2021**, *5*, pkaa098. [CrossRef]
75. Fischer, A.J.; Ghelardi, G. The Precautionary Principle, Evidence-Based Medicine, and Decision Theory in Public Health Evaluation. *Front. Public Health* **2016**, *4*, 107. [CrossRef]
76. Greenhalgh, T.; Howick, J.; Maskrey, N. Evidence based medicine: A movement in crisis? *BMJ* **2014**, *348*, g3725. [CrossRef]
77. Siegel, R.; Ma, J.; Zou, Z.; Zou, Z.; Jemal, A. Cancer statistics. *CA Cancer J. Clin.* **2014**, *64*, 9–29. [CrossRef]
78. Lilja, H.; Cronin, A.M.; Dahlin, A.; Manjer, J.; Nilsson, P.M.; Eastham, J.A.; Bjartell, A.S.; Scardino, P.T.; Ulmert, D.; Vickers, A. Prediction of significant prostate cancer diagnosed 20 to 30 years later with a single measure of prostate-specific antigen at or before age 50. *Cancer* **2010**, *117*, 1210–1219. [CrossRef]
79. Hugosson, J.; Carlsson, S.; Aus, G.; Bergdahl, S.; Khatami, A.; Lodding, P.; Pihl, C.-G.; Stranne, J.; holmberg, E.; Lilja, H. Mortality results from the Göteborg randomised population-based prostate-cancer screening trial. *Lancet Oncol.* **2010**, *11*, 725–732. [CrossRef]
80. Schröder, F.H.; Hugosson, J.; Carlsson, S.; Tammela, T.; Määttänen, L.; Auvinen, A.; Kwiatkowski, M.; Recker, F.; Roobol, M.J. Screening for Prostate Cancer Decreases the Risk of Developing Metastatic Disease: Findings from the European Randomized Study of Screening for Prostate Cancer (ERSPC). *Eur. Urol.* **2012**, *62*, 745–752. [CrossRef] [PubMed]
81. Etzioni, R.; Gulati, R.; Tsodikov, A.; Ms, E.M.W.; Penson, D.; Heijnsdijk, E.A.; Bs, J.K.; Draisma, G.; Feuer, E.J.; De Koning, H.J.; et al. The prostate cancer conundrum revisited. *Cancer* **2012**, *118*, 5955–5963. [CrossRef] [PubMed]

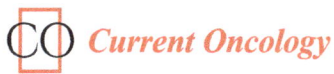

Case Report

Marrying Story with Science: The Impact of Outdated and Inconsistent Breast Cancer Screening Practices in Canada

Jennie Dale [1,*,†]**, Michelle Di Tomaso** [2,†] **and Victoria Gay** [2,†]

1. Independent Researcher, Toronto, ON, Canada
2. Independent Researcher, Vancouver, BC, Canada; michelleditomaso70@gmail.com (M.D.T.); victoria@victoriagayconsulting.com (V.G.)
* Correspondence: info@densebreastscanada.ca
† These authors belong to the non-profit organization Dense Breasts Canada.

Abstract: Behind the science of breast cancer in Canada, as well as globally, are the stories of thousands of women, their families, and their communities. These include stories from those who have died or those suffering from the realities of stage III and stage IV breast cancer due to late detection, misinformation, and dismissal. The reality for these women is that, whilst grateful for the latest developments in cancer research, much of this knowledge is not reflected in policy and practice. Canadian guidelines do not reflect the recommended screening by experts within the field and inequities in screening practices and practitioner knowledge exist in different areas within Canada. Told through the stories of women with lived experiences of late-stage breast cancer and supported by scientific evidence, this paper explores the impact of outdated breast cancer screening practices on the lives of women. Recent patient advocacy is driving changes, such as notifying women of their breast density in a few jurisdictions in Canada, but we call for the whole medical community to take responsibility and ensure breast screening is optimised to save more lives.

Keywords: breast; cancer; screening; dense; patient advocacy; breast density; breast density notification; Canada

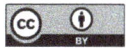

1. Introduction

Story 1. *In 2019, a 46-year-old finds a lump in her breast and speaks to her family doctor. She is referred for a mammogram and ultrasound, then booked in for a biopsy of an 8 cm lump; within a few weeks, she is diagnosed with Triple Positive de novo stage IV breast cancer. This is after being denied regular mammograms by her family doctor at the age of 40 because the screening program in the province where she resides, Alberta, requires a requisition for the first screen of patients in their 40s and only begins self-referral at the age of 50. This is also after being repeatedly monitored using mammography for one existing lump when she lived in British Columbia in her 30s, and after practitioners had paperwork showing that her Volpara Breast Density Score is D, meaning a decreased sensitivity of mammography to identify cancerous masses and an increased risk of breast cancer. If this woman had not moved from the province of British Columbia to Alberta, she could have self-referred for screening from the age of 40 and possibly learned she had cancer before the Triple Positive breast cancer had spread to her lymph nodes, spine, sternum, and ribs. She would also be aware of her breast density category and the risks associated with this, as they are reported on the patient-facing screening documentation. Therefore, it is unlikely she would have been given a 22% prognosis of living for the next five years. That was three years ago. She has 2 children, aged 5 and 8.*

Regrettably, this example of a lack of information on breast density, inconsistencies in screening practices between geographical jurisdictions (ten provinces and three territories) in Canada, and dismissal by the healthcare system is not unique. In North America, it is estimated that 5% of women with breast cancer will be diagnosed with de novo stage IV (metastatic) disease [1]. Statistics from the United States suggest that, of new diagnoses of metastatic breast cancer, 26% are de novo (12,966 in the US in 2013) [2]. Late-stage breast cancer (stages III and IV) results in increased morbidity, more intensive chemical and surgical treatment, and increased mortality (Table 1) [3–6]. With optimal screening practices and knowledge-sharing, combined with improved education and awareness between practitioners and patient communities, the number of late-stage diagnoses can be reduced.

Table 1. The relative 5-year survival of breast cancer patients by stage [6].

Stage	Relative Survival (%)
Stage I	100
Stage II	93
Stage III	72
Stage IV	22

Dense Breasts Canada is a national education and advocacy organisation committed to raising awareness about the risks associated with dense breasts, advocating for breast density notification and optimal breast cancer screening. Over the past six years, Dense Breasts Canada has collated the stories of women in Canada who were not informed of their breast density, denied mammograms, and dismissed by healthcare practitioners. These stories of screening, diagnosis, and treatment experiences represent an important component of the breast cancer landscape that we believe should be central to research, knowledge translation, guidelines, policy, and practice.

Concerningly, the stories shared with Dense Breasts Canada highlight five key shortcomings in the screening and diagnosis of breast cancer in Canada: (i) the impact of outdated screening guidelines from the Canadian Task Force on Preventive Health Care (Canadian Task Force); (ii) inconsistencies between the Canadian Task Force breast cancer screening guidelines and those of the jurisdictions across Canada, creating confusion for medical practitioners and patients; (iii) inequities in screening practices between jurisdictions in Canada, resulting in an increased risk for women in a few provinces; (iv) limited awareness among practitioners and the general public of breast density risks and screening options; and (v) the dismissal of women by medical practitioners.

This paper looks at these five issues through stories of women with breast cancer to bring a personal lens to the science and policy, and to highlight the pressing need for the medical community to collectively advocate for the current science to match the policy, knowledge, and practice.

2. Marrying Stories and Science

2.1. The Impact of Outdated and Inconsistent Screening Guidelines

Story 2. In 2020, a woman in Ontario feels a thickening of her breast tissue. She is 47. She thinks it is likely due to premenopausal changes. It develops into a dimple, so she visits her family doctor for an exam. He refers her for a mammogram. She is called back the next day for another mammogram and a biopsy. She has no history of breast cancer in her family and is shocked at the callback. The lumpectomy and sentinel node biopsy reveal stage I grade 3 breast cancer. Radiation treatment and tamoxifen are planned. At her preradiation CT scan, two additional tumours are found in her lungs and pancreas. She has an extensive Whipple procedure (pancreaticoduodenectomy) to remove the tumour in her pancreas, which also removes part of her small intestine, gall bladder, and pancreatic duct. The pathology reveals that the pancreas and lung tumours have metastasized from the breast cancer. Her diagnosis is updated to de novo stage IV breast cancer. It takes six months to recover from her surgery. She stops her career as an intensive care nurse and goes on long-term disability. She also has surgery to remove her ovaries, which pushes her into the menopause. She takes the drugs Letrozole and Ibrance, which cause *fatigue and mouth sores. She experiences ongoing digestive issues. She loses contact with many friends. Check-ups show that the cancer has stabilised. The median survival rate for women with metastatic breast cancer is three years. Her diagnosis was two years ago.*

The Canadian Task Force publishes guidelines for breast cancer screening [7]. The screening guideline for women aged 40–49 is significantly based on the Canadian National Breast Screening Study (CNBSS) [8,9], which concluded that mammography for women in their 40s did not reduce breast cancer deaths. This contributed to the recommendation that advised against mammograms for women in their 40s [7,10]. These guidelines were adopted by the Ontario Breast Screening Program, which is why this 47-year-old patient was not screened in her 40s.

Since the initial publication of the CNBSS, there has been a suite of evidence questioning the study protocol validity, particularly the likelihood of compromised randomisation [11–17]. Since its publication, the evidence has also shown the benefits of improved screening regimes. For example, Arleo and Hendrick [18] used modelling to demonstrate that the most lives are saved by annual screening starting at the age of 40; Coldman and Phillips [19] showed that women who screened between 40–49 years of age were 44% less likely to die of breast cancer than women who did not; Oeffinger [20] estimated that 27% of the total years of life lost to breast cancer were a result of cancers that are detectable between the ages of 40 and 49; and Webb and Cady [21] found that the median age at diagnosis of fatal cancers was 49 years and most deaths from breast cancer occurred in unscreened women. Even greater mortality risks are experienced by Black, Asian, Native American, and Hispanic women, with a younger age of onset (mid-to-late forties in comparison with mid-sixties for Caucasian women) and a higher incidence of aggressive breast cancer [22–24]. These studies suggest that, to maximise mortality reduction and life-years gained, regular screening needs to start before the age of 50.

As the Canadian Task Force guidelines consider only the results from randomised clinical trials [7] and it would not be ethical to assign women to a non-mammography control arm, these guidelines will remain unchanged until we successfully advocate for these guidelines to change or for the CNBSS to be retracted.

The Canadian Task Force also only considers mortality reduction as a benefit of screening. Looking beyond mortality, regular mammography screening from the age of 40 is associated with a decreased stage at diagnosis and the receipt of less extensive treatments as well as a reduced need for chemotherapy, reduced mastectomies, and increased breast-conserving surgery [3–5,25,26]. Considering this scientific evidence, and the significant surgical, chemical, and hormonal treatment the woman in this story had to endure due to the late diagnosis, it is essential that quality of life, treatment options, and surgery are also considered in screening recommendations [5].

The Canadian Society of Breast Imaging recommendations for optimal screening to reduce mortality and morbidity [27] (Table 2) vary considerably from the Canadian Task Force Recommendations. As these are the recommendations of the experts within the breast radiology community and are based on current scientific evidence, we recommend they be adopted.

2.2. Differences between Provincial and Canadian Task Force Breast Cancer Screening Guidelines Create Confusion for Medical Practitioners and Patients

Story 3. *A 50-year-old woman originally from Brazil moves to Canada at the age of 40. She is aware of her breast density, has a history of finding benign cysts in her breasts, and has had regular mammograms, starting at the age of 35, until she moves to Canada. On multiple occasions, she speaks to her family doctor in British Columbia about screening mammography, but is repeatedly discouraged and quoted the Canadian Task Force screening guidelines that recommend mammograms every 2 years from the age of 50, rather than the provincial guidelines in British Columbia, which allow for self-referral at the age of 40. She has had progressively worsening hip pain from the age of 47 and repeatedly visits the family doctor for this reason; she is referred to a physiotherapist and* *told to practice yoga. Upon a worsening of the symptoms and seeing a different physician, she has an X-ray then CT scans and biopsies, which reveal stage IV breast cancer with two nodules in her right breast, multiple lesions in the pelvic bones and greater destruction to the hip socket, iliac, and ischium bones as well as multiple nodules in her lungs.*

Although the Canadian Task Force breast screening guidelines currently do not recommend screening until the age of 50, screening varies considerably between the ten provinces and three territories of Canada. For example, in the province of British Columbia, women can self-refer every 2 years from the age of 40 [28], yet, as women do not receive invitation letters to the screening program, most are not aware of this opportunity. A survey of 2530 women in Canada showed that 42% of respondents were unaware of the age they were eligible for screening [29]. Conflicting messages between the Canadian Task Force and provincial guidelines, as well as the information available to practitioners and patients may have led in the above case to the diagnosis of de novo metastatic breast cancer.

Table 2. Comparison of breast screening recommendations from The Canadian Task Force on Preventive Health Care [7] and the Canadian Society of Breast Imaging recommendations [27].

Breast Screening Recommendations: Canadian Task Force on Preventive Health Care	Recommendations: Canadian Society of Breast Imaging and Canadian Association of Radiologists
Screening for women aged 40–49 is not recommended	Women aged 40–49 should screen annually with mammography
Women aged 50–74 should screen every 2–3 years with mammography	Women aged 50–74 should screen every 1–2 years with mammography
There are no recommendations for screening women over age 74	Women over aged 74 should screen every 1–2 years with mammography as long as they are in good health with life expectancy of ~7+ years
Supplemental screening is not recommended for women with dense breasts	Women with dense breasts can benefit from a supplemental screening
Risk assessment is not recommended	Risk should be assessed by age 25–30 to determine if early screening is appropriate
Clinical breast exam is not recommended	Mammography may miss breast cancers and a clinical breast exam is complementary to mammography
Breast self-exam is not recommended	Breast self-awareness is recommended

The Canadian Task Force emphasises the potential harms caused by "false-positives" (when women are recalled for further examination because of radiological signs on the screening examination that then turn out to be normal or benign), suggesting that screening leads to physical and psychological consequences that are a greater risk for women under 50 years of age [7]. A review of surveys concluded that the level of short-term stress that being recalled caused did not reach that of clinical anxiety [30], and many studies have shown no evidence of long-term distress in recalled women with "false-positive" mammograms [31–33]. A survey of women by the Canadian Task Force confirmed that reductions in breast cancer mortality outweighed any recalls or overdiagnosis [34], but this was dismissed by the authors, who suggested that the women surveyed did not have enough information to make this conclusion [35]. An emphasis on the harm of mammograms due to unnecessary anxiety ignores the reassurance received by the majority of patients and the scientific literature that underlines the benefits of regular screening. Yet, this is not widely translated to medical practitioners across Canada. This is also demonstrated in Story 3 and the 47-year-old diagnosed with stage IV breast cancer as well as in hundreds of stories from women across Canada collected in the recent survey by Dense Breasts Canada [29].

"Even with women being able to self-refer for mammograms between ages 40 and 50 in BC, I think that there needs to be more education, including and perhaps most importantly, of family doctors regarding symptoms, the need for an earlier baseline mammogram, breast density effects on not only reducing how effective mammograms can be at detecting tumours but also predisposing women to breast cancer, so that misguided information

will not end up leading to late diagnoses and deaths that could have been prevented."
50-year-old patient diagnosed with stage IV breast cancer at the age of 47.

2.3. Geographical Inequities in Screening across Jurisdictions Mean Several Women Risk a Late Diagnosis Based on Where They Live

Story 4. *A 50-year-old mother of three in Ontario finds a lump in her left breast before she is scheduled for her first mammogram, which is available for women in Ontario from the age of 50. She has previously inquired about mammograms in her 40s due to a family history of breast cancer (maternal and paternal aunts, and a first cousin who was diagnosed premenopausal), but has been informed that she "did not qualify under the rules and, by implication, should not worry". After discovering the lump, she has a mammogram, which detects a vague architectural distortion. She has an ultrasound that shows three masses and an MRI, which reveals five. The post-surgical pathology reveals that there are actually nine tumours in one breast. Cancer is also found in most of her lymph nodes on the same side. She is diagnosed with stage III breast cancer. She is never informed of her Category D density. She has a radical mastectomy of the left breast, a full nodal dissection on the left side, and chemotherapy. In addition to the scar tissue, irreversible tightness in the chest muscles, hair loss, nausea, and fatigue associated with chemotherapy, her treatment pushes her into the menopause, accelerating the effects of aging, reducing her peak cardio fitness, and increasing her risk of osteoporosis. She is required to take an aromatase inhibitor daily.*

Differences in provincial screening protocols across Canada result in women such as this 50-year-old being diagnosed with later stage breast cancer because of where she lived. Jurisdictional variations in screening for women between the ages of 40 and 49 vary dramatically [36] (Table 3). For example, women aged 40 who live in Nova Scotia can self-refer to the screening program for annual screening. If they lived in other provinces, such as Saskatchewan or Quebec, they would need a diagnostic requisition from their healthcare practitioner.

Table 3. Screening differences between jurisdictions in Canada for women aged 40–49 [36].

Province/Territory	Can Self-Refer at Age of 40	Can Self-Refer Annually in their 40s	Need a Requisition from Ages 40–49
British Columbia	Yes		
Nova Scotia	Yes	Yes	
Prince Edward Island	Yes	Yes	
Yukon Territory	Yes	Yes	
Alberta			1st screen only
Manitoba			Yes
New Brunswick			Yes
Saskatchewan			Yes
Ontario			Yes
Newfoundland			Yes
Quebec			Yes
North West Territories			1st screen only
Nunavut (no program)			

Had this woman lived in British Columbia, Nova Scotia, Yukon, or Prince Edward Island—where women can self-refer at the age of 40 and, for the latter three, annually (Table 3)—her cancer may have been found earlier.

Jurisdictional variations in screening relate not only to the age at which women are eligible for screening (40 or 50), but the age at which screening stops (69 in Quebec; 74 in other jurisdictions) and the frequency of screening (annual or biennial) as well as variations due to different risk factors, such as breast density.

Furthermore, there are no national guidelines for screening individuals at a "high risk" and screening protocols vary across jurisdictions [37]. The definition of a high risk of developing breast cancer also varies across Canada. It is up to the individual province whether women are considered to be high risk based on a lifetime risk of 20–25%.

Although the Canada Health Act suggests that people in Canada should have "uniform access to insured health services, free from financial or other barriers" [38], this is not the case; access to breast cancer screening—and, therefore, the risk of a late-stage diagnosis—varies depending on where women live in Canada.

2.4. Limited Awareness of Breast Density Risks and Screening Options

Story 5. *A 36-year-old woman finds a lump on her right breast. After a mammogram, it is deemed to be benign and disappears over time. She is informed that she has dense breasts, but given no information about what this might mean. She assumes it is positive and related to her healthy and fit physique. Eighteen years later, at fifty-four, she finds another lump in the same breast. She had a clear mammogram six months earlier as part of the biennial screening program in Ontario, but has not been informed of her breast density or any associated risks through either the screening mammogram results letter she received or at any screening appointments or follow-ups. Upon the examination of her lump, her family doctor refers her for a mammogram and ultrasound, followed by a biopsy. She has a lumpectomy and sentinel node biopsy, revealing Triple Negative stage III aggressive grade 3 breast cancer. Her diagnosing physician tells her that the cancer has probably been developing for quite a time, but was likely missed on the previous mammogram because of her heterogeneously dense breasts. She receives chemotherapy, the removal of 17 more lymph nodes, a prophylactic bilateral mastectomy, and 25 rounds of radiation. An aggressive treatment plan is designed to target the late-stage breast cancer, which may have been detected sooner if breast density had been considered and supplemental screening performed.*

Approximately 43% of women over the age of 40 have dense breasts [39]. Dense breasts are a risk factor of greater prevalence than family history [40] and pose two risks: an increased risk of breast cancer and an increased risk that the cancer will be masked on a mammogram by dense tissues [41]. Women with dense breasts are significantly more likely to be diagnosed with an interval cancer [42]. In Canada, only six jurisdictions provide information on breast density directly to all women having a screening mammogram (Table 4). In five jurisdictions, only women in Category D of density are informed, even though both Category C and D are considered to be dense and associated with an increased risk of breast cancer and difficulty in detection through mammograms. This means that a large percentage of women in Canada are still not being informed of their breast density and are denied the opportunity to be proactive about their breast health.

Table 4. Breast density notification differences between jurisdictions in Canada [36].

Province/Territory	All Women Having a Screening Mammogram Are Mailed Their Breast Density in Results Letter	Only Women in Category D Are Told Their Density	Women in Category D Are Offered Annual Mammograms
British Columbia	Yes		
Nova Scotia	Yes		
Prince Edward Island	Yes		Yes
Yukon Territory		Yes	Yes
Alberta	Yes		
Manitoba	Yes		
New Brunswick	Yes		
Saskatchewan		Yes	Yes
Ontario		Yes	Yes
Newfoundland		Yes	Yes
Quebec			
North West Territories		Yes	Yes
Nunavut (No program)			

Although it is encouraging that women in a few jurisdictions are now being told their breast density in the results letters mailed by the provincial screening programs, not all correspondence provides information on the associated risks of dense breasts. In addition, only six provinces offer annual mammograms for women with category D density. Seely and Peddle [43] compared interval cancer rates in provinces where mammography is performed biennially to provinces that recall women with the highest density annually. They showed that provinces screening women with dense breasts annually had fewer interval cancers.

In addition, only women in British Columbia and Alberta have relatively accessible supplemental screening. Evidence since 1995 has shown that an ultrasound finds additional cancers missed by mammograms [44–46] and reduces the interval rates and rates of late-stage disease [47,48]. Wu and Warren [49] found 7 additional cancers per 1000 women via a screening ultrasound in women with dense breasts. Of those, 40% of the cancers were in women with no family history and 60% were in women with category C density.

Had the above-mentioned woman lived in British Columbia or Alberta, where women with dense breasts are informed of their breast density and can access a screening ultrasound more easily, her cancer may also have been found much earlier. The differences in breast density notifications in the jurisdictions across Canada, combined with the gaps between the scientific evidence and practices, are likely impacting on the lives of women.

2.5. Dismissal of Women

Story 6. *A 42-year-old woman in Alberta starts experiencing back pain whilst walking. It does not improve. She has an X-ray, which comes back clear, and is referred to a physiotherapist and chiropractor. The pain persists and worsens over the next year to the extent that she has to stop work. During physiotherapy exercises, she hears a popping noise and experiences excruciating pain. She is referred for another X-ray, which shows arthritic changes, but with no explanation as to the cause. She does not think it could be breast cancer as she was dismissed by her family doctor as "too young" when she requested a mammogram. Serendipitously, she reads an article about a woman with metastatic breast cancer with no obvious symptoms apart from back pain. She does a self-exam and finds a lump. In quick succession, she has a mammogram, ultrasound, biopsy, and MRI (privately paid). She learns that the breast cancer has metastasized throughout her bones, liver, and lymph nodes. She is diagnosed with stage IV Invasive Ductal Carcinoma, hormone negative, and Her2-positive cancer. She has surgery to insert rods in both of her femurs, spends six weeks in the hospital, and has radiation targeting her pelvis and femurs as well as six rounds of chemotherapy. She has ongoing targeted therapy every three weeks. She uses a wheelchair and a walker. She is 46. She has three teenage children.*

Although not explored widely in the literature, the dismissal of women with breast cancer symptoms can be inferred in the number of malpractice cases for delays in breast cancer diagnoses. It represents a major number of malpractice claims in the UK [50]. In the USA, it is the second most common cause of legal medical malpractice suits and the largest total indemnity pay-out by medical insurance companies; two-thirds of these claims involve women aged 50 and younger [51–54].

Murphy et al. [55] reviewed 264 cases of litigation about breast cancer care, of which 59% related to delays in diagnosis. Allen and Petrisek [51] investigated the evidence of dismissal by healthcare practitioners upon common signs of breast cancer, such as the identification of lumps and nipple discharge. Several women in this study indicated that "physicians failed to recognize symptoms, neglected to perform diagnostic procedures and provided erroneous information because they were unwilling to believe that younger women were likely to experience this illness" [51]. According to a systematic review, this is a common reason for a delayed diagnosis in premenopausal women [56]. Stories such as these are also explored by Dense Breasts Canada [29] and mirror the case study provided in this section.

Delays in diagnoses are not always attributable to practitioners. The reasons for women delaying the seeking of a diagnosis after the identification of symptoms have also been explored [56–59] and are estimated to represent a minority of cases of 20–30% [60]. However, a previous dismissal, lack of respect, and symptoms not taken seriously by healthcare practitioners for breast-related or other health issues in the past have been contributing factors in many cases [58]. A delayed diagnosis due to repeated practitioner dismissals has been demonstrated for other health issues of women, including endometriosis, with an average of 7–10 years to diagnosis [61,62], and premenstrual dysphoric disorder, with an average of 20 years [63], as well as a spectrum of other medical conditions explored by Dusenbery [64]. Such dismissal is commonly attributed to the perception of medical issues of women being influenced by emotional factors [65,66].

Although the persistent dismissal of the health issues of women is a much larger issue, it is evident that there is a considerable need to address delays in breast cancer diagnoses related to gaps in the current knowledge and communication between healthcare practitioners and patients.

3. Discussion

The stories and issues presented in this paper are emblematic of the flaws in the screening policies in Canada. The 46-year-old diagnosed in Story 1 with de novo stage IV breast cancer who was denied a mammogram in her 40s due to the specific screening practices within her province was dismissed on multiple occasions by her family doctor and was not informed of her breast density. Women in their 40s are not acceptable losses, particularly considering that 17% of breast cancer cases occur in this age group [67]. Many of these women have young children, are caring for aging parents, and are contributing to the economy.

Dense Breasts Canada has successfully advocated for patient notification of breast density, and ten jurisdictions (Table 4) have made changes to their practice over the past six years, but, as the stories demonstrate, more must be done to ensure access to the early detection of breast cancer for all women in Canada. We are asking for support from the medical community in advocating for: (a) updated guidelines for breast cancer screening; (b) sharing current evidence with all healthcare providers; and (c) tracking the incidence of metastatic breast cancer.

Updated policies in Canada based on scientific evidence of reduced mortality and morbidity would include: self-referral for annual mammograms across jurisdictions starting at the age of 40; directly informing all women having a screening mammogram of their breast density and the associated risks of dense breasts; and offering annual supplemental ultrasound screening (in addition to mammograms) to all women with dense breasts (Category C and D), regardless of family history. Additionally, high-risk women should be identified and offered supplemental MRI where available.

Furthermore, although this study focuses on Canada, we recommend that internationally updated guidelines be based on the latest scientific evidence. The documentation suggests that breast screening policies in other countries have been influenced by the outcomes of the CNBSS, which is cited in screening guidelines and recommendations for the US [10], UK [68], Europe [69,70], and Australia [71]. The CNBSS study has been discredited [12] and should be retracted from the medical literature. Oncologists and other breast cancer specialists globally can advocate for updated screening guidelines.

We recognise that advocacy will not change outdated screening guidelines and practices overnight. To reduce the incidence of stage IV breast cancer, medical professionals, advocates, and patients need to be presented with the benefits and limitations of screening based on current evidence. This specifically includes: directly addressing gaps in education relating to breast density; the benefits of screening at the age of 40 and breast cancer in younger women; and an increased awareness of eligibility of women for screening. Advocacy is the responsibility of all stakeholders in the breast cancer community. Contradictions in the guidelines compared with the latest evidence can be presented at local, national, and international conferences of medical practitioners; specifically, nurses and family practitioners. Information can be included in the content for continuing medical education sessions. Importantly, whilst women are referred to oncologists at the stage of breast cancer identification and treatment, conversations with patients are essential to highlight the latest evidence of screening.

Finally, we need to track the incidence of stage IV breast cancer across the jurisdictions in Canada to actively support the development of policies and practices that target a reduction in the incidence of late detection. This has recently been implemented in the province of Quebec where the incidence of stage IV breast cancer is being tracked to support research into screening, diagnosis, manifestation, and treatment [72].

Our article includes six stories from women with stage III and de novo stage IV breast cancers to demonstrate the significant impacts of misguided policies as well as misinformation among the medical community and patients. These stories were chosen as they exhibit the impacts of late diagnosis, but there are also many positive stories of screening and early detection.

> **Story 7.** *A 41-year-old woman living in Prince Edward Island self-refers for a mammogram, which leads to the detection of stage I Invasive Ductal Carcinoma. It is confirmed by the general practitioner and surgeon that the tumour could not have been identified by a physical examination. She has surgery to remove the tumour and sample the lymph nodes, 21 rounds of radiation, and hormone therapy scheduled for the next 5–10 years. She knows that access to self-referral for screening from the age of 40 in her province allowed her breast cancer to be found early.*

> **Story 8.** *A 40-year-old woman from British Columbia is encouraged by her family doctor to have a screening mammogram to obtain a "baseline" and understanding of her breast density. Her breasts are identified as dense, and an abnormality is detected. She has a diagnostic mammogram, ultrasound, and then biopsy and is diagnosed with stage I breast cancer 17 days after her initial screening mammogram. She has a lumpectomy, completes 20 rounds of radiation, and receives hormone therapy, which is scheduled for the following 5 years. She is grateful to have been able to self-refer for screening at the age of 40, and that her proactive family doctor recommended her to go.*

4. Conclusions

Using a series of case studies, we have highlighted the impacts of suboptimal cancer screening on the lives of women. We highlighted stories of late diagnosis due to: outdated and inconsistent screening guidelines from the Canadian Task Force; inconsistencies between those guidelines and those of individual jurisdictions, creating confusion for medical practitioners and patients; geographical inequities in screening between jurisdictions, resulting in an increased risk for women in a few provinces; limited awareness of both medical professionals and patients of the risk of dense breast; and the dismissal of women by medical practitioners.

We ask for the medical community to advocate for better policies by: (a) individually and collectively asking for breast screening guidelines to be updated to reflect the latest scientific evidence; (b) information-sharing between the medical community and patients; and (c) the national and provincial collection of stage IV breast cancer incidences.

Action from our whole community to advocate for optimal screening practices will help to reduce mortality from breast cancer as well as reduce the incidence of stage III and de novo stage IV breast cancers, reduce aggressive treatment and surgery, lessen the need for chemotherapy, and increase the quality of life for women with breast cancer.

Author Contributions: Conceptualisation, J.D. and V.G.; data curation, J.D.; writing—original draft preparation, V.G.; writing—review and editing, J.D., V.G., and M.D.T. All authors have read and agreed to the published version of the manuscript.

Funding: This research received no external funding.

Institutional Review Board Statement: Not applicable.

Informed Consent Statement: Written informed consent was obtained from the patients to publish this paper.

Data Availability Statement: Not applicable.

Acknowledgments: We offer our sincerest thanks to the women whose stories are shared within this manuscript, and the many women who have shared their stories with Dense Breasts Canada over the years.

Conflicts of Interest: The authors declare no conflict of interest.

References

1. Tao, L.; Chu, L.; Wang, L.I.; Moy, L.; Brammer, M.; Song, C.; Green, M.; Kurian, A.W.; Gomez, S.L.; Clarke, C.A. Occurrence and outcome of de novo metastatic breast cancer by subtype in a large, diverse population. *Cancer Causes Control* **2016**, *27*, 1127–1138. [CrossRef] [PubMed]
2. Mariotto, A.B.; Etzioni, R.; Hurlbert, M.; Penberthy, L.; Mayer, M. Estimation of the number of women living with metastatic breast cancer in the United States. *Cancer Epidemiol. Prev. Biomark.* **2017**, *26*, 809–815. [CrossRef] [PubMed]
3. Ahn, S.; Wooster, M.; Valente, C.; Moshier, E.; Meng, R.; Pisapati, K.; Couri, R.; Margolies, L.; Schmidt, H.; Port, E. Impact of screening mammography on treatment in women diagnosed with breast cancer. *Ann. Surg. Oncol.* **2018**, *25*, 2979–2986. [CrossRef] [PubMed]
4. Barth, R.J., Jr.; Gibson, G.R.; Carney, P.A.; Mott, L.A.; Becher, R.D.; Poplack, S.P. Detection of breast cancer on screening mammography allows patients to be treated with less-toxic therapy. *Am. J. Roentgenol.* **2005**, *184*, 324–329. [CrossRef]
5. Yaffe, M.J.; Jong, R.A.; Pritchard, K.I. Breast Cancer Screening: Beyond Mortality. *J. Breast Imaging* **2019**, *1*, 161–165. [CrossRef]
6. Canadian Cancer Society. Survival by Stage. Available online: https://cancer.ca/en/cancer-information/cancer-types/breast/prognosis-and-survival/survival-statistics (accessed on 20 April 2022).
7. Klarenbach, S.; Sims-Jones, N.; Lewin, G.; Singh, H.; Thériault, G.; Tonelli, M.; Doull, M.; Courage, S.; Garcia, A.J.; Thombs, B.D. Recommendations on screening for breast cancer in women aged 40–74 years who are not at increased risk for breast cancer. *CMAJ Can. Med. Assoc. J.* **2018**, *190*, E1441–E1451. [CrossRef]
8. Miller, A.B.; Baines, C.J.; To, T.; Wall, C. Canadian National Breast Screening Study: Breast cancer detection and death rates among women aged 40 to 49 years. *CMAJ Can. Med. Assoc. J.* **1992**, *147*, 1459.
9. Miller, A.B.; To, T.; Baines, C.J.; Wall, C. The Canadian National Breast Screening Study-1: Breast cancer mortality after 11 to 16 years of follow-up: A randomized screening trial of mammography in women age 40 to 49 years. *Ann. Intern. Med.* **2002**, *137*, 305–312. [CrossRef]
10. Siu, A.L. Force UPST. Screening for breast cancer: US Preventive Services Task Force recommendation statement. *Ann. Intern. Med.* **2016**, *164*, 279–296. [CrossRef]
11. Boyd, N.F. The review of randomization in the Canadian National Breast Screening Study: Is the debate over? *CMAJ Can. Med. Assoc. J.* **1997**, *156*, 207–209.
12. Yaffe, M.J.; Seely, J.M.; Gordon, P.B.; Appavoo, S.; Kopans, D.B. The randomized trial of mammography screening that was not—A cautionary tale. *J. Med. Screen.* **2022**, *29*, 7–11. [CrossRef] [PubMed]
13. Boyd, N.F.; Jong, R.; Yaffe, M.; Tritchler, D.; Lockwood, G.; Zylak, C. A critical appraisal of the Canadian National Breast Cancer Screening Study. *Radiology* **1993**, *189*, 661–663. [CrossRef] [PubMed]
14. Kopans, D.B.; Feig, S.A. The Canadian National Breast Screening Study: A critical review. *AJR Am. J. Roentgenol.* **1993**, *161*, 755–760. [CrossRef] [PubMed]
15. Tarone, R.E. The excess of patients with advanced breast cancer in young women screened with mammography in the Canadian National Breast Screening Study. *Cancer* **1995**, *75*, 997–1003. [CrossRef]
16. Seely, J.M.; Eby, P.R.; Gordon, P.B.; Appavoo, S.; Yaffe, M.J. Errors in Conduct of the CNBSS Trials of Breast Cancer Screening Observed by Research Personnel. *J. Breast Imaging* **2022**, *2*, 135–143. [CrossRef]
17. Seely, J.M.; Eby, P.R.; Yaffe, M.J. The Fundamental Flaws of the CNBSS Trials: A Scientific Review. *J. Breast Imaging* **2022**, *4*, 108–119. [CrossRef]
18. Arleo, E.K.; Hendrick, R.E.; Helvie, M.A.; Sickles, E.A. Comparison of recommendations for screening mammography using CISNET models. *Cancer* **2017**, *123*, 3673–3680. [CrossRef]
19. Coldman, A.; Phillips, N.; Wilson, C.; Decker, K.; Chiarelli, A.M.; Brisson, J.; Zhang, B.; Payne, J.; Doyle, G.; Ahmad, R. Pan-Canadian study of mammography screening and mortality from breast cancer. *J. Natl. Cancer Inst.* **2014**, *106*, dju261. [CrossRef]
20. Oeffinger, K.C.; Fontham, E.T.; Etzioni, R.; Herzig, A.; Michaelson, J.S.; Shih, Y.-C.T.; Walter, L.C.; Church, T.R.; Flowers, C.R.; LaMonte, S.J.; et al. Breast cancer screening for women at average risk: 2015 guideline update from the American Cancer Society. *JAMA* **2015**, *314*, 1599–1614. [CrossRef]
21. Webb, M.L.; Cady, B.; Michaelson, J.S.; Bush, D.M.; Calvillo, K.Z.; Kopans, D.B.; Smith, B.L. A failure analysis of invasive breast cancer: Most deaths from disease occur in women not regularly screened. *Cancer* **2014**, *120*, 2839–2846. [CrossRef]
22. Rebner, M.; Pai, V.R. Breast Cancer Screening Recommendations: African American Women Are at a Disadvantage. *J. Breast Imaging* **2020**, *2*, 416–421. [CrossRef]
23. Yaffe, M.J. Looking at breast cancer through the ethnic and racial lens-one size definitely does not fit all. *Cancer* **2021**, *127*, 4356–4358. [CrossRef] [PubMed]

24. Hendrick, R.E.; Monticciolo, D.L.; Biggs, K.W.; Malak, S.F. Age distributions of breast cancer diagnosis and mortality by race and ethnicity in US women. *Cancer* **2021**, *127*, 4384–4392. [CrossRef] [PubMed]
25. Coldman, A.J.; Phillips, N.; Speers, C. A retrospective study of the effect of participation in screening mammography on the use of chemotherapy and breast conserving surgery. *Int. J. Cancer* **2007**, *120*, 2185–2190. [CrossRef] [PubMed]
26. Herrmann, C.; Morant, R.; Walser, E.; Mousavi, M.; Thürlimann, B. Screening is associated with lower mastectomy rates in eastern Switzerland beyond stage effects. *BMC Cancer* **2021**, *21*, 229. [CrossRef] [PubMed]
27. Seely, J.; Alhassan, T. Screening for breast cancer in 2018—What should we be doing today? *Curr. Oncol.* **2018**, *25*, 115–124. [CrossRef]
28. BC Cancer Screening: Breast. Available online: http://www.bccancer.bc.ca/screening/breast/get-a-mammogram/who-should-get-a-mammogram (accessed on 9 February 2022).
29. Dense Breasts Canada. Failing Canadian Women. 2021. Available online: https://densebreasts.ca/wp-content/uploads/2021/09/Failing-Canadian-Women.pdf (accessed on 20 July 2021).
30. Bond, M.; Pavey, T.; Welch, K.; Cooper, C.; Garside, R.; Dean, S.; Hyde, C. Systematic review of the psychological consequences of false-positive screening mammograms. *Health Technol. Assess* **2013**, *17*, 1–170, v–vi. [CrossRef]
31. Lampic, C.; Thurfjell, E.; Bergh, J.; Sjödén, P.O. Short- and long-term anxiety and depression in women recalled after breast cancer screening. *Eur. J. Cancer* **2001**, *37*, 463–469. [CrossRef]
32. Ellman, R.; Angeli, N.; Christians, A.; Moss, S.; Chamberlain, J.; Maguire, P. Psychiatric morbidity associated with screening for breast cancer. *Br. J. Cancer* **1989**, *60*, 781–784. [CrossRef]
33. Alter, R.C.; Yaffe, M.J. Breast Cancer Screening and Anxiety. *J. Breast Imaging* **2021**, *3*, 273–275. [CrossRef]
34. Pillay, J.; MacGregor, T.; Hartling, L. *Breast Cancer Screening: Part, B. Systematic Review on Women's Values and Preferences to Inform an Update of the Canadian Task Force on Preventive Health Care 2011 Guideline*; Canadian Task Force on Preventive Health Care: Edmonton, Canada, 2017.
35. Appavoo, S. Imaging, Paternalism and the Worried Patient: Rethinking Our Approach. *Can. Assoc. Radiol. J.* **2022**, *73*, 121–124. [CrossRef] [PubMed]
36. My Breast Screening. Breast Screening in Canada Tool. Available online: https://mybreastscreening.ca/ (accessed on 3 October 2021).
37. Canadian Partnership Against Cancer. Breast Cancer Screening in Canada. Environmental Scan 2019-Last Updated 13 January 2021, 43. Available online: https://s22457.pcdn.co/wp-content/uploads/2021/01/breast-cancer-screening-environmental-scan-2019-2020-Jan132021-EN.pdf (accessed on 20 April 2021).
38. Government of Canada. Health Care Act. Canada. Available online: https://laws-lois.justice.gc.ca/eng/acts/c-6/page-1.html (accessed on 12 January 2022).
39. Sprague, B.L.; Gangnon, R.E.; Burt, V.; Trentham-Dietz, A.; Hampton, J.M.; Wellman, R.D.; Kerlikowske, K.; Miglioretti, D.L. Prevalence of Mammographically Dense Breasts in the United States. *JNCI J. Natl. Cancer Inst.* **2014**, *106*, dju255. [CrossRef] [PubMed]
40. Engmann, N.J.; Golmakani, M.K.; Miglioretti, D.L.; Sprague, B.L.; Kerlikowske, K.; Consortium, B.C.S. Population-attributable risk proportion of clinical risk factors for breast cancer. *JAMA Oncol.* **2017**, *3*, 1228–1236. [CrossRef] [PubMed]
41. Boyd, N.F.; Guo, H.; Martin, L.J.; Sun, L.; Stone, J.; Fishell, E.; Jong, R.A.; Hislop, G.; Chiarelli, A.; Minkin, S.; et al. Mammographic density and the risk and detection of breast cancer. *N. Engl. J. Med.* **2007**, *356*, 227–236. [CrossRef] [PubMed]
42. Boyd, N.F.; Byng, J.W.; Jong, R.A.; Fishell, E.K.; Little, L.E.; Miller, A.B.; Lockwood, G.A.; Tritchler, D.L.; Yaffe, M.J. Quantitative Classification of Mammographic Densities and Breast Cancer Risk: Results from the Canadian National Breast Screening Study. *JNCI J. Natl. Cancer Inst.* **1995**, *87*, 670–675. [CrossRef]
43. Seely, J.M.; Peddle, S.E.; Yang, H.; Chiarelli, A.M.; McCallum, M.; Narasimhan, G.; Zakaria, D.; Earle, C.C.; Fung, S.; Bryant, H.; et al. Breast Density and Risk of Interval Cancers: The Effect of Annual Versus Biennial Screening Mammography Policies in Canada. *Can. Assoc. Radiol. J.* **2022**, *73*, 90–100. [CrossRef]
44. Gordon, P.B.; Goldenberg, S.L. Malignant breast masses detected only by ultrasound. A retrospective review. *Cancer* **1995**, *76*, 626–630. [CrossRef]
45. Berg, W.A. Supplemental screening sonography in dense breasts. *Radiol. Clin. N. Am.* **2004**, *42*, 845–851. [CrossRef]
46. Weigert, J.M. The Connecticut Experiment; The Third Installment: 4 Years of Screening Women with Dense Breasts with Bilateral Ultrasound. *Breast J.* **2017**, *23*, 34–39. [CrossRef]
47. Ohuchi, N.; Suzuki, A.; Sobue, T.; Kawai, M.; Yamamoto, S.; Zheng, Y.-F.; Shiono, Y.N.; Saito, H.; Kuriyama, S.; Tohno, E.; et al. Sensitivity and specificity of mammography and adjunctive ultrasonography to screen for breast cancer in the Japan Strategic Anti-cancer Randomized Trial (J-START): A randomized controlled trial. *Lancet* **2016**, *387*, 341–348. [CrossRef]
48. Corsetti, V.; Houssami, N.; Ghirardi, M.; Ferrari, A.; Speziani, M.; Bellarosa, S.; Remida, G.; Gasparotti, C.; Galligioni, E.; Ciatto, S. Evidence of the effect of adjunct ultrasound screening in women with mammography-negative dense breasts: Interval breast cancers at 1 year follow-up. *Eur. J. Cancer* **2011**, *47*, 1021–1026. [CrossRef] [PubMed]
49. Wu, T.; Warren, L.J. The Added Value of Supplemental Breast Ultrasound Screening for Women with Dense Breasts: A Single Center Canadian Experience. *Can. Assoc. Radiol. J.* **2022**, *73*, 101–106. [CrossRef] [PubMed]
50. Andrews, B.; Bates, T. Delay in the diagnosis of breast cancer: Medico-legal implications. *Breast* **2000**, *9*, 223–237. [CrossRef] [PubMed]

51. Allen, S.M.; Petrisek, A.C.; Laliberte, L.L. Problems in doctor-patient communication: The case of younger women with breast cancer. *Crit. Public Health* **2001**, *11*, 39–58. [CrossRef]
52. Osuch, J.R.; Bonham, V.L. The timely diagnosis of breast cancer: Principles of risk management for primary care providers and surgeons. *Cancer* **1994**, *74*, 271–278. [CrossRef]
53. Zylstra, S.; Bors-Koefoed, R.; Mondor, M.; Anti, D.; Giordano, K.; Resseguie, L.J. A statistical model for predicting the outcome in breast cancer malpractice lawsuits. *Obstet. Gynecol.* **1994**, *84*, 392–398.
54. Mitnick, J.S.; Vazquez, M.F.; Kronovet, S.Z.; Roses, D.F. Malpractice litigation involving patients with carcinoma of the breast. *J. Am. Coll. Surg.* **1995**, *181*, 315–321.
55. Murphy, B.L.; Ray-Zack, M.D.; Reddy, P.N.; Choudhry, A.J.; Zielinski, M.D.; Habermann, E.; Jakub, L.E.; Brandt, K.R.; Jakub, J.W. Breast Cancer Litigation in the 21st Century. *Ann. Surg. Oncol.* **2018**, *25*, 2939–2947. [CrossRef]
56. Ramirez, A.J.; Westcombe, A.M.; Burgess, C.C.; Sutton, S.; Littlejohns, P.; Richards, M.A. Factors predicting delayed presentation of symptomatic breast cancer: A systematic review. *Lancet* **1999**, *353*, 1127–1131. [CrossRef]
57. Barber, M.D.; Jack, W.; Dixon, J.M. Diagnostic delay in breast cancer. *Br. J. Surg.* **2003**, *91*, 49–53. [CrossRef]
58. Granek, L.; Fitzgerald, B.; Fergus, K.; Clemons, M.; Heisey, R. Travelling on parallel tracks: Patient and physician perspectives on why women delay seeking care for breast cancer symptoms. *Can. Oncol. Nurs. J. Rev. Can. Soins Infirm. Oncol.* **2012**, *22*, 101–106. [CrossRef] [PubMed]
59. Granek, L.; Fergus, K. Resistance, agency, and liminality in women's accounts of symptom appraisal and help-seeking upon discovery of a breast irregularity. *Soc. Sci. Med.* **2012**, *75*, 1753–1761. [CrossRef] [PubMed]
60. Bish, A.; Ramirez, A.; Burgess, C.; Hunter, M. Understanding why women delay in seeking help for breast cancer symptoms. *J. Psychosom. Res.* **2005**, *58*, 321–326. [CrossRef]
61. Ballard, K.; Lowton, K.; Wright, J. What's the delay? A qualitative study of women's experiences of reaching a diagnosis of endometriosis. *Fertil. Steril.* **2006**, *86*, 1296–1301. [CrossRef]
62. Nnoaham, K.E.; Hummelshoj, L.; Webster, P.; d'Hooghe, T.; de Cicco Nardone, F.; de Cicco Nardone, C.; Jenkinson, C.; Kennedy, S.H.; Zondervan, K.T. Impact of endometriosis on quality of life and work productivity: A multicenter study across ten countries. *Fertil. Steril.* **2011**, *96*, 366–373.e8. [CrossRef] [PubMed]
63. Osborn, E.; Wittkowski, A.; Brooks, J.; Briggs, P.E.; O'Brien, P.M.S. Women's experiences of receiving a diagnosis of premenstrual dysphoric disorder: A qualitative investigation. *BMC Women's Health* **2020**, *20*, 242. [CrossRef] [PubMed]
64. Dusenbery, M. *Doing Harm: The Truth about How Bad Medicine and Lazy Science Leave Women Dismissed, Misdiagnosed, and Sick*; HarperCollins: New York, USA, 2018.
65. Bernstein, B.; Kane, R. Physicians' attitudes toward female patients. *Med. Care* **1981**, *19*, 600–608. [CrossRef] [PubMed]
66. Hoffmann, D.E.; Tarzian, A.J. The girl who cried pain: A bias against women in the treatment of pain. *J. Law Med. Ethics* **2001**, *29*, 13–27. [CrossRef]
67. Howlader, N.; Noone, A.; Krapcho, M.; Miller, D.; Brest, A.; Yu, M.; Ruhl, J.; Tatalovich, Z.; Mariotta, A.; Lewis, D.; et al. (Eds.) *SEER Cancer Statistics Review, 1975–2017*; National Cancer Institute: Bethesda, MD, USA, 2021.
68. Marmot, M.; Screening, T.I.U.P.O.B.C.; Altman, D.G.; Cameron, D.A.; Dewar, J.A.; Thompson, S.G.; Wilcox, M. The benefits and harms of breast cancer screening: An independent review. *Br. J. Cancer* **2013**, *108*, 2205–2240. [CrossRef]
69. Daneš, S.D.; Fitzpatrick, P.; Follmann, M.; Giordano, L.; Rossi, P.G.; Gräwingholt, A.; Hofvind, S.; Ioannidou-Mouzaka, L.; Knox, S.; Lebeau, A.; et al. *European Commission Initiative on Breast Cancer (ECIBC): European Guidelines on Breast Cancer Screening and Diagnosis Evidence Profile*; European Commission Joint Research Centre: Sint Maartensvlotbrug, The Netherlands, 2017.
70. Colzani, E.; Daneš, J.; De Wolf, C.; Duffy, S.; Fitzpatrick, P.; Follmann, M.; Giordano, L.; Rossi, P.G.; Gräwingholt, A.; Hofvind, S.; et al. *ECIBC Recommendation on Mammography Screening for Women Aged 40–44: Evidence Profile*; European Commission Joint Research Centre: Sint Maartensvlotbrug, The Netherlands, 2016.
71. Irwig, L.; Glasziou, P.; Barratt, A.; Salkeld, G. *Review of the Evidence about the Value of Mammographic Screening in 40–49-Year-Old Women*; NHMRC National Breast Cancer Centre: Sydney, Australia, 1997.
72. Canadian Cancer Society. The Canadian Cancer Society and the McPeak-Sirois Group Team up to Improve Metastatic Breast Cancer Research and Care. Ontario. Available online: https://cancer.ca/en/about-us/media-releases/2022/ccs-and-the-mcpeak-sirois-group-team-up-to-improve-metastatic-breast-cancer-research-and-care (accessed on 15 March 2022).

MDPI
St. Alban-Anlage 66
4052 Basel
Switzerland
Tel. +41 61 683 77 34
Fax +41 61 302 89 18
www.mdpi.com

Current Oncology Editorial Office
E-mail: curroncol@mdpi.com
www.mdpi.com/journal/curroncol

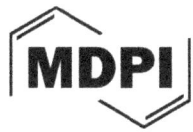

www.ingramcontent.com/pod-product-compliance
Lightning Source LLC
LaVergne TN
LVHW070411100526
838202LV00014B/1437